THE HEALER'S POWER

HOWARD BRODY, M.D.

THE HEALER'S POWER

YALE

UNIVERSITY

PRESS

NEW HAVEN

AND LONDON

Designed by Sonia L. Scanlon
Set in Berkeley type by Rainsford Type,
Danbury, Connecticut
Printed in the United States of America by
Edwards Brothers, Ann Arbor, Michigan.

Library of Congress Cataloging-in-Publication Data
Brody, Howard.
    The healer's power / Howard Brody.
        p.   cm.
    Includes bibliographical references and index.
    ISBN 0-300-05174-3
    1. Medical ethics.   I. Title.
    [DNLM: 1. Ethics, Medical.   2. Physician-Patient Relations.
    3. Power (Psychology)   W 50 B8643h]
    R724.B77   1992
    174'.2—dc20
    DNLM/DLC
    for Library of Congress   91-24291
                                                        CIP

The paper in this book meets the guidelines
for permanence and durability of the Committee
on Production Guidelines for Book Longevity
of the Council on Library Resources.

10 9 8 7 6 5 4 3 2 1

The dream of reason did not take power into account.

—Paul Starr, *The Social Transformation of American Medicine*

Our townsfolk were not more to blame than others; they forgot to be modest, that was all, and thought that everything was still possible for them; which presupposed that pestilences were impossible. They went on doing business, arranged for journeys, and formed views. How should they have given a thought to anything like plague, which rules out any future, cancels journeys, silences the exchange of views. They fancied themselves free, and no one will ever be free so long as there are pestilences.

—Albert Camus, *The Plague*

CONTENTS

This book owes its birth to Linda Garcia-Shelton and Anne Hudson Jones. In September 1986, Linda, the behavioral science coordinator for the St. Joseph Hospital Family Practice Residency in Flint, Michigan, organized a conference for the residents on literature, ethics, and medicine. She invited Anne, her friend and former colleague at the University of Texas Medical Branch in Galveston, to cover the literature beat, and I was asked to participate as the "ethicist." Linda and Anne chose the literary selections the residents would read prior to the conference, including Dostoevsky's "The Grand Inquisitor," Vonda McIntyre's "Of Mist, and Grass, and Sand," William Carlos Williams's "The Use of Force," and Richard Selzer's "Brute."

I had read these works before, except for McIntyre's. But reading them conjointly for this conference brought into sharp focus themes that I had missed on earlier readings. It now seemed that my job as ethicist would be to discuss the use and abuse of the physician's power—for that was what these readings seemed to be about. And this topic seemed a logical and indeed obvious thing to discuss. Yet I had the impression of treading on new ground. I could not recall another conference that had called up this topic in this particular way. Indeed, I had the impression that my years of reading in medical ethics had left me poorly equipped to address this topic.

Why did the word *power* draw such a blank? Perhaps my memory was faulty. I pulled all the books on medical ethics off my shelves and started to search the indexes and tables of contents. *Power* was scarcely to be found.

As a long-time devotee of Sherlock Holmes, I began to wonder if *power* might be medical ethics' dog that didn't bark in the night-time. I wondered first why *power* was missing and second what medical ethics would look like if it were put back. Hence this book.

The parallelism of this book's title with that of Eric Cassell's 1976 volume, *The Healer's Art*, is intentional. I have benefited greatly from Cassell's insights into the physician-patient relationship and the nature of suffering and healing. It is appropriate that this volume should reflect that debt. The parallelism may serve another purpose as well. If physicians are comfortable talking about the *art* they practice but uncomfortable talking about the *power* they wield, then one of the themes of this book will be given additional support.

In this book I try to break some new ground in medical ethics and show that a new language and a new approach will provide fresh insights on some old topics. For this reason the book is intended to be a beginning to a line of conversation, not a finished analysis of what the physician's power consists of or how it should be employed. If the conversation seems fruitful, others will have to take up the discussion. I do not, for the most part, attempt to refute or reject accepted ways of thinking about medical ethics. Therefore the most obvious rejoinder to this book will be, "It is interesting and diverting, but we really do not need to talk about power and to reach whatever valid conclusions you offer; the standard tools and principles of medical ethics would have taken us to the same place just as well." Accordingly, I will try both to defend my conclusions as valid and to show why this rejoinder is implausible.

This book also marks a personal departure. For a number of years I have pursued a dual career in medical ethics and in family practice. Because family practice allows a physician to see patients of all ages and sexes and to gain experience with a wide variety of diseases and conditions, it would seem in many ways an ideal specialty for one interested in medical ethics. Yet it would also seem that being a family physician would not alter one's view of medical ethics in any fundamental way; after all, it is hardly plausible to suggest that ethical principles or moral rules differ substantially among medical specialties. With this book, I try to make the case that there *is* something ethically significant and unique about family practice (or, more generally, primary medical care). I do not mean that family physicians are more ethical than other practitioners but that the concept of good primary care ought to occupy a central place in medical ethics and ethical medicine.

I do not think that it was accidental that reading a collection of short stories first set me to thinking about the importance of power in medical ethics. The standard intellectual and analytic tools of one's discipline tend to erect and reinforce barriers to looking at things in different ways, whereas imaginative literature may force one to realize for the first time that the barriers are there, and what lies on the other side. Therefore, I try in the first two chapters particularly to use literary material and examples to illustrate why the theme of power is worth investigating.

Chapter 1, admittedly an unusual way to begin a book on medical ethics, is an extended literary exercise, the full import of which may become clear only upon reading chapter 2. It confronts the reader in what I hope is a compelling way with many of the themes that will be raised later.

Chapters 2 and 3 offer an overview of the kinds of power the physician possesses, how power can be used and abused, and why medical ethics has largely avoided talking about this. At the end of chapter 3, I offer three general rules for the responsible use of power, with the cryptic labels of owned power, aimed power, and shared power. These will provide useful points of departure in the later chapters.

Chapter 4 focuses on the physician-patient relationship and looks at the issue of sharing power. The argument for the ethical importance of primary care is made here. There are also some introductory comments on virtue in medical ethics, which will be taken up more extensively in chapter 16.

Chapters 5 through 13 address topics commonly found in books on medical ethics, in each case trying to show how a power approach high-lights dimensions of the problem that are obscure or puzzling within the more usual framework. Chapters 6 and 7 on informed consent; chapter 8 on truthful disclosure and confidentiality; chapter 10 on substituted judg-ment, best interests, and quality of life; and chapter 12 on cost containment all address traditional issues of medical ethics. By contrast, chapter 5 ("Care versus Work"), chapter 9 ("The Rescue Fantasy"), chapter 11 ("The Power to Determine Futility"), chapter 13 ("The Physician's Income"), and chapter 14 ("The Social Power of Expert Healers") raise new issues that are com-monly excluded from books on medical ethics or radically reframe familiar issues. In these chapters I have selected for discussion especially those areas of medical ethics where I thought a power approach would be most useful. But I have also tried to include some standard material from medical ethics where it could be argued that the power approach offers very little beyond what we know on the basis of the more usual modes of analysis. This is done primarily to test the scope and limits of the power metaphor. (Chapters 8 and 12 are perhaps the best examples.)

Where the chapter titles or approaches seem unusual for a work on ethics, it is often because the concepts employed would seem more relevant to medical psychology or sociology. One of my theses is that *power* was excluded from the lexicon of medical ethics because it was associated with the social sciences, not with ethics. If power is brought back into ethics, one advantage will be increased awareness of the overlap between ethical and social-science investigations into medical issues. Now that medical ethics has succeeded in establishing itself as an active discipline—and hence need not fear that its methods will be misunderstood or derided—it has everything to gain and nothing to lose by looking to the social sciences for insights.

Chapter 15 begins the process of concluding the book by discussing some aspects of ethical theory. New ways of thinking about ethical reasoning and knowledge within medicine allow discussion of power issues which complements other ethical principles and concepts. Chapter 16 readdresses questions of virtue and character first raised in chapter 4 and emphasizes the importance of the virtue of compassion and a subsidiary virtue, labeled *empathic curiosity*, for guiding the responsible use of power. Finally, Chapter 17 summarizes what has been done in this book and what has yet to be accomplished.

I have presented some of the ideas in this book in various lectures and seminars for the past several years and am grateful to the many people who offered criticisms and requests for clarification. Memory will not allow me to note every one by name, but I had particularly valuable opportunities to present these ideas in the medical humanities seminar at Hiram College (Ohio) conducted by Carol Donley and Martin Kohn and at a bioethics seminar at the University of Virginia conducted by John Fletcher. Linda Garcia-Shelton, Ronald Simons, Jack Coulehan, Roger Sider, Tom Tomlinson, and Leonard Fleck each read and commented on portions of the manuscript. I owe a special debt to James and Hilde Lindeman Nelson, who read the entire manuscript and offered especially timely and helpful suggestions and encouragement.

I have been aided throughout this work by my many colleagues in the departments of Family Practice and Philosophy and the Center for Ethics and Humanities in the Life Sciences at Michigan State University. Michigan State continues to offer unique benefits for interdisciplinary scholarly work in medical ethics and humanities, and my opportunities to interact with interested faculty in the liberal arts, the social sciences, allopathic and osteopathic medicine, nursing, and veterinary medicine have (I hope) left their stamp on this book. During the last stages of work on the book, I was partially supported by the Center for Meaning and Health, a joint project of Michigan State University and the Fetzer Institute of Kalamazoo.

As always, Gladys Topkis and the staff of Yale University Press have been most helpful and encouraging. Richard Miller expertly separated wheat from chaff in the final editing.

As an academic career that seeks to combine medical practice with teaching, research, and administration becomes ever more hectic, a book like this can only be written on time that is stolen from family activity. I am deeply grateful to Daralyn, Sheila, and Mark for their patience and understanding.

THE HEALER'S POWER

A ltogether they had made a terrible hash of things. It was not that they were bad doctors. The two internists, though in private practice, were allowed to admit their patients to the hospital's teaching service and to supervise residents and medical students involved in their patients' care. But this case went wrong from the start. A man in his late forties had become ill—nothing specific or worrisome, but the results of some of the laboratory studies were out of the normal range, and the doctors decided to admit him to the hospital for further evaluation. Then a few more tests yielded abnormal results and the internists, while still having no solid diagnostic clues, felt compelled to follow up with some more invasive procedures. Eventually they decided to do a liver biopsy. It went badly; there was serious bleeding, and then other complications set in. Now the patient was not just somewhat ill—he was seriously ill, and as the complications started to cascade, his condition worsened day by day.

The internists, horrified by this result—and still not knowing precisely what the underlying medical condition was—proceeded to make things worse for themselves. Fearing that the liver biopsy and its complications could be grounds for a lawsuit, they ordered the residents and the medical student who were following the case not to give out any information to the patient or his family about the deteriorating course and its causes. All questions were to be referred back to the internists—and they gave only the most superficial answers, hurrying on and trying to avoid the family as much as possible. As doctors typically do when terrified of malpractice suits, they acted so as to maximize the chances that they would be sued.

The residents adapted to this pattern easily; they had work to do on other patients, and they had long ago realized that questioning the authority of the attending physician was a useless exercise. It was different for the medical student. As medical students typically do, she spent much more time with the patient and could not help encountering the family in the corridor of the intensive care unit. And she was fresh from a different sort of medical training, at a school where students were taught a good deal about talking to patients and families; about emotional reactions to illness and impending death; about frank disclosure of information, even if the news was bad, even if one did not know the truth. And this student took this training very much to heart. Her teachers at medical school had warned her that in her third year she would encounter attending physicians and residents trained in the old way, who prized technical skill and scientific knowledge above sensitivity to patients, and that it would be a struggle for her to hang onto her values.

For four days, as the patient got worse, the student upheld her loyalty to the physicians in charge and managed to suppress her own thoughts. On the fifth day she could no longer manage it. She encountered the family—anxious, questioning, frustrated, angry, scared—in the hallway. They again beseeched her to tell them what was happening; they could no longer place any faith in the obviously insincere reassurances of the internists. This time the student could only do what she had been trained to do. She looked at them kindly and sadly, took their hands, and said: "Your father is dying. You need to be with him so that you can say goodbye to him."

And so the case came before the Chief of Medicine. The plight of the internists was a sorry one, but the hospital had ways of handling that. Maybe there would be a lawsuit; more likely things would be smoothed over. The bad outcome itself was sufficient punishment. Comments would be whispered in the conference rooms and lounges. There would eventually be a formal case discussion with postmortem review. Others would impersonally but ruthlessly expose and discuss the internists' defects in technique and judgment. The internists would have to participate and would have to act scientific, as if being flayed in this fashion were an invigorating learning experience for them, one in which shame and guilt played no part. And by their having to put on such a front, having to deny any real feelings about the death, their punishment would be rendered even more excruciating. If they returned to their usual, competent style of medical practice, the case would be forgotten after a few months, and they would be restored to their former status.

But with the medical student it was different. Her case was one of insubordination, direct violation of clear instructions from a superior. She had no license to practice medicine; she had no permission to exercise independent judgment; her presence at the patient's bedside was at the pleasure of the attending physicians. Yet she had dared to hurl her values—values emanating from a new medical school of little credibility and reputation—directly into the teeth of this long-established hospital. This behavior could not be tolerated. And since she was assigned to the internal medicine service, it was the Chief of Medicine who would have to deal with her.

The Chief of Medicine had practiced in the hospital for forty years. He was an endocrinologist of legendary diagnostic skill, and his prodigious laboratory research had earned him an enviable reputation. Unlike other hospitals, where surgery paid the biggest share of the bills and surgeons dominated the power structure, here internal medicine remained supreme, and the Chief of Medicine was king.

In his large office, its windows looking out over the city, the Chief of Medicine hurried to clear his desk of routine matters before interviewing the student, his last duty of the day. His thin frame looked physically unimposing behind the desk. But when he stood, despite his slight stoop, his height commanded respect.

He did not act obviously excited, but he was beginning to realize that this was to be a special interview. He gradually became aware that he had deliberately manipulated his schedule so as to make the interview come at the close of the day, when he and the student could be alone in this office without being overheard or interrupted. He was looking out the window, his back to the room, when the student entered.

He turned, and they faced each other. She was very slight, with a freckled face and sandy brown hair cut short. Her eyes, though, were open, frank, questioning.

"I have been waiting for you to come," he began. "I have known for a long time that you were going to come. It was ten or twelve years ago that I saw the first signs. People were saying that medicine would have to change, that we should start dealing with patients in different ways, that our science, our technical skill, our clinical judgment, were no longer good enough. And other things were happening at the same time. Young people began to question authority, to protest; they began to talk about their rights and to imagine that anyone in power was a threat. They started looking inside themselves and thinking that what they found there was more profound than anything taught by those who were wiser and more experienced.

"Meanwhile, the medical school you attend was founded, and your professors seemed to think that these things were more important than gross anatomy and biochemistry and that you students were a rich lode waiting to be mined instead of blank slates waiting to receive of knowledge. Now you have come to me, as I knew you must.

"Tomorrow morning I will call your dean of students and make sure that you are dismissed and will never practice medicine in this country. The school will resist this, because they will have the silly, sentimental idea that you were justified and are being treated unfairly. But ultimately they cannot ignore the will of the Chief of Medicine of this hospital; and so you will be dismissed. That is tomorrow morning. But tonight we will talk. I have many things to say to you, things that have been in my mind for years, as soon as I began to be sure that you would come. And you will listen so that you will know why what you have done is so repugnant to those of us who care about medicine and who must protect it and carry it forward."

The student spoke quietly and matter-of-factly. "So, because you disagree with the faculty of my medical school about how students should be taught, you will make me suffer for it."

"Do not speak—by your actions you have already had your say! This one last time you must stand here and listen to the voice of medicine, of those of us who must carry out the work that your coming has threatened, to learn why we who believe in healing must use whatever power we have to stamp out what you represent."

His voice gradually grew quieter, more reflective. "You have come to learn how to heal. You would offer hope and comfort to the sick and dying. But you offer these great goods only to a privileged few. Are you shocked at this? Did you not think you had come to serve all the people, the poor and illiterate as well as the rich and educated? But what I tell you is so. For you offer your particular brand of healing and hope to the few who, in sickness, want to think and act on their own behalf. You seek out the rare person who desires the power to make choices when his own life and death hang in the balance, and the even rarer person who, having been given that power, has any idea what to do with it. Your skills at communicating, educating, informing—all those faddish pursuits that intrigue the fools who presume to instruct you—those skills are aimed at the privileged few. And while you would offer comfort and hope to those privileged hundreds or thousands, the millions or billions would go to their graves shut off from the hope and comfort they need. For you cannot have it both ways. What is hope for the privileged few is the deepest despair for the masses. The millions fear sickness and death and want the doctor to abolish those fears. The doctor who tells them that they have the power to choose in the face of sickness and death, and who encourages them to choose, fills them with anguish. The message of freedom, for the millions, is empty and hopeless. They have no confidence in their own wisdom, their own resources, to pull them through. They look to the doctor to have all the power, to make all the choices, to be free to act for them. The doctor who insists that the power, choice, and freedom are not his destroys the last hope of the millions of sufferers.

"Now, I am not claiming that people are going to come to us for advice on what to eat or whom to marry or how to carry on their lives. I know full well that the patient who nods sagely at my lecture on the evils of cholesterol and promises to follow my instructions to the letter is thinking about where to buy his next greasy hamburger before he is out the door. The millions are very happy to consider themselves free and to hold tight to their own choices and their power to make them despite our advice— but only so long as they feel and act healthy. I happen to know that you have never been seriously ill and that your contact with the sick has been very limited. Those of us who have spent our lives working among the sick know the truth of my description. We know the look of anguish that comes over the sick on being asked to make the simplest of choices and the look of relief when the doctor appears to exercise power over sickness.

"I know what you are thinking. I have heard the attacks coming from the privileged few who cannot identify with the millions, or indeed from the millions who are healthy at present and fondly assume that they will feel equally capable when they are sick. They say that we doctors have an unbridled arrogance, that in modern society we strive to drape the priest's mantle over our own shoulders.

"These attacks are on target. It is indeed the priesthood that we seek, and must seek if we are to help the millions. You have been taught that the history of medicine is a history of ignorance and naked plays for power, and you have adopted that as an excuse to learn nothing about the history of medicine. But religion and medicine issue ultimately from the same source. Do you really think that we have advanced that much beyond primitive society, in which priest, soothsayer, and medicine man were all embodied in the same person? Can you look at recent examples of contagious epidemic diseases in our society—the society that thought it had outgrown epidemics and contagion—and seriously say that we are not ready to burn witches at the stake, to sacrifice victims to appease the gods, once the fear is upon us?

"Medicine and religion spring from the same well deep within the human spirit, and they have much in common. They try to address the most profound fears of humanity, and ultimately there are two ways to do this—through meaning or through magic. The human race is drawn to discover the meaning of events surrounding our lives and our deaths. Religion has responded to this need by constructing holy mythologies of God and afterlife; medicine has responded by providing a scientific theory of health and sickness. The privileged few want this meaning as their preferred way of dealing with all of life's travails; and the millions want this meaning, at least in small doses, so long as they are healthy and comfortable. But in times of great need and fear, the millions do not want meaning; they want magic, and the more potent the better. The great religions of the world recognize this deep need and try to accommodate it by making sure there is enough magic in the ritual and cant to satisfy the unsophisticated millions. If they fail in this, they are soon challenged, and evangelists and faith healers who can provide the magic that the people seek soon spring up to attack the church's authority.

"And so we who would accept the priesthood of healing the sick must have our magic too. The magic comes in three forms—miracle, mystery, and authority. You were taught at your school that this is not how medicine should be practiced. You were taught that medicine is about solving practical problems, that patients' questions are to be answered fully and frankly, and that the physician should share power with the patient. They taught you this, at the new place with its new ideas, and then they sent you here—as if this were the wilderness, the place of old-fashioned and barnacle-ridden medicine, where you would be tempted to give up your new and correct ideas, and where withstanding the temptation would be a test of your goodness.

"And so you were tempted, but you were a good student, and you held fast to the ideas that you were taught. And of course you did not bother to think that in rejecting miracle, mystery, and authority, you rejected the only means to heal the millions and became the enemy and the obstacle of those of us who would truly do the healing work.

"Here you have seen the power of miracle. We do not, it is true, perform miracles routinely. Often we are powerless in the battle against disease and death, even if we win a skirmish or two along the way. But the patients seize hold of those occasional victories and blow them up into miracles, for it is ultimately miracles they want of us. Of course, when they fancy themselves and their loved ones healthy, they say smugly that they realize medicine cannot do everything, that man is not immortal, that they respect a doctor who can admit frankly that he is not omniscient. But when they think they stare death in the face or think their wives or children or parents do, they want miracles, and they want doctors who look and talk like people who perform miracles. They do not want psychiatrists or thanatologists with their five scientifically validated stages of dealing with the dying process, and they do not want to talk about dying, unless the talk itself is its own kind of magic—as if saying the words will make the fears go away.

"People are not supposed to be able to understand miracles; and so a place in which they can hope for a miracle must be a place shrouded in mystery. Did you think it was an accident that most hospital buildings are mazes of corridors, at different levels and in different wings, broken by unexpected ramps and stairways and blank walls? No visitor and hardly any patient can find their way around, but those who work here are people who have penetrated these mysteries. Our talk must be mysterious; our writing must be mysterious and illegible as well. We must walk down the hall as if we were always pondering mysteries or on our way to perform miracles; no one must be allowed to ask us a question or engage us in light conversation without worrying whether some other poor mortal is being allowed to creep a bit closer to the brink of death because our tasks were interrupted.

"The human body, the human brain, is hard-wired for mystery. You have seen a suffering patient experience profound relief from pain and sleep soundly for the first time in weeks after getting an injection of sterile water, under the impression that it was a potent narcotic. You have seen a patient unable to sit still at the start of an interview leave the examining room calm and placid, simply because the physician has mouthed some meaningless mumbo jumbo of a diagnosis that sounds impressive and scholarly. You have seen a patient sent for a series of diagnostic X rays who does not know their purpose but tells the physician later how grateful he is for the relief he has got as a result of the 'treatments'. And these people do not simply feel better; their pulse goes down, their blood pressure goes down, their serum catecholamines go down, their secretory antibodies go up—their entire body tells us of the power of mystery to heal, and of the terrible harm we will do to those who trust us if we ever try to make too much sense to them.

"You have seen the power of authority, the white coat, the upright posture of the doctor looking down on the recumbent figure in bed. The chief of service, the fellows, the residents, the intern, and the medical student all assume their places in the pecking-order procession through the ward. Yet even patients who know full well that you are just a medical student still want to call you *doctor* and want to think of you as a doctor, and they are disappointed when you, with your silly scruples, refuse the title.

"If you would think about it, instead of rejecting authority because it is arrogant and paternalistic, you would see that patients have a need to recognize authority and bow down to it. It is not simply that they trust the person in authority to work miracles for them. It is more basic. To be sick is to feel dependent and childlike, to feel unwhole, broken, defective. To be sick is to be robbed of basic self-esteem, to feel powerless to do what everyone else can do without hesitation or effort. To be sick is to be embarrassed before all onlookers. They say that we doctors reduce our sick patients to dependence and passivity by our arrogance and authoritarianism. But why should we bother when the sickness has already done it for us?

"And so we make a choice. We can stand forth as people of authority and make the patient feel that despite all the anguish and embarrassment, there is something fitting and acceptable in his miserable state. For is it not appropriate to feel childlike and dependent in the face of the majestic authority we represent? Or we can look uncomfortable with authority, try to put ourselves at the level of the patient, reject any attempt to place us on a pedestal. And if we do this, we render the patient truly miserable; for in the presence of a fellow human being his less-than-human helplessness and inadequacy are hurled back into his face. By acting as people of authority, we offer a balance for the way the sickness has diminished the patient, and in this balance we offer the patient a glimmer of the human contact he feared he had lost forever. By refusing to accept authority, we place ourselves out of the reach of our patients, we double their embarrassment and anguish, and we shout at them that they are not of the human community, that they have been cast out.

"You were taught, at that place of the new medicine, that it was the traditional, authoritarian physician, not the disease, that was the patient's enemy. Then you were sent here, to the wilderness, to be shown how to take care of patients. Most of your fellow students soon came to accept our way and to look back on what they had been taught in the classroom as unrealistic, ivory-tower nonsense. But you stood firm and rejected the temptation—and never for a moment did you guess that in rejecting it you were rejecting the secret of healing, the power to heal the millions.

"Now, let me tell you something else that is just beginning to occur to you. You will be thinking: 'This fanatic, this incredible egotist, has in his ravings revealed the utter inconsistency of his claim. For he functions in this hospital as head of the medical service, as the top scientist in a department of medical scientists dedicated to using the latest scientific knowledge and techniques to diagnose and treat disease. The attitude of the scientist must be that of detached reason; there can be no room for quasi-religious fervor, for appeals to magic and mystery. When he throws around scientific terms, he wishes to appear the exponent of objective reason; and so he cannot hope to be taken seriously when he tries to wrap himself in the priest's mantle.'

"That is what you will be starting to think, and it shows that you do not yet understand the enormity of what it means to heal the sick. For I now say to you: if the priest's mantle, once made explicit for what it is, reveals the sham of the scientist, then I accept and admit that sham. Most physicians are content to practice a useful and ultimately soul-preserving self-delusion; they can act both like priests and like scientists, as the mood strikes them or as circumstances call for, and never acknowledge the contradiction, never realize that they are anything more or less than the model scientist-physician. But a few among us are not permitted the luxury of this delusion. We must look our shamming squarely in the face; we must go about our work in full consciousness of it; and we must stifle all our natural feelings of shame under this burdensome knowledge so that we may continue our job of healing.

"Yes, we do realize that our scientific and objective posturing is a sham and that the priesthood is our real business. I say again: do you think I know nothing of the history of medicine? Do you think I have not read carefully through treatises from a hundred years ago and reflected on the primitiveness of the science, the many gaps in knowledge, the quaint but erroneous conclusions? And do you think I am so blind as not to realize that today's texts will appear just as quaint and primitive to our successors? Those men of a century ago healed because they believed their incantations; their so-called science provided the ceremonial backdrop and special effects, needed to inspire, awe, and ultimately heal the multitudes. Do you think I would fail to see that our lasers, scanners, and computerized toys are just a finer and richer set of stage props? The only difference is that our predecessors may have truly believed. I cannot believe; I know too much. It is my burden to go on shamming, keeping my awful secret to myself. This burden, this lie—from which you would turn away so self-righteously— is what I must bear if I am to continue to heal. And I will continue, for the millions need me. The thousands may condemn me, or would if they knew; but I must go on, for the love of the millions."

He had been pacing frantically; but then he stopped. "I understand you better than you know. For I see in you a good deal of myself when I was young. I too was going to withstand the temptation in the wilderness, remain pure and minister to the thousands. I too was going to treat my patients as my equals, admit my doubts openly, be an educator and not a performer of miracles. Fortunately, I saw the light and returned to the true path of healing.

"It was an older physician than I am now who first taught me the possibility of a new kind of medicine and urged the new ways on me. He became my revered mentor. I saw how he spoke to his patients, how he spent time with them, and I resolved to live up to his standard. And when I began my practice here at the hospital, one of his long-standing patients became one of my own first patients. This man had greatly trusted my mentor and transferred that trust to me.

"This man smoked heavily, and even then some of the medical journals were hinting at the dangers of cigarettes. I saw from my mentor's chart notes that he had frequently raised the issue of smoking with this man. I knew from his style that he would have given medical information and offered assistance in order to persuade him to quit. But he would not, and indeed could not, have manipulated, blustered, or lied. He would have treated this man as an adult and expected him to make an adult decision, whether or not he agreed with the outcome.

"The first few times I saw this patient, I followed my mentor's example. Then about a year later something happened—I am still not sure what was different about me that day. But I talked to this man, who was there simply for a regular checkup, and was suddenly overwhelmed by a feeling of anger and frustration. Strange, unaccustomed words began to pour out of my mouth. I was demanding, insisting, ordering that he quit smoking. I was aghast at how I had abandoned my principles and hardly dared guess what his reaction would be.

"The man thanked me sincerely. He said that all the time that my mentor had been educating and informing him, and for the brief time that I had been doing the same, he had wondered just how serious we were about this smoking business. Now, finally, he knew that it was a matter of urgency and importance. Once his doctor had given firm instructions, he had no doubt that he would quit immediately and permanently. And indeed from that minute he never smoked again.

"About two years later I became worried about his coughing and weight loss and ordered a chest X ray, which showed a mass like a golf ball in his right lung. I know that had I told him to quit on his first visit, this mass would still have appeared when it did. But I also know that had my mentor ordered him to quit years earlier, the man might have been spared.

Because I revered my mentor's approach, I accepted his work with this patient as my own work; and between us, with our scruples and principles, we had cost this trusting man his life. It took him another eighteen months to die in great agony, and every day of those months was a rebuke to me. The millions trust us as that man trusted us back then, and you can see how shabbily I repaid that man's trust. I have learned my lesson. I will not betray the trust of the millions. I will keep my horrible knowledge to myself and do what needs to be done to heal them."

It was now totally dark outside. His passion seemed spent. He avoided looking at the student. "You may go now. I will never see you again. Indeed, both of us must make certain that I never see you again. But I will not have you removed from medical school. I do not mean you any harm personally. It is just that you must stay out of my way and not hinder my work."

What happened at this point is not clear. One version has it that the student kissed him before she left the room. But that version is probably apocryphal.

I t will not be difficult, I trust, to recognize chapter 1 as a modification of "The Grand Inquisitor," a "prose poem" that appears in Dostoevsky's novel *The Brothers Karamazov* ([1880] 1950). It may be more difficult to see why a book on medical ethics should begin with this sort of amateur literary exercise and why I will be referring to several other short stories in this chapter.

My central argument is that medical ethics is about power and its responsible use. For several reasons, however, the word *power* is essentially absent from the vocabulary that scholars of medical ethics have constructed for their discipline and that has been accepted by almost everyone who does work in the field or tries to apply medical-ethics insights to the clinical context. I wish to show that with *power* put back into the vocabulary, a few puzzling issues in medical ethics begin to make more sense and the enterprise as a whole starts to hang together in a more enlightening way.

The existing vocabulary, which constitutes the standard view of modern medical ethics, seems to be all-inclusive, offering a category or label for almost every imaginable ethical dilemma. It is hard to make a convincing argument that something basic is missing so long as the argument remains confined within that vocabulary. But if we approach medical ethics from a new angle, we may bypass the rationalizing and intellectualizing defenses of the scholarly approach and become aware of a glaring incompleteness. I find that literary texts offer precisely this sort of fresh look at an old subject.[1] And so in this chapter I shall employ some analyses borrowed from literature to clear the way for further inquiry in later chapters. I will

---

1. For a representative review of the uses of literature to inform discussion of medical ethics, see Brock and Ratzan 1988.

begin by offering an analysis of "The Grand Inquisitor" to show why it leads legitimately to a medical application.

The Grand Inquisitor's Argument

Dostoevsky's Grand Inquisitor is an elderly cardinal of the Spanish Inquisition. He confronts Christ, who has returned to earth to be among His suffering people, and threatens to burn Him at the stake as a heretic. The major portion of the story is a theological argument in monologue (with Christ as the silent listener) in which the Grand Inquisitor expounds on the temptations offered to Christ by the Devil in the wilderness. Whereas Christ thought He was preserving His holiness and integrity by refusing the temptations, the Grand Inquisitor asserts that the Devil was showing Him the true and only way in which He could have aided suffering humanity. The church of the Middle Ages, in fact, was following the way of the Devil and not the way of Christ, but by so doing it was carrying out Christ's function for the masses far more effectively than had it followed Christ's example and teachings. The Grand Inquisitor's demand of Christ is that He take Himself away and not hinder the church in its necessary work.

That, in brief outline, is the theology. The dramatic power of the story, I think, comes from the fact that the Grand Inquisitor at first seems to be a melagomaniac and a hypocrite. The reader thinks: it cannot possibly be for the good of suffering humanity that he seeks the power to commit his atrocities; it can only be for his own selfish ends. But the passion and frenzy of the Grand Inquisitor to explain himself, to confess himself to Christ, is ultimately compelling. (It is no accident, for the story's internal logic, that Christ happens to have come down to earth at that time; it is only to Christ that the Grand Inquisitor could possibly confess. The steadfastness with which he keeps his horrible secret from all human ears— that he is following the way of the Devil in the name of Christ—is a key part of his self-justification.) The climax of the story is when the reader arrives, surprised, at the realization: *however abominable I may find the Grand Inquisitor's arguments and position, I have to grant that he might just possibly be sincere.*

What does all this have to do with the Chief of Medicine in the last chapter and with medical ethics? Making this clear will require stepwise analysis of the Grand Inquisitor's argument. I take the argument to go as follows:[2]

2. I have adopted this seven-point analysis from a seminar presentation by Martin Benjamin.

1. The most important duty of the clergy is to promote the happiness and well-being of the greatest number of people. (The Grand Inquisitor, it will be seen, is a thoroughgoing utilitarian.)

2. Two approaches have been offered to the clergy to promote happiness and well-being. The first, the way of Christ, is to encourage people to assume greater freedom and responsibility over their own lives. The second, the way of the Devil, is to offer people a life of subjugation to the forces of miracle, mystery, and authority.

3. Most people are made happy by subjugation to miracle, mystery, and authority and become profoundly unhappy when challenged with freedom and responsibility. (As the Grand Inquisitor puts it, Christ through His way has offered salvation to the the elite thousands while condemning the millions to abject misery.)

4. Most people, however, feel a duty to follow the way of Christ and avoid the way of the Devil; they would be unhappy if their leaders admitted explicitly that they were adhering to the Devil's advice.

5. Therefore, it must be the duty of the clergy to subjugate the populace to miracle, mystery, and authority while explicitly declaring that in so doing they are following the way of Christ.

6. The implicit irony and contradiction of point 5 can be resolved in two ways. The average clergy will simply be unable to confront the contradiction squarely and so will employ various rationalizations to convince themselves that miracle, mystery, and authority represent Christ's way. They will be honest (if shallow and lacking insight) when ministering to the masses. The rare, courageous clergy, however—the Grand Inquisitors— will be unable to dodge the full force of the contradiction. They will face it squarely but will keep it to themselves as their own terrible secret, knowing how much unhappiness would be caused if they were ever to reveal it.

7. Therefore, the Grand Inquisitors show that their love for humanity is greater even than Christ's in two distinct ways. First, they refuse to follow the teaching of Christ and follow instead the teaching of the Devil, for only in that way can they *effectively* accomplish Christ's purported ends. Second, they make an immense personal sacrifice in carrying out their first task, for they forego the natural impulse toward confession. They wear their terrible secret knowledge of the hidden contradiction of the church like their personal crown of thorns, which constantly pricks but has to be borne for the good of suffering humanity.

This is a long and convoluted argument and could be challenged on many points. But I think, however, that the average modern reader would be inclined first to reject point 3. This is the fundamental reason that the Grand Inquisitor seems to be an agent of evil: he holds an irredeemably cynical view of the common people and their ability to handle the challenge of freedom. True, a few people wish to give up their freedom in order to have the comfort of mystery and authority throughout their lives. And most of us, under particular stress or threat, will temporarily seek safety in subjugation to authority. But in the long run we prize our freedom too much to remain entranced by miracle, mystery, and authority. And so the Grand Inquisitor is simply wrong. He has not got his psychology of human nature straight.

This objection to point 3 is likely to arouse the sympathy of any student of ethics: after all, if this premise is accepted, it is hardly worth the effort to talk about ethics. Hence it is important to see that point 3 could be modified so as to appear, on the surface at least, much more plausible and psychologically accurate:

3*. Most people, *when well*, are fully capable of assuming freedom and responsibility. But these same people, *when sick*, can be comforted only through subjugation to miracle, mystery, and authority.

Please note that the point is not that 3* is true, only that it is, on its face, more plausible than 3. Its plausibility has for centuries fueled the unquestioned paternalistic attitude of physicians toward patients.[3] It led, for example, to the pious statements of the physicians interviewed by Oken (1961), who in the name of kindness routinely withheld the diagnosis of cancer from their patients. Yet these same doctors confirmed that they would want to know their own diagnoses if they themselves were seriously ill, countering that they were physicians and so were made of sterner stuff. One or another version of 3* has arisen even in the wake of the "new" medical ethics, which views physician paternalism as a sin on a par with matricide and child abuse. Eric Cassell (1976) has cited the results of Piaget-type experiments to demonstrate that the sick regress to a more infantile state of cognitive capacity; and Edmund Pellegrino (1979) asserts the "fact of illness," by which he means primarily the patient's psychological vulnerability in the face of "ontological assault," as a fundamental truth underlying all of medical ethics.

It does not matter whether Cassell and Pellegrino, who are avowedly antipaternalistic, have succeeded in distinguishing their psychological arguments sufficiently from the "old" paternalism of the simple-minded physician. The point is that one can erase much of what makes the Grand

---

3. On the issue of physician paternalism, its definition and possible justifications, see Childress 1982; Brody 1985.

Inquisitor seem *obviously* evil or hypocritical by replacing the premise in 3 with that in 3*. But if we do so, instead of the story of the Grand Inquisitor we get the story of the Chief of Medicine.

Three Kinds of Power

The Chief of Medicine presents a certain image of the physician, his power, and his use of that power. It is enlightening to compare that image with the one presented in a very different story, "Of Mist, and Grass and Sand," by Vonda McIntyre (see Appendix).[4]

Medical sociologists over the past decades have analyzed the physician's power or authority and have concluded that it is a compound of several distinct elements. (I will deviate from the standard sociological usage by using the term *power* only, for simplicity. *Authority* I take to be socially legitimated power.) They differ among themselves on minor points of how to label the various elements and how many there are. What follows is my own set of labels, which nevertheless draws heavily from the work of Paterson (1966), Siegler and Osmond (1973), and Starr (1982). I propose that the physician's power can be divided into three components—Aesculapian, charismatic, and social.[5]

Aesculapian power refers to the power the physician possesses by virtue of her training in the discipline and the art or craft of medicine. The power arises from the healer's possession of the knowledge of a body of obscure and complex facts and theories, a variety of practical skills for manipulating instruments and body parts, and experience in the application of this knowledge and skill in a range of practical settings. To the extent that the art or craft of medicine is defined to include psychological needs and vulnerabilities and how best to deal with these problems, Aesculapian power will also derive from knowledge of and experience in those elements of the psychology of illness. Aesculapian power is an impersonal power; it is transferable from any physician to any other of comparable skill and experience. It is also independent of social status or class.

Charismatic power is based on the physician's personal qualities and cannot readily be transferred. We presume that these qualities—courage,

---

4. This story first appeared in the science fiction magazine *Analog* (vol. 92, no. 2 [October 1972], pp. 73–91). It was reprinted in *Women of Wonder: Science Fiction Stories by Women about Women*, edited by P. Sargent (New York: Vintage, 1975) and appears unchanged as the first chapter of McIntyre's novel *Dreamsnake* (Boston: Houghton Mifflin, 1978). For an excellent analysis and discussion of the story, see Jones 1983.

5. For a complementary discussion of the aspects of the physician's power, see Drane 1988, p. 87.

decisiveness, firmness, kindness, and so on—are personality characteristics of the physician independent of the disciplinary knowledge and skill that give rise to Aesculapian power.

The origins of the term *charisma* suggest that the source of power of this type is divine grace or gift. My use of the label is agnostic; it neither rules out nor requires that divine grace be a source of the physician's personal power.[6]

Social power arises from the social status of the physician. One source of it is an implied contract between the medical profession and society which turns over to that profession the authority to determine what counts as medical knowledge and medical truth (Freidson 1970). Ordinarily, physicians are delegated the authority to rule on who is sick and who is well, and whether a particular person's misfortune is to be deemed a true disease or something else; the physician's word on the subject is sufficient to set in motion various social roles and practices (such as the "sick" role) in a way that no word from a lay person could do (Parsons 1978; Brody 1987d, pp. 34–38). It is possible that physicians could possess and wield this aspect of social power even while occupying a very low rung of the socioeconomic class scale (such as the Greek slave physicians of the Roman Empire). If we needed to set this aspect of power apart from other types of social authority, we could call it *cultural power*.[7]

The more common case in today's Western medicine, however, suggests that society generally accords high status in other ways to those to whom

6. Moskop (1981) has a slightly different account of charismatic power. He notes that the physician is commonly involved in events of great importance to people—birth, death, trauma—and that "because physicians work in these existentially charged situations, they are in a unique position to provide guidance and comfort to patients and families. . . . We expect the good physician to exhibit strong interpersonal skills and psychological strength as well as technical competence and commitment to patient welfare" (p. 40). I have elected to label certain interpersonal and psychological skills as a type of technical competence and hence to subsume those skills under Aesculapian power. Still, it is worth noting that Moskop has identified a source of personal power (due to the subject's frequent encounter with highly charged events) that need not be confused with charisma either in the sense of divine grace or in the sense in which a politician or pop star is said to be charismatic.

7. A physician struggling with how much to tell an elderly patient about his poor prognosis indicates an awareness of cultural power: "So you can look at it from the viewpoint that I feel incompetent because I can't fix it, or you can look at it from the viewpoint of the power that I have—*knowing* that I can't fix it. . . . What I feel is the power that I have in telling him something that's so horrible" (Barnard 1986, p. 36). The physician feels this terrible sense of power because, through a combination of knowledge and socially delegated authority, he can *make something be the case simply by saying it is so*, a power not shared by many other professional groups. (For more discussion of the case study from which this quotation is drawn, see chapter 13.)

it entrusts the cultural power to define medical truth and knowledge. If physicians either are drawn from the higher socioeconomic and educational classes or rise to them upon undertaking medical practice, then cultural power will be mixed with the power gained from high social status alone. That power will appear most prominent when the patient is of relatively low socioeconomic status. The physician will live in a certain neighborhood, wear certain clothes, drive a certain car, and use language in a way that tends to cause others in society to defer to her wishes, even when the influences of cultural, charismatic, and Aesculapian power are corrected for.

There is one other reason for not insisting that cultural power should be recognized as a distinct form of physician's power. How one classifies that power will depend on how positivistic a view one takes of medical science. I agree with the sociologists that although facts may be real, there is no knowledge without interpretation of the facts; all knowledge therefore is by nature a social construction, medical knowledge included. But others might insist that medical knowledge simply describes what is true about the world, that the reason we believe a physician and not a chimneysweep about health and illness is that the physician knows what's true and the chimneysweep doesn't; there is no "social construction" about the matter at all. To the positivist, then, the power I have called cultural power is neither a distinct form of power nor related to social power in any way but is instead a manifestation of Aesculapian power. However interesting this debate might be in other contexts (Caplan, Engelhardt, and McCartney 1981), it need not occupy us for purposes of this book, and so subsuming cultural power under the heading of social power may be a good way to avoid getting sidetracked.

Armed with this classification scheme, we can now see why the conceptions of the healer presented by the Chief of Medicine and by Snake, the healer in McIntyre's story, are so different. Just as the Grand Inquisitor is willing to grant the theological emptyness and corruption of the church, the Chief of Medicine is willing to grant that Aesculapian power is a hollow shell. He'll take what he can get out of medical knowledge as it now exists; but he is too smart, or too cynical, to rely on that knowledge as a base for power; he knows it has too many cracks and patched-over sections, and there is still so much that the best physicians and scientists don't know. For him, the power to heal lies primarily in the physician's charismatic and social power. Sometimes these sorts of power will indeed heal, by stimulating the placebo response or whatever we wish to call the body's self-healing mechanisms (Brody 1980, 1987d). Sometimes the patient will die or will fail to improve, and in those cases the exercise of charismatic and social power reassures sufferer and onlookers that "everything possible is being done." Aesculapian power may be empty in substance, but it is grand for enhancing the physician's charismatic and social power. Someone who can stop a human heart and then start it again after surgery, or twirl the dials on a magnetic resonance imaging machine, must indeed be the sort of person to whom one speaks with awe and respect.

The skillful use of charismatic and social power kept medicine successful over the centuries when Aesculapian power was relatively empty of effective interventions. The combination still works well today, when more than half the patients coming to see a physician do not have a clearly diagnosable disease and most of those who do will either get better by themselves or cannot be cured. But in spite of his power and the magnificent success it has achieved, the Chief of Medicine suffers from a basic insecurity. He is convinced that he would lose his considerable social and charismatic power, and hence his ability to heal, if the public came to know the real deficiencies of Aesculapian power. Just puncture the myth of the omnipotence of modern scientific medicine, and all will be lost. It is not at all clear that the Chief of Medicine is right in thinking this. The advocates of the "new" medical ethics of patient autonomy and informed consent have bet the rent that he isn't, and so far the data seem to be on their side, not his.[8]

But Snake presents a very different image. We do not know what was in Vonda McIntyre's mind when she wrote the story, but the result is almost as if she consulted the classification scheme above and said, "Let's see what it would be like to have a healer who could rely only on Aesculapian power, with no recourse to charismatic or social power." For Snake, Aesculapian power is no metaphor; she relies literally on the sacred serpent of the Greek god of medicine for her own healing practices. But while we are familiar with the irony of "the operation was a success but the patient died," the story presents us with a novel irony: the patient is cured but the healer slinks away, a failure in her own eyes. So great was her lack of charismatic and social power that she herself was almost killed in the process.

To see how McIntyre has created the image of the healer as relying on Aesculapian power only, we need to analyze how Snake understands her failure and why she is reasonably certain that her teachers will deal harshly with her when they hear the story. The family of the sick child was fearful and hostile, and this led to the death of one of the three snakes. But their fear, hostility, and lack of understanding of her art are no excuse. She feels that she should have dealt more adequately and forthrightly with those

8. See chapter 6 on patients' desire for full disclosure of medical information.

feelings and done more to make the family her allies instead of her ad-versaries. That is, the psychological skill necessary to understand and dis-arm their fear and hostility is an inseparable part of the body of knowledge and skills that makes her a healer. She failed to use those skills, probably because she was tired and weak from hunger; but her failure is analogous to that of the surgeon performing a delicate operation when weak and hungry whose instrument slips and damages a vital structure as a result.

The function of the small snake, Grass, has been to bring relief from pain and to comfort those who cannot be helped by more aggressive measures. His death leaves intact the two snakes who have the power to cure disease. But Snake never imagines for a minute carrying on her healing duties with those two snakes alone. Clearly, in her view of her healing art, the power to cure without the power to relieve suffering and pain is not worth having. Despite her use of one of the most primitive metaphors for healing, the magic serpent, McIntyre's conception is holistic in the broadest sense of that often misused term.

In sum, these two stories offer between them a survey of the different types of power a physician may use in the name of healing. Neither story, however, deals *directly* with the misuse or abuse of that power (even though we suspect that abuse of power is precisely what characterizes the Grand Inquisitor and his medical cousin). To get a clear idea of how that aspect of the physician's power affects the physician-patient relationship, we will have to move on to a different train of argument, and to different stories.

The Dark Side of the Force

It seems axiomatic that the use of power must go hand in hand with its potential misuse. ("Power tends to corrupt" is, after all, the first portion of Lord Acton's famous maxim.) Some misuses of physician power are both obvious and analytically uninteresting—for example, the physician prac-ticing fee-for-service medicine who enriches himself by ordering unnec-essary tests and procedures. But I wish to argue that the patient's response to the physician is influenced by a deep-seated fear of the misuse of medical power—much as is illustrated by the boy's family in the story of Snake. To see why this might be so, we will have to delve beneath the more obvious misuses of power to aspects of medical practice and medical at-titudes that are seldom discussed under the heading of ethics.

In the movie *Cobra*, actor Sylvester Stallone plays a macho cop who engages in the violent and bloody elimination of criminals. Though he is mostly a man of few words, he does manage to say to one of his victims, "You're the disease and I'm the cure." It is worth asking why, in that world of mayhem, a medical metaphor should have suggested itself. The answer to this question may show how and why the misuse of power must be explicitly addressed in medical ethics.

I offer speculation, not argument or data, for here we are dealing with a sensitive area of the human soul that few people, physicians or not, are willing to expose fully to daylight. I speculate that somewhere in our more primitive depths is a lust, half childish, half sadistic, to use whatever power we might have to victimize others less powerful, *and to enjoy it*—to glory in the fact that they and not we are the victims, and to escape for a moment into the fantasy that since we can avoid their victimhood through our power, we are invulnerable and need never again feel fear.[9]

But we are civilized, and the influences of culture and society force this dark lust down into our subconscious most of the time, if we are normal. We seldom have the chance to act out this impulse. But the impulse does not go away, and somewhere deep down it gnaws at us, seeking expression.

Now, think for a moment of the circumstances that would be required for us both to act out this impulse, savoring our use of power over a helpless victim, and to get away with it without social condemnation or ostracism. One possibility is that we could unleash this power only when engulfed in the anonymity of a mob; but even there we might have pangs of conscience. The ideal, it would seem, would be for the prospective victim somehow to be labeled as totally and irretrievably *evil*. This would make it socially impossible for anyone to identify with the victim or take his side.

Next we would have to ask, who is it that has the social authority to brand something as evil? The answer is the physician. For our present purposes, labeling a biological state of affairs as a disease can be seen as declaring that we are in the presence of an evil that ought to be eliminated;[10] no right-thinking person could declare that he was on the side of the

9. Doerflinger (1989) notes "a fact of human nature: Human beings are tempted to enjoy exercising power over others; ending another person's life is the ultimate exercise of that power" (p. 19). Doerflinger is here arguing against legalization of assisted suicide or active euthanasia. I suggest that he narrows the issue of "the human will to power" too much by tying it to the killing of patients. As the short stories reviewed below indicate, the will to power may reveal itself in many more mundane ways.

10. On the connection between the concept of disease and the notion of evil, see Clouser, Culver, and Gert 1981; Brody 1987d, pp. 22–26. It may seem an overstatement to ascribe this power exclusively to physicians. Under various circumstances, political leaders and clergy can authoritatively pronounce someone or something evil; indeed this routinely occurs when war is declared. However, the statements of these leaders are viewed by American society as at least debatable, whereas the pronouncements of physicians appear to be grounded in unassailable biological facts.

disease and not that of the sufferer. To label some state of affairs as con-
stituting a disease and then diagnose individual patients as having the
disease or not having it are ordinarily seen as well within the legitimate
authority of the physician.[11] Little wonder, then, that Stallone's cop would
like to see himself as having the social authority to declare what (or who)
is a disease and what is not.

All of us wish to be able to depend on physicians to come to our aid
when we fall ill. So we tell ourselves over and over again that physicians
do indeed have this great power, which includes the power to call something
evil and, in effect, declare war on it. But of course they are totally benevolent
in their use of that power. They will always assiduously observe the distinction between the disease and the person who has it. Never would they
use this awesome power to declare that the *person* is evil, or in any way
direct their forces against the individual who suffers at the same time that
they attack the disease. Naturally, mistakes sometimes happen. But when
the individual medical equivalent of the Vietnam War tragedy occurs and
the physician reports that he had to destroy the village in order to save it,
we assume that the intention was benign. But this comforting story denies
that physicians too are human and that they have buried within them this
same impulse to relish the unresisted use of power. For further discussion,
I will borrow another movie phrase, from George Lukas's *Star Wars* trilogy,
and refer to this impulse in the physician as "the dark side of the force."

John Ladd says that the physician's power "presupposes trust and confidence; it also begets fear, distrust and resentment" (1980, p. 1129).[12]
Because trust and confidence are necessary to get the medical enterprise
off the ground—and because medical power is used for beneficent purposes
almost all the time—we tell ourselves the comforting story. But the fear,
distrust, and resentment remain because we are unable to believe it totally.
As patients, we suspect that physicians, if they were optimally insightful

11. The positivist would see this purely as an outgrowth of Aesculapian power, whereas
the sociologist or anthropologist would see it as falling under what I have called cultural
power.

12. Leon Kass (1989) recounts the Greek myth according to which Athena took blood
from the dead Gorgon, Medusa, and made from it two powerful drugs: the blood drawn from
the left side of the monster's body provided protection against death, whereas that from the
right produced a deadly poison. Versions of the myth vary over which Athena then gave to
Asclepius, the founder of medicine—vials of both drugs or a vial of the left-sided drug only.
The former version captures perfectly the point of this section—first, that patients have reason
to fear the destructive side of medicine at the same time that they seek its aid; and second,
that the destructive power and the healing power spring from the same source.

and candid, would declare, along with Dr. Walter Franz in Arthur Miller's *The Price*:

> You start out wanting to be the best; and there's no question that you do need a certain fanaticism; there's so much to know and so little time. Until you've eliminated everything extraneous—including people. And of course the time comes when you realize that you haven't merely been specializing in something—something has been specializing in you. You become a kind of instrument, an instrument that cuts money out of people and fame out of the world. And it finally makes you stupid. Power can do that. You get to think that because you can frighten people they love you. Even that you love them.—And the whole thing comes down to fear. (Miller 1985, p. 82)[13]

In Vonda McIntyre's story, the sources of society's distrust and resentment are obvious because Snake's medical power is linked directly to a vehicle that would ordinarily be seen as deadly to innocent people. In the everyday physician-patient relationship, the sources of fear and distrust may be much harder to discern.

This line of speculation will make the average physician uncomfortable and defensive. How dare I even think of comparing the hardworking, compassionate physician to Stallone's sociopathic killer? To glimpse how the dark side of the force may be present just beneath the surface, we again require the offices of literature, which can lull us into an attitude of intellectual defenselessness and then hit us with a message that our rationalizations would ordinarily deflect. And since we would reject a cautionary message about doctors as stemming from paranoia or jealousy if it were penned by a layman, we also require a physician-author who is honest and brave enough to bare his soul in this way.

Two splendid revelations of the dark side of the force are the short stories "The Use of Force," by William Carlos Williams ([1933] 1984), and "Brute," by Richard Selzer (1982). Each depicts a physician vulnerable to loss of control: an underpaid and overworked Depression-era pediatrician making a lonely house call and a house surgeon up all night in the emergency room. Each depicts a patient who needs treatment and disdainfully

---

13. Admittedly, Miller seems here to be alluding to a search for money or fame rather than the impulse to use power purely for its own enjoyment and release. I will address the definition of the dark side of the force in the next chapter.

rejects it: a five-year-old who won't let the physician look in her throat for diphtheria, and a drunk who won't lie still to let the doctor suture the gash in his scalp. Each depicts a situation where the justification for treatment is clear, the consequences of noncompliance are grave, and the patient's ability to make a rational decision is nonexistent. Eventually, the pediatrician forces open the girl's mouth and discovers that she does indeed have diphtheria; the surgeon sews the drunk's ears to the cart, tells him that if he moves he'll tear his own ears off, and thus is able finally to repair the laceration. Looked at from the outside, the actions of the two physicians seem defensible, if crude. "After all, they did it for the patient's own good," would be the natural reaction. We know that the actions are indefensible, that the dark side of the force has been loosed, only because the two physician-authors are candid enough to lay bare the characters' thoughts.

Literary analysts routinely regard "The Use of Force" as describing what is, for all intents and purposes, a rape.[14] The narrator makes it clear that he begins the encounter somewhat angry and alienated but basically in control of his rational faculties; but as he responds to the pure, animal fury of the resisting girl, "the worst of it was that I too had got beyond reason. I could have torn the child apart in my own fury and enjoyed it. It was a pleasure to attack her. My face was burning with it" (Williams [1933] 1984, p. 59).

Selzer's surgeon sews down the drunk's ears, looks him squarely in the face to announce that he will now have to hold still or else tear his ears off—and grins at him. At the end of the story, recounting the incident for the benefit of the "young surgeon" to whom the volume is addressed, the older physician makes it clear that it is primarily the grin that he now regrets. The sewing down of the ears might be excused; the grin was an extra, purely for the pleasure of self-release. The beautiful ambiguity of the story's title is now clear. At the start, it seems to the reader that "Brute" must refer to the physically splendid but torn and raging creature lying on the cart. At the end, it seems rather that the brute might be the surgeon

14. On the implications of this story for medical ethics, see Bell 1984; Terry and Williams 1988. More generally, Ross (1989) has argued that this impulse to use power for its own sake is hinted at by the prevalence of war and military metaphors in medical language. So long as we are invited to view disease as a moral outrage rather than as a natural, biological phenomenon, we find ourselves obligated to respond aggressively. Quoting Susan Sontag, Ross adds that to label a nonmedical phenomenon with the name of a dreaded disease, such as cancer, is virtually an incitement to violence against it. Furthermore, "Contemporary medicine's focus on fighting disease (in contrast to caring for sick patients) has made war metaphors much more viable" (Ross 1989, p. 42).

who grinned, who allowed the dark side of the force to take command, knowing that he was safe from retribution or censure.

These two stories might be thought of as aberrations—unusual events selected precisely for their literary interest.[15] To see the dark side of the force in action in a more mundane fashion, we might turn instead to Samuel Shem's scatalogical novel of the internship experience, *The House of God* (1978). Much of the dark humor of the novel is intended to provide emotional release for the beleaguered house staff at the expense of the patients; it is the neediest and most pitiful patients, the "dirtballs" and "gomers," who are the butt of the most outrageous jokes. The interns are placed in a fundamentally inhumane situation without any power over their destinies. Their patients are really their fellow victims; but to feel this kinship fully would be to admit in a terribly painful way both their own powerlessness and their own vulnerability to aging and death. Their only way (they think) to avoid feeling victimized and helpless is to avoid identifying with the patients, to see the patients instead as their tormenters and then to unleash their angry humor at the patients. Ideally, the anger would have been directed at the true tormentors, such as the medical educators who gloried in and perpetuated the internship system and who showed, by their righteously horrified letters of condemnation to the editors of medical journals, how uncomfortable the book had made them.

15. Roger Sider, reviewing an early draft of this chapter, commented that the dark side of the force is consistent with the more general view of human nature as containing inherent possibilities for evil. He added that he saw a corresponding feature on the patient's side of the equation, in the self-destructive behaviors and habits many patients display. These comments suggest that the dark side of the force is widespread.

CHAPTER 3

THE DARK

SIDE OF

THE FORCE:

CLINICAL

EXAMPLES

A further illustration of "the dark side of the force" might show both how it could arise in practice and why the concept is a useful one to introduce into medical ethics. Consider the issue of whether physicians should have sexual relations with their patients. That almost all textbooks of medical ethics exclude this issue suggests implicitly that it is not a subject requiring ethical analysis. This position has a good deal to be said for it. The American Academy of Psychiatry, for example, condemns the practice in no uncertain terms; and there seem to be no informative or interesting ethical arguments that can be given on the opposing side (Webb 1986).

Since sex with patients is strongly condemned and no persuasive ethical justification can be offered for it, several facts become striking. First, a significant number of psychiatrists (a better-studied population than other specialties, though no data indicate that they are more frequent offenders) engage in it—about 5 to 10 percent according to various surveys. Second, these physicians are unlikely to admit moral impurity or lack of will; instead they offer various justifications for such behavior. One is that the practice may be therapeutic (presumably helping patients shed low self-esteem or neurotic inhibitions, for example); survey respondents characterized their sexual encounters as "caring" and "helpful" much more often than "harmful" or "exploitative." Another major justification was love—a startling 92 percent of offenders described their patients as being in love with them at the time of the incident (Gartrell, Herman, Olarte et al. 1986).

We have already made note of Williams's story "The Use of Force," which describes a physician engaged in what seems the symbolic equivalent of a rape. It is generally agreed today that rape is not primarily a sexual act; instead it is an act of violence. The urge underlying a rape is not an urge for sexual release but rather an urge to dominate powerfully another human being. In everyday society, this fact may be concealed by treating rape as a sexual act that gets out of hand; we then are tempted to attribute to rape things we think are true about other sexual acts (for example, that the woman who was raped must have done something to encourage or entice the rapist). This in turn helps us deny what rape shows us about the power relationships between men and women in our society. In medicine, we generally consider sexual relations with patients unprofessional; it will not do to excuse this behavior simply as an expression of sexual urge or a form of sexual release. But we can accomplish the same thing within medicine that the rape-as-sex reasoning does in society if we pretend that sex with patients somehow falls under the rubric of therapy. The therapeutic mantle cloaks the act in an assumption of altruism and beneficence and denies the power differential between physician and patient that effectively renders any such sexual act an act of dominance and victimhood (Karasu 1980).

Indeed, this mode of reasoning subtly increases the physician's self-image of power even as it denies that power plays a role in the genesis of the action. For a physician who engages in sex with a patient might be seen as giving in to temptation and hence as less powerful in relation to the patient. But a physician who can successfully control his sexual urges so as to use sex as a sort of therapy presumably shows that he is in even better control than most of us are and thus possesses an even more powerful therapeutic armamentarium. This mode of self-justification seems to clinch the argument that the need to exercise power for its own sake—the dark side of the force—is what underlies having sex with patients.

The second justification offered for sexual relationships with patients—that the patient must be in love with the physician—leads to further speculation about how the dark side of the force may exist just below the surface even in the more usual physician-patient encounter. There is a small but compelling literature on what causes physicians to dislike certain patients (Klein et al. 1982; Smith and Zimny 1988). Although the issue is rather complex, a reasonable generalization is that physicians especially dislike and try to avoid alcoholics, drug abusers, those seeking compensation benefits, chronic complainers, angry and hostile patients—that is those who cannot or will not display gratitude for the physicians' care and services. Now, if we say this baldly, the average physician will firmly deny the charge because it runs counter to his self-image to be dependent in any way on patient gratitude. The physician is supposed to be scientifically objective and professionally detached. His patients are supposed to be dependent on him; the idea that he might be in any way dependent on them is a blow to his professional ego. But if we get beyond this rather macho self-image and ask instead about the truth, we would find, among physicians secure enough to be honestly insightful, a confirmation of the role of gratitude in their own mental well-being. The physician who turns to alcohol or other drugs or becomes depressed is often the one whose practice offers few such emotional rewards. The unimpaired physician will admit that a single unexpected expression of thanks from a grateful patient is enough to make his day.

What I have just put forth—admittedly with less-than-thorough documentation—is a two-part assertion: physicians to some degree depend on the gratitude of their patients, and they have a need to deny this dependence.[1] Further speculation is needed to link these phenomena to the notion of power and the dark side of the force. The first point, regarding the need for gratitude, is analogous to a point made by feminists about men's need to see women as perpetually grateful to men for the attention and material well-being with which men provide them. The argument is that the relationship between men and women is basically a disparity in power, with men having the social status and control necessary to maintain their privileged power status and prevent women from getting uppity. However, men wish to deny the existence of this power and their own need to maintain it, partly because if it were made explicit the power disparity could not be long maintained in a society like ours, and partly because men's self-image of beneficence is inconsistent with it. The myth of perpetual, bottomless feminine gratitude serves this purpose of denial well.[2] The average man will argue (subconsciously): those who are dominated by the unjust power of others are never grateful to their persecutors; women are grateful to men; therefore the relationship between men and women must be that of beneficence and not that of domination. (It is worth recalling that 92 percent of the psychiatrists who admitted having sex with patients

1. Jack Coulehan argues that this is too broad a generalization. Physicians may dislike alcoholics, workers' compensation claimants, and other categories of patients out of narrow-mindedness and lack of empathy; the patients' inability to express gratitude may be lower on the list of undesirable attributes.

2. For an example of this line of analysis—turned to the specific question of (male-dominated) society's difficulty in dealing rationally or consistently with women who murder men—see Jones 1981, pp. 176–237; Ketchum and Pierce 1981. The following passage indicates how a feminist approach to ethical issues in medicine leads to a line of inquiry like the one I pursue in this book: "The ethical questions discussed . . . include patient autonomy, informed consent, and nonmalfeasance, but they are placed in a feminine context in which empowerment is central. These ethical themes are tied to the power theme because it is through authentic participation in decision making that patients in fact become powerful" (Ratcliff et al. 1989, p. 7).

asserted that the patients were in love with them at the time; moreover, the vast majority of the offending psychiatrists were male.) I speculate that, in an analogous way, the physician's need for the patient's expressed gratitude partly arises from a subconscious awareness of the power differential—an awareness that the dark side of the force lurks always beneath the surface—and a need to keep that awareness subconscious.

The second matter, the physician's need to deny the need for gratitude, is a bit more straightforward. Again taking an analogy from feminism, the power possessed by those in the dominant role may be threatened in two ways. One is by being made too obvious and explicit; hence the need to have it covered up with expressions (or myths) of gratitude. But the other is by empowering those in the submissive role so that they can challenge the power of the dominant ones. This is what is threatened by acknowledging that physicians need their patients' gratitude, for patients would then have the clear prerogative of selectively giving or withholding this gratitude, thus exercising power over the physician.[3] But that would be too much of a threat to the physician's power. The threat can be averted neatly (though at the cost of some dishonesty) by adopting a shared self-image that denies the physician's need for gratitude.

My argument is that physicians need occasional expressions of gratitude from patients partly to deny their own power over patients and its possible misuse, and they need to deny their need for this gratitude partly because openly acknowledging it would suggest a loss of physicians' power. (I insist on *partly* because I have no desire to cut physicians off from the rest of humanity; all people, I suppose, need occasional expressions of gratitude from others if they are to enjoy optimal psychological equilibrium.) The argument is speculative and hence cannot serve as proof of the existence of what I have been calling the dark side of the force. I offer it only as an additional illustration, which if true confirms the basic concept and shows its applicability to common doctor-patient encounters.

The point, for purposes of our inquiry, is not that physicians are brutes in saints' clothes. They are not. The point is that the dark side of the force always exists as an impulse, usually kept well under control but always

---

3. An interesting way to remove the patient's power and choice in the matter is to insist that the patient has a duty to be grateful to the physician; this is what Stephens (1989a) suggests is done in the first (1847) code of ethics of the American Medical Association. The relevant passage states: "A patient should, after his recovery, entertain a just and enduring sense of the value of the services rendered him by his physician; for these are of such a character, that no mere pecuniary acknowledgement can repay or cancel them" (American Medical Association 1848).

remaining not far below the beneficent surface. Patients sense this, and the power of the physician gives rise to more or less fear, distrust, and resentment depending on how far below the surface the impulse is felt to be and how strong or weak is the control that holds it in check. To suggest that the language of medical ethics must take the concept of power seriously is to call for a medical ethics that deals forthrightly with these feelings, not one that denies their very existence.

Until now I have been using the term *the dark side of the force* as if it were synonymous with any abuse of the physician's power. I have been interested in arguing that this dark side is a real phenomenon and underlies patient reactions to encounters with the physician: otherwise Vonda McIntyre could be accused of literary license in depicting the fear and anger that the family directs toward the healer, who has endured tremendous suffering in trying to save their child's life. But the use of power against the patient, motivated by the pleasure and release of being able to use one's power and control without social repercussions—the dark side—is only one form of abuse of power. There are at least two others.

The most obvious and least interesting abuse of power is that which is intended for the physician's selfish material benefit. The physician under a fee-for-service system who performs unnecessary procedures and the "gatekeeper" physician in a prepaid plan who supplements his bonus by underserving patients are examples I will discuss in later chapters. That this is a clear abuse of the physician's power is one of the reasons that (as I will argue later) the income of the physician deserves to be regarded explicitly as an ethical issue in medicine.

Another form of power abuse is what is meant when the physician is accused of playing God. Erde (1989) shows that the term *playing God* is most often used to stop debate or to beg the question and thus is an undesirable addition to the vocabulary of medical ethics. In at least one situation, however, there is some meaning that can be given to the term. Erde argues that its use suggests a worldview that entails the concept of the great chain of being, which in turn holds that God created the world in such a way as to include everything that ought to be included and exclude everything that ought to be excluded. To offer oneself as the architect of an improved world is to display hubris, a disrespect both for God and for the content of His creation. Now, if a physician makes use of the power of medical science to try to remodel the world—for instance, by altering life forms through genetic manipulation, or by eliminating classes of infants from birth by genetic screening and selective abortion, or by euthanasia of those considered unfit—she is guilty of precisely this sort of hubris. It is an abuse of power in two ways. First, it is the use of medical and scientific power to force her own view of the ideal world onto others, who may not share her conception. Second, it is the subterfuge of undertaking God-like work while wrapping herself in the physician's mantle, as if the good motives normally attributed to physicians who aim solely to heal the sick could be used to justify these other acts by implication.

In many instances, as Erde points out, there is no obvious dividing line between redesigning the world, in the sense that offends the proponent of the great chain of being, and simply trying to heal the sick. After all, God created sickness and sick people, and if one tries to help them, is one not interfering in God's plan? But in at least some cases it might be clear when a physician has stepped out of bounds and attempted to use medical power to push for a personal view of how the world ought to be instead of submitting his views on these matters for open discussion in the appropriate public forum. And if that occurred, we could appropriately consider it an abuse of power of the sort to which playing God ambiguously refers.

An Objection

This analysis of the three kinds of power and discovery of "the dark side of the force" set up one of the major objections to the thesis of this book. This objection is that the core of medical ethics has to do with the proper use of Aesculapian power. The dark side of the force, the misuse and abuse of power, has to do primarily with the physician's charismatic and social power—more often the latter. But there is nothing about charismatic or social power that is necessary for the physician to be able to diagnose and treat illness. The physician in the "pure" role of physician requires only Aesculapian power. The problem of the abuse of power arises from the multitude of other social roles physicians play in complex societies like ours; and those can be clearly separated from the physician as healer.[4] Medical ethics can deal quite well with the proper use of Aesculapian power, utilizing its comfortable analytic vocabulary; the physician's abuse of power in economic and political terms can be left to the sociologists and others to deal with. Hence the absence of the term *power* from the vocabulary of medical ethics signals nothing amiss.

4. McCullough, in a paper that otherwise anticipates much of what I wish to say about shared power in later chapters, hints at this position when he notes the "distinction between the morally authoritative use of power and raw power in the physician-patient relationship" (McCullough 1988, p. 461). By "raw power" he presumably has in mind what I have called the dark side of the force. McCullough seems to see this distinction as fairly obvious and straightforward, whereas for me it is an overly optimistic portrayal.

Indeed, even though I have quoted John Ladd as one of the few philosophers willing to conceptualize medical ethics as a problem of power, other writings of Ladd's suggest that he holds a view similar to this. He argues that the power of the physician to occupy and keep a high socioeconomic status, and to impose her will on patients individually and collectively, is a matter separate from the Aesculapian power the physician needs to heal.[5] The solution, then, is a simple political one: allow the physician to keep Aesculapian power, strip her of undeserved social power, and all will be well.

The question, then, is how easy it is to bracket charismatic and social power off from Aesculapian power. If the bracketing is easy in real-life medical contexts, then medical ethics can be excused for focusing solely on Aesculapian power and avoiding consideration of other, messier power problems. If the bracketing is difficult or impossible, then medical ethics has no choice but to take *power* into the fold of its essential vocabulary. What arguments can be made to show that the bracketing is difficult or impossible?

At this point it should become clear why I have elected to begin this book with stories drawn from literary sources. Three of the stories cited— "The Chief of Medicine," "The Use of Force," and "Brute"—suggest that the bracketing of Aesculapian power is an illegitimate and impoverished way to understand the physician-patient encounter, both when it works (as in "The Chief of Medicine," presumably) and when it goes wrong (as in "The Use of Force" and "Brute"). The Chief of Medicine, parroting the theology of the Grand Inquisitor, insists that his ability to heal derives primarily from charismatic and social power. The "brutes" in Williams's and Selzer's stories can do their deeds and get away with them because of their social status and because of how they have learned to carry themselves in those social roles. The point of both stories is the fine line between the dark side of the force and "he was only doing it for the patient's own good"; but to see that point, it is necessary to see the physician's Aesculapian, charismatic, and social power as inextricably intertwined. For example, we have to accept his knowledge of how serious diphtheria is and how likely

5. On this score compare Ladd 1980, quoted here and in the previous chapter, with Ladd 1979, 1982. Ketchum and Pierce (1981) criticize Ladd's later position: "A physician cannot relinquish at will the power that is his qua physician. Moreover, to deny or ignore one's power, when one actually does have it, is not the likeliest road to morality" (p. 278). But even Ketchum and Pierce err in focusing solely on the institutional aspects of medicine and thus reducing the issue of power to one of social power only. For other uses of the term with strictly social connotations, see Erde 1980; Daniels 1984.

it is that this girl has it, given her symptoms. We also have to accept his skill in getting children and their parents to cooperate with physical examination in order to know what is a reasonable use of force and what is not. (If pediatricians did not routinely employ charismatic and social power, few children would ever get examined!) Unless we understand these things, we will assume that Williams's pediatrician stepped over the line at the very outset of the encounter, and not only when the animal fury took over.

The story "Of Mist, and Grass, and Sand," is unique in showing us a healer for whom Aesculapian power predominates over charismatic and social power. But the story's uniqueness reinforces the main argument. Maybe in a world of science fiction, healers could be more like Snake and less like the Chief of Medicine. But it is hard to recognize in Snake any idea of a healer that seems relevant to our own world, even if all the reforms in medical practice that we would like to see were accomplished. At the very least, Snake could have gotten her work done more easily and efficiently, and certainly at much less cost and danger to herself, had she possessed a bit more social and charismatic power. Yet her ability to reassure the young boy while at the same time stating flatly that she is going to hurt him suggests considerable charisma; and the way the family and the tribe react to her suggests that anyone who carries around trained snakes has achieved a sort of social power, whether of her own seeking or not. If we recall that Snake accepts as an inherent part of her Aesculapian ability the social and psychological skill necessary to comprehend and disarm the patient's and the family's fear and anger in the face of illness and death, we see that it is almost impossible to draw lines between Aesculapian, charismatic, and social forms of power.

The blurred lines between the different sorts of power are further suggested by the discussion of the hybrid or derivative "cultural power." I suggested in chapter 2 that one could subsume that variety of power under the more general heading of social power, primarily so as not to get mixed up in a debate between biological positivism and social construction. But it is also well to recall that the exercise of the physician's cultural power—to designate certain biological states as diseases and certain individuals as sick—ideally draws heavily on the proper exercise of Aesculapian power and could be justified by reference to the physician's Aesculapian knowledge. Now, cultural power seems an excellent example of a power whose use and abuse are separated by a fairly slim margin. When sick, we want the physician to have the authority both to explain what is happening to us, why our body seems not to submit to our will, and to prompt our family and friends toward a posture of understanding, concern, and practical support (Cassell 1976). The physician accomplishes this by providing a disease label for our suffering, to show both ourselves and others that we are not to blame, that we are not being merely lazy or disloyal, and so forth. But the power to label, and so to mobilize social resources on behalf of the sufferer, is not far from a power to define homosexuality as a disease or (among Soviet psychiatrists) to define political dissent as mental illness. It is precisely this potential abuse of medical power, subtly manifested as the "medicalization" of various aspects of society, that has fueled the criticisms of Ivan Illich (1976) and others. And if I am correct in suggesting that cultural power has deep roots in Aesculapian power (even though its consequences may be social), then we cannot avoid concerns over medical abuse of power by focusing our attention on Aesculapian power only.

The Chief of Medicine rests a good deal of his case on his understanding of the placebo effect. I have argued at length elsewhere (Brody 1980) that the placebo phenomenon needs to be seen as all-pervasive in medicine and may play some role in almost every healing encounter. Patients indeed get better because of specific cures worked through the application of medical science, and they get better because the natural history of the disease process tends toward spontaneous recovery; but they also get better, a good deal of the time, because of the symbolic aspects of the healing encounter and because the meaning of the experience of being ill has been rendered more positive and less frightening. This occurs, in turn, when the patient receives a satisfactory explanation of the illness, when those around him respond with care and support, and when he regains a sense of mastery or control over the illness (Brody 1980). A skilled healer can facilitate all these changes; but she can best do so if she has a fair amount of cultural, charismatic, and social power in addition to pure Aesculapian power.

As a further illustration of the intertwining of the different sorts of power, consider the viewpoints expressed in letters to the *Journal of the American Medical Association* in response to the article "It's Over, Debbie" (1988), describing an apparent instance of active euthanasia in the United States. A number of physicians wrote to condemn both the physician for killing the patient and *JAMA* for publishing the article. Their moral stance was that doctors should never kill, period, and that active euthanasia should not be debated or discussed but condemned outright. Yet several non-physicians wrote to suggest that they feared a lingering death due to over-zealous use of medical technology more than they did active euthanasia at the hands of an untrustworthy physician.[6] And public opinion polls generally show that a majority of American citizens favor active euthanasia in some circumstances.

This seems to be an example of a divergence of opinion between what physicians and patients think of as proper uses and abuses of medical power. From the physicians' side, to use medical power (presumably Aesculapian) to end a patient's life is an obvious and indefensible instance of abuse of power; patients will be adequately reassured about the morality of medicine only if all right-thinking physicians totally condemn active euthanasia. The assumption seems to be that if patients fear generally the misuse of medical power, this is what they fear above all else. But for many patients abuse of medical power is inappropriate prolongation of life in terminal illness—again, an example of Aesculapian power. By contrast, for the physician to use medical power to relieve the symptoms of dying and return control to the patient—even if that means active intervention to shorten life—would be seen as a fully defensible use of Aesculapian power. We have here a fundamental dispute about the use of medical power, whether for or against the patient; and it involves almost solely Aesculapian power. We do not have to see charismatic or social power as contaminating Aesculapian power in order for questions of the misuse and abuse of power to arise.

To summarize, I agree with the Chief of Medicine that healing may come through the exercise of social and charismatic power as well as through the use of Aesculapian power. I agree with him that both physicians and patients are prone to overestimate the Aesculapian component of curing and to underestimate the charismatic and social components, and that this misperception, when it occurs, serves sometimes to enhance the placebo response. I disagree with him that the physician's power to cure cannot survive a greater degree of disclosure to the patient about the real limitations of Aesculapian knowledge and skill. And I disagree with him most profoundly when he suggests that anything that increases the power of the

---

6. The "Debbie" article describes active euthanasia carried out by a gynecology resident on a young woman with terminal ovarian cancer, under highly questionable circumstances. For the range of viewpoints expressed in letters to the editor, see *Journal of the American Medical Association* 259 (April 8, 1988): 2094–98. The strongest condemnation by a physician of both active euthanasia and its open discussion is in Gaylin et al. 1988; for more balanced discussions, see Vaux 1988; Lundberg 1988. For a review of the practice of euthanasia in the Netherlands, see Pence 1988; Fenigsen 1989; Rigter 1989. The "Debbie case" is discussed further in chapter 5 below.

patient within the healing encounter must simultaneously decrease the healing power of the physician—that the power relationship between physician and patient is a zero-sum game. It is this mistake specifically that I will address in the remainder of this book.[7]

How Was Power Excluded from Medical Ethics?

The argument I have been framing thus far can be summarized as follows: *The central ethical problem in medicine is the responsible use of power. Physicians have considerable power to alter the course of illness. But this same power can, with only subtle redirection, be used against the patient instead of against the disease on the patient's behalf. The problem is to empower physicians for the performance of their essential tasks while protecting the patient from the potential misuses and abuses of power.*

Nothing about this formulation seems especially striking or original; John Ladd (1980) has made precisely this same point. Then why is it possible to read page after page of scholarly works on medical ethics, to scan their tables of contents and indexes, and never encounter the word *power*?[8]

An answer may be found by returning to the development of medical ethics as we now think of it—in the late 1960s and early 1970s, when analytic philosophy became intrigued by this subject and wrested it away, for a time, from the theologians and religious ethicists who had had the field to themselves in the previous two decades. The answer will be uncomfortable for those steeped in the analytic mind-set, who wish to think that the concepts and vocabulary of medical ethics, as they developed them,

---

7. Ratcliff et al. (1989, p. 7) note similarly that power distribution among people is not necessarily a zero-sum game. They give as an example the way that a hospice program can empower both the patient and the provider. Freed from the restrictions of the hospital setting, both are better able to shape the use of technology to their particular ends.

8. I have not done a word-by-word analysis of the medical ethics literature but have tried to attend carefully to that literature since 1972. In the course of working on this book I reviewed the indexes and tables of contents of thirty-eight volumes on medical ethics; only two mentioned the term *power*, and neither used it in the way I do here. A later volume that does discuss power in several contexts is Drane 1988. See also Staum and Larsen 1981. The exceptions to the general lack of discussion of power within works on medical ethics tend to prove the main thesis. For example, Karasu (1980) makes very effective use of the power concept in discussing the ethics of psychotherapy; but as a psychiatrist he would be viewed as on the border between medicine and the social sciences. Waitzkin and Stoeckle's paper (1972) on communication of information to patients includes a section entitled "The Problem of Uncertainty and the Problem of Power." This reflects primarily a social-science orientation and cites many works by sociologists. Since I completed the early drafts of this book, *power* seems to be finding its way back into the ethics lexicon; see for example McCullough 1988, 1989; Callahan 1989; Doerflinger 1989.

are eternal truths that reflect the nature of the subject and were not shaped or colored by the events going on in the world at the time the analytic philosophers were carrying on their work. For I think it is precisely in the work world of the analytic pioneers in medical ethics that we find why *power* was excluded from the vocabulary.[9]

Modern medical ethics began in the world of medical education. Some thoughtful medical educators, their consciousness of ethical matters raised by pioneering religious authors such as Joseph Fletcher and Paul Ramsey, decided that the training of physicians ought to include ethics. The first to address this need, in the 1960s, were concerned chaplains and clergy working within medical schools; by the 1970s a few analytic philosophers became interested in applying their ethics training in this area. These philosophers endured a fair amount of ostracism from their straight-philosophy colleagues, who thought that to direct one's career into "applied ethics" was the kiss of death for any respectable intellectual.

The philosophers found that one of their first tasks would be to explain to the clinician-educators exactly who they were and what they were doing there. The clinicians thought they knew this already. For, some time previously, medical education had had its first influx of "outsiders"—behavioral and social scientists—imported to deal with large gaps in medical education having to do with the emotional, cultural, and social aspects of illness and of sick people. And so it was natural for the clinicians to assume that the new Ph.D.s were simply more of the same. When the philosopher explained that he wished to explore the ethical issues in withholding life-prolonging treatment from terminally ill patients, the clinician nodded and said, "Oh, yes, you are going to talk about the psychology of grief and Kubler-Ross's five stages of the dying process."

Being classed among the behavioral scientists had significant drawbacks, as the philosophers quickly realized.[10] The obvious one was a confusion in the methodology of scholarship and research. Philosophers simply do

9. Again, I base this generalization in part on personal experience. I am also indebted to Gerald Osborn's unpublished master's thesis (Cambridge University, 1985) on the history of medical ethics in the United States since the 1960s. See also Jonsen et al. 1978.

10. For a fairly typical (though unusually insightful) statement of these issues, see Clouser 1973. Clouser carefully distinguished the methods and subject matter of ethics from those of law, religion, social sciences, counseling, and psychiatry. He rejected any connection between the study of ethics and moral exhortation in fairly radical terms: "The discipline itself will not provide the motivation to live by it any more than the study of political science will motivate one to become a politician" (p. 789). For a later and, I believe, more mature assessment of how the study of ethics should alter the behavior of medical students, see Culver, Clouser, Gert, et al. 1985.

not attack problems the way sociologists and psychologists do, by gathering empirical data in order to test their hypotheses. It was hopeless to try to teach any methodology of ethics in medicine unless this difference was made clear from the start.

There was another, more subtle reason to avoid being identified with the earlier wave of behaviorists. Coming into medical education with little appreciation of the needs of medical students and of clinical medicine, these behaviorists naturally taught from their own discipline's major texts and articles and proceeded as much as possible as if medical students were graduate students in sociology, anthropology, or whatever. This pedagogy antagonized the students and obscured the utility of certain behavioral concepts for medical practice. Perhaps even more important, these behaviorists had, in conducting their own research, bitten the hand that fed them. Physicians' tribal customs and strange rites, the hidden feelings aroused by patients—all these were exciting and perfectly acceptable research topics from the perspective of the social scientists. But such work was viewed quite differently by the clinicians. It seemed like "doctor bashing," the inappropriate use of special privilege (having been invited within the temple to see the secret rites performed) to make a name and sell one's book by holding the priests up to public ridicule.

At this point the philosopher-pioneers had to make a strategic decision. They could insist that properly carrying out the task of scholarly inquiry required maintaining assiduously the same sort of critical distance from the clinicians that the social scientists had employed.[11] This would allow medical ethics to be free from the taint of favoritism or special pleading and would also insure that physicians, now wary, would exclude them from many of the contexts of medical care where the most difficult and complex decisions were made. Alternatively, they could insist that they were not doctor bashers and represented no threat whatever to their clinician colleagues. In general, they chose the latter course. This is illustrated by the statement that went out early from leading ethicists, and remained unchallenged, that they were not and never would be the moral police

11. For a particularly good statement of the reasons for this critical distance in ethics, see Churchill 1978. It is important to recognize, however, that this distance was viewed as an attitude of analysis and was not intended to rule out collegiality and cooperation between "ethicists" and physicians. The fact that Churchill felt it necessary to remind the ethicists of the need for distance illustrates how high the level of cooperation and identification had already become: "Ethicists who teach in professional schools work very hard for the trust and acceptance that allows them to function with ease and effectiveness in their institutions. I do not want to minimize the importance of such acceptance" (p. 15).

(Clouser 1975). It was not their intent to root out bad behavior and punish it; supposedly the mechanisms that professional medicine had developed for policing itself would have to suffice (however inadequate those mechanisms may have been). Their intended audience was not the morally defective physician who needed reform; it was the morally well-intentioned physician who wanted to do the right thing but was confused as to what the right thing was.

This strategic decision has generally worked very well. It allowed the philosophers to get on with their work in a stunningly successful fashion, so that the philosophical vocabulary for defining and analyzing moral problems is now part of almost every medical curriculum and has figured in prominent national reports, guidelines, and court decisions. Most clinicians view medical ethics as an attempt to be genuinely helpful and accept the idea that to be considered minimally knowledgeable in medical ethics, one must show one's familiarity with the accepted vocabulary.

But a small side effect of this strategy was the unself-conscious decision to exclude *power* from the vocabulary, for it was a social scientist's word.[12] The physician's power and authority, their origins, how they often exceeded the real knowledge that medicine claimed for itself, how physicians often used them for their own selfish gain—this was the stuff of sociological and psychological analysis of medicine and of physician behavior. But physicians want to be seen by patients as benevolent; and the word *power* applied to the physician himself (instead of to the impersonal science and technology the physician claims to represent) suggests the specter that I have referred to as the dark side of the force, never far from the physicians' consciousness despite their best efforts to deny it. And so the philosophers learned early and well that if they analyzed ethical issues in terms of power relationships, they ran the risk of being seen as social scientists and as doctor bashers.

Another reason might be suggested for the exclusion of *power* from the medical-ethics lexicon. I think this reason is less important, but it will sound more respectable to the philosophers. It starts by noting the ease with which the terms *power* and *force* may be confused. The political philosopher Thomas Hobbes defined power as one's present means to obtain some future good; and he listed a variety of natural powers (such as bodily strength, knowledge, prudence, and eloquence) and instrumental

12. For a discussion of power by Hobbes, a social-political philosopher, see below. Another often-cited discussion is May 1972, pp. 99–119. A good example of the use of the term in an analysis of medicine by social scientists is Gilligan and Pollak 1988.

powers (such as riches, reputation, and friendship) (Hobbes [1651] 1962, chap. 10, pp. 66–74). Now, we would tend to have very different moral judgments about using strength and riches to get what one wants, as opposed to using reputation and eloquence. Power defined in this way is ethically neutral. In ordinary speech, however, power tends to be restricted to the negative end of this spectrum of means; unless carefully specified, power suggests the employment of unfair or unequal means to get what one wants and also the relative inability of others to object to this, even though they might have good reasons to do so.

Philosophers attending specifically to questions of political power will be as careful as Hobbes in distinguishing different cases; but philosophers discussing ethics more generally are prone to the ambiguity and distortion of ordinary usage. If a philosopher is asked, "What is ethics?" it would be very natural for her to reply that ethics is providing sound reasons to justify one's behavior. She would add, by way of illustration, that this could be contrasted with an appeal to force, where who is right is determined by who is stronger or better armed and not by who has the most persuasive reasons. She would go on to say that a world that routinely employs force to settle disputes has no use for ethics, but a world that seeks to avoid the use of force will inevitably turn to ethics. The lesson, of course, is that where force is, ethics is not. But when in ordinary language force and power are used almost synonymously, it is easy to conclude that appeals to power constitute rejections of ethical reasoning and that to discuss power issues must be to discuss something other than ethics. Stated openly in this fashion, these conclusions are of course incorrect. The person who is best able to provide good reasons and argue cogently for her position may be the most powerful person around for that very reason. But if the question of power is not explicitly examined and remains implicit, it is quite easy to fall into this trap of thinking that power-talk cannot be ethics-talk.

I have now reviewed two possible reasons why *power* has been banished from the vocabulary of medical ethics. But regardless of which reasons were operating and when, medical ethics has nevertheless developed a rich, complex, and useful body of work. In what way, then, has the taboo status of *power* made any important difference? Why now declare a need to welcome it back to the fold? The remainder of this book is intended to address this question, but here I can briefly sketch an answer.

Without a concept of power, medical ethics proceeded by postulating several basic moral principles that ought to guide ethical inquiry. Ethical dilemmas were seen as arising primarily when these principles came into conflict with one another. A standard list of the most important principles might be autonomy, beneficence (and/or nonmaleficence), and justice (Beauchamp and Childress 1983, 1989).

These principles are both valuable and illuminating, but they can also be quite misleading when used in a context that denies the relevance of the issue of power. Autonomy has been analyzed and used in a variety of ways, some of them congenial to the issues I shall address below. But one popular way of viewing autonomy—seeing it as fundamentally opposed to unacceptable medical paternalism—has been to think of autonomy as taking power away from the physician and returning it to the patient. This is never said—the vocabulary is that of autonomy, paternalism, rights, and contracts, never of power—but it is implied. And this implication therefore ignores the basic reason patients seek the help of a physician in the first place. Surely the physician should be stripped of inappropriate power that works toward her personal advantage rather than toward the patient's health; but just as surely any diminution of the physician's power runs the risk of robbing the patient of *his* most valuable resource. Which is which? A vocabulary of autonomy that disallows any reference to power cannot say.

The principle of beneficence correctly depicts the primary motivator of the physician's helpful interventions; and the principle of justice suggests an impersonal distribution of the available medical resources according to greatest need or merit. Both, thereby, implicitly deny the possibility of abuses of power. They tend to refute not only what I have called "the dark side of the force" but also less dramatic issues like the physician's income, social status, academic and professional stature, and immunity from legal liability and administrative inconveniences. Both patients and politicians, who were not born yesterday, know how power can be used selfishly and approach professional protestations of benevolence and public-spiritedness with at least some skepticism. By eliminating *power* from the lexicon of medical ethics, we force ethics to be less sophisticated than the patients and the politicians.

Guidelines for the Responsible Use of Power

The language of ethical principles—autonomy, beneficence, and justice, among others—has been justifiably popular in medical-ethics circles because it promises fairly straightforward, practical rules or guidelines. And this promise has been largely fulfilled, in documents such as the reports of the President's Commission (1983) and more recently in a set of guidelines (1987) on life-sustaining treatment produced under the aegis of the Hastings Center. Power-talk is unlikely to be welcomed into the field unless it has at least some similar promise of providing practical guidelines. Before launching into an analysis of specific problem areas in medicine, we might ask whether there are some model guidelines for the responsible use of power in medicine. If so, we can keep them in mind during later discussion and test them out against specific cases and problems, refining them as we go along.

John Ladd concluded his brief article on the subject of power analysis (1980) by suggesting three components of the responsible exercise of power:

> *Realism*: being aware of the true consequences of one's acts or omissions
> *Accountability*: being ready and able to give an explanation of one's use of power; this eventually leads to broader participation in medical decisions
> *Purposiveness*: having a specific end toward which the power is directed, rather than simply drifting along with it because it is there or employing power merely for its own sake[13]

This list is a good starting point, but some modifications may be in order. My earlier discussion suggests that purposiveness is a useful guideline, since it is violated directly in the dark side of the force. The word, however, is clumsy for continued reference.

Realism is no doubt important in medical thinking, but it is already widely accepted that a physician cannot make a good ethical decision without knowing the likely consequences of her interventions or the prognosis of the patient's illness with and without treatment. This is true whether one wishes to speak in terms of ethical principles or in terms of power. The particular sort of realism I am most concerned about in this book is being explicitly aware of power struggles and power disparities when they occur in medical settings; if we use the other guidelines, which cause us to refer explicitly to power issues, then realism of this sort will be promoted anyway. For these reasons it seems superfluous to continue to refer to realism as a necessary guideline for the responsible use of power.

Accountability, as described by Ladd, has two components—candor and mutual participation. He thinks the first will inevitably lead to the second, but as we will later see, several features of medical practice could prevent this development. It seems worth keeping the two ideas distinct, at least for a preliminary survey.

13. For additional comments on medical power, see Ladd 1981 and chapter 13 below. For a somewhat similar list of ethical "signposts" for responsible physician behavior, see Campbell and Higgs 1982, p. 106.

Taking note of these comments on Ladd's list leads to the following proposal:

We can have the highest degree of confidence that the healer's power is being used ethically and responsibly when that power can be described as *owned power, shared power*, and *aimed power*.

Owned is here used in the sense of *acknowledged*; it suggests both candid admission of a fact and acceptance of personal responsibility for the state of affairs admitted.

Although these guidelines will have to be tested out against actual medical issues, some preliminary considerations indicate that shared power may turn out to be the most basic or central of the three. First, it is possible to own or disclose one's power without sharing it (as one popular T-shirt slogan reads, " 'Cause I'm the mommy, that's why"). And it is also possible to aim one's power at a particular goal without sharing it. But it is quite difficult to share power without candidly disclosing it and without aiming it (or, better, allowing the other party to help aim it). Second, shared power tends to promote a degree of self-correction that prevents abuse and victimization. One can own one's power and make mistakes in its use; indeed, those who are victimized may be dissuaded from complaining precisely because the power has been candidly disclosed. One can also aim one's power at the wrong end. But if one shares the power precisely with the person in greatest danger of being victimized, the potential for self-correction of error seems greatest. As Ladd commented, "One of the best ways of avoiding the corruption of power is to share it" (1980, p. 1129).

T he new or autonomy-centered medical ethics has one thing in common with the old, which Robert Veatch (1981) has termed the Hippocratic or beneficence-centered medical ethics: much writing on the subject has been devoted to the physician-patient relationship. In the old ethics, the discussion was on how to discern and implement what is good for the patient, with and sometimes without the patient's cooperation, all the while maintaining amicable relations with patient, family, and professional colleagues. The new ethics has focused on how to promote patient autonomy and contain or eliminate physician paternalism. Only recently have some writers begun to ask whether other aspects of the relationship deserve at least as much attention as the autonomy-paternalism dimension (Brody 1987b). These recent criticisms provide a good foundation for assessing how we could look at the physician-patient relationship if power were a more basic component of our ethics vocabulary.

Basic Obligations of the Physician

How medical ethics came to discover patient autonomy, how it tried to ground an autonomy-centered model of the physician-patient relationship in deeper ethical theories (such as social-contract theory), and how it next came to critique the overemphasis on autonomy and justify a more active role for the physician have all been reviewed extensively (Brody 1985, 1987b, 1989c). It is still useful to have a list of basic conditions for an ethically sound physician-patient relationship as a springboard for further discussion. I have not found a better list than the four "rights in personal care" proposed by Charles Fried (1974).

The choice of Fried's approach as a starting point may seem unusual.

Fried wrote his book on human experimentation near the beginning of the first wave of the new ethics. His selection of the term *rights in personal care* suggests a legalistic, potentially adversarial approach to the physician-patient relationship. Indeed, that relationship was not the primary focus of Fried's inquiry: he developed his list only as a point of contrast with the relationship between investigator and subject in the experimental setting. Nonetheless, Fried's approach seems to have withstood the test of later criticism.

I will restate the components of Fried's list, retaining his titles but expressing them as physician obligations rather than as patient rights:

Lucidity: The physician has the obligation to disclose the nature of the patient's illness as well as the nature of any proposed treatment, along with any viable alternative treatments.

Autonomy: The physician has the obligation to allow the patient to make important medical-care decisions on his own behalf and to defer to the patient's competent wishes even when he feels that the course chosen may not be in the patient's best interest.

Fidelity: The physician has an obligation to act in a trustworthy fiduciary manner and to view himself as the patient's agent in health-care matters.

Humanity: The physician has an obligation to treat the patient with compassion and sensitivity, especially bearing in mind the increased emotional vulnerability brought about by illness and fear of death.

Putting these thoughts together, Fried regards the physician essentially as "the servant, not of life in the abstract, but of the life plan of the patient" (1974, p. 99). The physician is not the "servant of the patient," obligated to honor his every whim. But where the issue is the patient's life plan—his enduring preferences, values, and projects, which help determine who he is—the physician is obligated to use medical technology in the way that best furthers that life plan, even if she thinks this would not be in the patient's long-term interest.[1]

Fried's formulation of the four basic obligations could be viewed as playing a pivotal role in the development of the new ethics, partly looking backward at the Hippocratic tradition, partly encapsulating the primary concerns of the new ethics, and partly anticipating the most recent criticisms of the new ethics. It contains important Hippocratic elements in the obligations of fidelity and humanity. The physician clearly must try to do

1. On the concept of a life plan and its relationship to illness and the meaning of illness for the patient, see Brody 1987d, esp. chap. 3 and 5.

what is best for the patient and not do anything to harm the patient or his vital interests. Moreover, the physician must view the patient's plight with compassion and sensitivity—and that includes discerning when fear, depression, or other consequences of illness might render the patient less able to decide rationally what is best for him. But the inclusion of those Hippocratic elements does not constitute a defense of medical paternalism, for they go hand in hand with the centerpiece of the new ethics—autonomy, and the full disclosure required for autonomy to be exercised to the best advantage. There is no defense in Fried's view for the paternalistic physician who benignly withholds bad news from a patient or imposes his own view of the patient's interest without consulting the patient. Still, autonomy is not the sole or the primary moral value in this list but is simply one of four. Fried thus foreshadows recent criticism of the new ethics as over-emphasizing autonomy.

Clearly, according to Fried, the physician has a duty to disclose the diagnosis and proposed treatment frankly to the patient and then to be guided by the patient's wishes. What of the physician who fears that the patient will be crushed by the diagnosis of an incurable disease and who therefore builds up to the final disclosure over a day or two instead of blurting it out at once? This physician may have fudged a bit on lucidity, but he did so in the name of humanity. What of the physician who withholds the dread diagnosis from a patient who has told him consistently in the past that he fears bad news and wants to be spared any such knowledge? The physician has violated the duty of lucidity but has preserved fidelity and autonomy, since the patient himself authorized that course. What of the physician facing an acutely ill patient who is acting irrationally but who minimally meets the criteria for mental competence and is refusing lifesaving treatment? If the physician finds a way to manipulate the patient into starting treatment, he may be violating the duty of autonomy but preserving fidelity and humanity. Moreover, if the patient is really somewhat irrational when he refuses treatment, and assuming that his life goals would best be served by avoiding an early death, then the physician, in temporarily setting aside respect for autonomy, is better serving the basic role of "servant of the life plan of the patient."

Fried's list of obligations, derived from an analysis of patient rights within an ethically acceptable physician-patient relationship, also coheres well with views of medical ethics that arise from a non-rights-based framework. For example, Pellegrino (1979) has insisted that medical ethics must be based in a philosophical elaboration of the nature of medical practice, not simply in an analysis of the rights of autonomous individuals. To Pellegrino, the roots of the ethics of the physician-patient relationship lie in what he calls "the act of profession and the fact of illness." To my reading, much of Pellegrino's "act of profession" could be linked conceptually to Fried's obligation of fidelity; and if we read the obligation of humanity to encompass a sensitivity to the unique vulnerability induced by sickness in otherwise competent and rational individuals, then "the fact of illness" is included as well. Pellegrino and Thomasma (1981) have argued further that medicine is best viewed as a skilled craft which aims to apply general scientific knowledge to individual cases for the purpose of a right and good healing action on the patient's behalf. The explicit inclusion of "right and good" is intended to signal medicine's value-laden nature. But this view of medicine seems to cohere reasonably well with Fried's concept of the "servant of the life plan of the patient." The main lesson of this comparison is that Fried has succeeded at looking not just at the rights of autonomous individuals but at rights *in personal (medical) care*. That is, without downplaying rights and autonomy, he has kept in sight the nature of the physician-patient relationship, what circumstances give rise to it, and what its ultimate objectives must be.

Though Fried eschewed explicit recourse to the term *power* in analyzing the relationship, his list of obligations fits nicely with Ladd's (1980) criteria for the ethical use of power. Fidelity requires that the physician always use her power on the patient's behalf and not to his detriment. Humanity requires that the physician always take into account the relative powerlessness of the sick patient while still preserving a human-to-human relationship. Autonomy requires that the physician be prepared always to share decision-making power with the patient. Lucidity requires that the physician be accountable for how she has used her power. In short, Fried's list of obligations is fully consistent with the idea that the goal of the physician-patient relationship is the ethical use of power on the patient's behalf, where the physician has a power advantage over the patient and neither of them wants to see that power advantage erased.

Finally, we should note that Fried, by discussing his obligations under the heading of *personal* care and by focusing on the life plan of the patient (which presumably requires an extended and in-depth relationship before the physician can be said to know it well enough to serve it), appears to tilt his analysis in the direction of a relationship more typical of primary medical care than of a subspecialty or in-hospital setting. When Fried wrote, few thought that medical ethics might require different treatments for primary and other sorts of care. It now appears that there are some important distinctions between these two aspects of medical practice that require systematic, if subtle, ethical differentiation. I will return to this point in a subsequent section but first must address the problems of the dominance of autonomy in the new ethics.

The Limitations of Autonomy

The phase roughly corresponding to much writing on medical ethics between 1969 and 1983 might also be labeled—to borrow another term from Robert Veatch (1984)—"autonomy's temporary triumph." The triumph was temporary for many reasons, but two are of special interest here. One is the need, underemphasized by the new ethics, to balance autonomy against other ethical principles of arguably equal weight. The second is the pervasiveness, under the influence of the new ethics, of some basic misunderstandings about what autonomy itself entails.

Almost all commonly consulted textbooks and theoretical works on medical ethics during the "new" phase provide a list of moral values and ethical principles and explicitly state that autonomy is in many cases the deciding one, but not the only one (Beauchamp and Childress, 1983). The possibility that in a particular case other principles might be more compelling than autonomy was always left open. Still, the implicit message that most readers probably derived was that autonomy was really what the new ethics was all about. This view was quite natural; after all, values like beneficence and nonmaleficence were recognized in antiquity, and autonomy was the only really novel principle under discussion. Moreover, which principle is most important depends in large part on who your enemy is, whose position you are struggling against. And the new ethics was univocal on that point: the enemy of ethical medicine was the paternalistic physician. The only way to do battle with the paternalistic physician, in the realm of reasoned argument, is to employ the concept of autonomy.

The new ethics had as its good outcomes both heightened respect for the rights and interests of patients in practice and deeper and more sophisticated analyses of the concept of autonomy in theory. But increasingly, thoughtful philosophers and physicians found it necessary to apply brakes to the autonomy bandwagon. Symptomatic of the problem was a discussion that appeared in a medical journal about the physician's limited duty to accede to requests from patients for treatment that the physician considers futile or harmful (Brett and McCullough 1986). The new ethics had clearly promulgated the message that any competent patient has the right to refuse any medical treatment and that the physician must honor that refusal in the name of respect for autonomy. The logic seemed clear that the physician was equally obligated to provide any treatment the competent patient demanded, so long as risks and alternatives were disclosed openly. But that logic ignored the possibility that beneficence might play a role in determining the physician's duty in such cases. And it ignored the possibility that medicine has inherent values defining what good practice consists of and that those values should not be readily sacrificed to the whims of patients. Specifically, it ignored the fact that patients autonomously request (or autonomously refuse) *medical care*; yet medical care might effectively disintegrate if patient autonomy were the only value permitted to define its scope and limits (see chapter 11 below).

If the focus on autonomy-talk eventually led to an incomplete understanding of the physician's duty to the individual patient, the tilted emphasis of the new ethics became even more obvious as issues of resource allocation and cost containment became increasingly apparent in the early 1980s. Principles of distributive justice were required to deal with allocation and rationing issues, but an ethics that had trained almost exclusively on autonomy discovered that those other muscles were notably flabby. A few optimists argued that medical costs could easily be controlled if only patients were given the freedom to refuse treatments they didn't want. But most analysts concluded that when we added expanded patient autonomy to a setting that already included exploding medical technology, widespread use of third-party payment mechanisms, and a capitalist free-market ideology, major cost overruns were the inevitable result. Inevitably, effective responses to problems of cost and resource allocation entailed placing restrictions on individual patient autonomy (Thurow 1984).

The need to see autonomy as only one of a constellation of ethical principles is consistent with an adequate understanding of what autonomy means. But a second, more subtle problem that began to emerge when the new ethics was subjected to closer critical examination was precisely the question of how autonomy is to be interpreted. Again the problem can be traced to the assumption about who is the enemy. So long as the bogeyman is the paternalistic physician, the message of the new ethics is that respect for autonomy is a negative, hands-off enterprise. Almost any physician behavior apart from full disclosure of all relevant information runs the risk of limiting patients' freedom of choice. And so (went the lesson most commonly drawn from the new ethics) the physician had better be neutral and dispassionate, simply noting to the patient, "All I can do is provide you with the facts; the decision is yours to make, not mine."

When this view of autonomy is stated so baldly, its indefensible nature is apparent. It is indefensible because it wants to sit on both sides of the fence as far as the reality of patients' autonomy is concerned. On one hand, it wants to hold that the autonomous choice of an informed patient is a robust, substantial matter that appropriately determines medical decisions. On the other hand, it wants to hold that the choice of an informed patient is such a weak reed that it will snap under the slightest pressure—the way the physician raises an eyebrow, or the color of his tie. Clearly we cannot have it both ways. If autonomy is to be respected, physicians must be permitted to use reasonable persuasion, just as people are permitted to do in other aspects of life where autonomy is assumed (Ackerman 1982; Brody 1985). If patients cannot be expected to stand up in the face of physician persuasion, then what we need to protect patients is a new army of benevolent paternalists, not respect for autonomy.

Of course, the view that the physician respects autonomy by taking a negative, hands-off stance was seldom stated so bluntly or extremely and hence for a long time escaped explicit discussion and refutation. This was particularly true because, at least at first, anyone calling this view into question was assumed to be trying to defend the old paternalism. It was some time before physicians and philosophers with confirmed antipaternalist credentials could find ways to criticize this view while working within the accepted vocabulary of the new ethics.

It is now asserted with increasing frequency that both the narrow, negative view of autonomy and the emphasis on autonomy to the neglect of social justice arise from the new ethics' mistaken tendency to view morality in individualist terms and to neglect social and community concepts (Callahan 1984; Brody 1987b). Medical ethics shares this individualist bias with most recent work in Anglo-American ethics and social philosophy. The bias tends to view rights as among the more robust and persuasive moral constructs and assigns rights to the individual human being. Whenever possible, such social concepts as the legitimate power of the state to govern are reduced to the sum of individual rights or of the free actions of individuals in isolation. It is a small jump from these tendencies to the idea that autonomy requires individual self-sufficiency and freedom from the interference of others. Social, cultural, and community influences on individual choice are also suspect because none of us autonomously chose which society or community to be born into or grow up in. (It is hard not to see in these tendencies of thought a reflection of the social unrest and civil rights disputes of the 1960s.)

In contrast to the negative view of autonomy, more recent authors have provided a view that encourages a more positive, active role for the physician. Ackerman (1982) pointed out that the illness, not the physician, may be the most potent barrier to autonomous choice and behavior; the physician should work actively with the patient to identify and remove those barriers and not be content with providing information and then standing back to allow the patient to choose. Tomlinson (1986) noted further that the isolated individual making a choice free from outside influence is simply not a desirable or sensible model of true autonomy. Most of us when faced with an important decision naturally turn to family, friends, and other trusted associates before finally committing ourselves to a choice and making it our own. When these important correctives are pointed out, it is easy for the new ethicist to reply, "Of course, that is what I meant by autonomy all the time. I never intended for it to be misunderstood in the way you have described." But the "negative" misunderstanding was precisely the picture of autonomy that many, if not most, observers took away from the new ethics as the object lesson, regardless of the intent of the originators (Brody 1985).

The difference between negative and positive views of autonomy is in part a difference between seeing autonomy as a side constraint and as an end constraint.[2] In the negative view, autonomy constitutes a boundary around our privileged rights and interests, and it is morally prohibited for others to cross that boundary without our consent. All this side-constraint view tells others is what they are prohibited from doing; it is silent on how they might best assist us in pursuing our interests and goals (Callahan 1984). Autonomy as end constraint describes a desirable state worth pursuing as a morally valued end, along with (or sometimes in conflict with) other valued ends. In the side-constraint view, benefit alone does not grant moral license to override autonomy and cross its boundary. In the end-constraint view, one of the ways a person benefits another is by enhancing her capacity for autonomous choice and behavior and removing reversible barriers that stand in the way of her autonomy. At times these two conceptions of autonomy may directly conflict: a standard example is the alcoholic who might be much more autonomous in the future if we could now succeed, by coercion or manipulation, in getting him into a good treatment program, but that coercion or manipulation would violate the limited degree of autonomy he now possesses. The side-constraint view would oppose forced treatment; the end-constraint view would tend to sanction it (Komrad 1983).

Side constraints must be respected in any society that values individual

2. This distinction is clearly drawn by Christie and Hoffmaster (1986, p. 65), who employ the terminology "autonomy as moral principle" versus "autonomy as a value"; I have translated this into the language of Nozick (1974).

rights. The problem comes when we try to build an ethical system for an enterprise like medicine out of side constraints only. This leads to Callahan's (1984) observation that autonomy (as the new ethics has characterized it) is a dumb, brutish thing, valuable for chasing away bullies but useless as a wise or friendly counselor. If medicine is fundamentally something to which people come specifically for wise counsel and support, then an ethics for medicine will have to include a generous dose of an end-constraint conception of autonomy. It cannot do completely without a side-constraint view, for paternalism and other violations of rights remain ever-present dangers; but the overall emphasis must be better balanced.

It is difficult to describe what is at stake here within the vocabulary of the new ethics so long as that vocabulary excludes *power*. As we saw in the last chapter, the side-constraint view entails a loss of the physician's power, since under the old Hippocratic ethics the physician was granted the power to cross the border with impunity so long as the justification was the patient's benefit. But that view is silent on whether the physician retains other powers or assumes any new ones. The implicit message of the side-constraint view, coupled with the identification of physician paternalism as the primary threat to patient rights, is that any physician power is dangerous to the patient and is likely to be put to unethical uses.

By contrast, the end-constraint view calls for using the physician's power to aid the patient by removing barriers to the patient's autonomy. If removing those barriers leads to enhanced power for the patient, thanks in part to the effective use of power by the physician, then we can see the outlines of a shared-power conception of the physician-patient relationship. But even the positive or end-constraint view, as it has been articulated thus far, fails to flesh out that conception by showing how the power is shared and which sorts of power are at issue.

The Call to Virtue

As we have seen, medical ethics may be shaped by trends peculiar to medicine (such as the prevalence of paternalistic attitudes and the need to combat them) and also by trends in philosophy and ethics generally (such as the individualist bias). A recently emerging "outside" trend is a call for a return to an ethics based on virtue as a corrective to the post-Enlightenment ethics, which has stressed rights and duties. In its strongest form, as propounded by MacIntyre (1981), this argument holds that post-Enlightenment ethics is incoherent and can be rendered meaningful only through a virtue-based approach. In less ambitious forms, it asserts merely that an ethic of rights and duties is incomplete without a consideration of virtue.

For MacIntyre, a coherent ethics requires three elements: a view of human nature as it now exists, a view of human nature as it would appear if human beings realized their true ends or goals (the Greek *telos*), and a set of virtues as the means of transition from present, imperfect human nature to the ideal human nature. The Enlightenment (according to MacIntyre) rendered ethics incoherent by rejecting the telos, trying to base ethics only on human nature as it actually exists, and thereby reducing virtues to prudential maxims that are optional rather than essential to ethical theory. What got lost in the Enlightenment's fascination with rights, duties, and consequences as they pertain to individual human actions considered in isolation was a view of practices—complex, organized, enduring patterns of behavior—and of the excellences that define and constitute those practices. To act virtuously means to act so that one's present action coheres with a train of actions that stretches into both past and future, and so that one's action conforms to a conception of excellence that emerges over time and does not yet exist fully realized. When we ask whether an action respects or violates rights and duties, and whether the consequences of the action are good or bad, we necessarily take actions singly and lose sight of the much larger organization of human behavior and human endeavor that is required to see those actions in their true context.

This is not the place for a detailed critique of MacIntyre's theory of ethics. His theory seems to come very close to rejecting any coherent ethics for a pluralist society and calling instead for the emergence (or imposition?) of a monistic conception of the good for human beings and human society. In a world concerned with the doings of such people as the late Ayatollah Khomeini, this proposal is likely to sound reactionary and unsatisfactory, even if post-Enlightenment ethics stands guilty as charged. The question for us is whether some lessons can be gleaned from the virtue-based criticism of the mainstream ethics which might then be applied to medical issues.

To the question "How can I be moral?" the virtue-based approach seems to suggest an answer like the following: "From all human activities, discover which are essential, and then discern the goals or ends toward which those activities are directed. Determine the sorts of excellences in your behavior and attitudes that would lead you, over time, to contribute maximally to the accomplishment of those ends and goals. Finally, seek to make your present behavior conform to the pattern suggested by those excellences." The approach of the mainstream of Anglo-American ethics of the post-

Enlightenment period would give the answer "Follow the rules." Depending on the particular ethical theory one favors within that general body of tradition, "follow the rules" might be taken to mean "respect the rights of others," "do your duty," or "strive to produce the greatest happiness for the greatest number." The major differences are that "follow the rules" encourages us to consider actions singly, rather than in the context of larger, organized activities, and in isolation from the identity and the personality of the actor.

How, then, does the virtue-based approach appear different when addressed to issues in medical ethics? A helpful summary was provided by Smith and Newton (1984), who suggested that the follow-the-rules approach to the physician-patient relationship (such as an ethics that stresses autonomy in the negative sense) amounts to an attempt to render that relationship doctor-proof. That is, it tries to provide a basis for ethical medicine that ignores the integrity and character of the physician. The concepts *integrity* and *character* are fully at home in the virtue-based approach but are foreign to the rule-based approach, since they address the cohesion and integration of behaviors and attitudes over time and the extent to which one defines one's own identity partly on the basis of those behaviors and attitudes and their coherence and integration.

The new ethics' dismissal of integrity and character, and the search instead for a doctor-proof set of rules, may again be seen as arising from the bogeyman of physician paternalism. The traditional Hippocratic physician (according to the new ethics) is not bound by any substantial rules when it came to ignoring or overriding the patient's expressed wishes. In that setting, the patient's only security is the physician's good character: since the physician alone gets to define what is a benefit and what isn't, and the patient's views on the matter are dismissed as irrelevant, one hopes at least that the physician is a decent person and will not take advantage of this power imbalance. But the security provided by good character is of little use, because everyone agrees that the person who violates my rights and interests but does so out of a sincere desire to benefit me is of sound and commendable *motivation* regardless of the wrongness of his actions. The paternalist is unrestrained by appeals to integrity and character because he sees himself as already well-endowed in that department. Only hard rules will put a spoke in his wheels and protect the rights of the patient. And so to the new ethics, any insistence that ethical medicine requires attention to the physician's moral integrity and character is likely to sound like a call for a return to paternalism.

The end point of a doctor-proof relationship, which assumes that we can wring morally acceptable actions out of any physician no matter how good or how bad his motives if only we have the right rules for him to follow, is precisely what I identified in the previous section as the outcome of the negative view of autonomy. We have an excellent sense of what the physician is not supposed to do in the process of helping the patient but virtually no sense of what he is supposed to do. The doctor-proof model presumes that the physician's power comes in two clearly designated and differentiated categories: power that helps fight illness and power that can be used to violate the patient's rights. The rules supposedly prevent any exercise of the second category of power while leaving the first intact, so no talk of integrity or character is needed. My view, as explained in the earlier chapters, is that no easy distinction is possible; the same sorts of powers can easily be redirected in either way. The physician, in that view, has to be a moral user of power in a realm where firm rules are extremely blunt instruments. Therefore, discussions of integrity and character cannot be excluded from a full analysis of medical ethics.

I stated above that Fried combines elements of both the new ethics and the more recent criticism of the new ethics. At first glance, Fried's list of physicians' obligations sounds like a follow-the-rules approach to the physician-patient relationship, and this impression is partially correct. A deeper analysis, however, will show that concerns for integrity and character, though not as explicit as we might wish, nevertheless seem more at home in Fried's conception than in the statements of many of his contemporaries. The obligations of lucidity and autonomy are in fact fairly straightforward examples of rule-governed conduct. But the obligations of fidelity and humanity are more open to nuances of interpretation and would defy any reduction to protocol or algorithm. Moreover, the physician's goal is not to follow all those obligations singly but to balance them among themselves and to resolve conflicts; and that again would seem to defy a simplistic, rules-based approach. The physician who consistently and sensitively applies the obligations of fidelity and humanity and is able to balance the four obligations when they conflict would seem *necessarily* to be someone of integrity and character. Finally, we should recall that Fried's schema derived not from a list of rules but from an attempt to get to the root of the concept of personal medical care. That is, Fried identified the essential ends of a specific human activity and then proceeded to derive his obligations from what would count as excellence in furthering that activity. Fried's reaction to the tradition of paternalistic medicine was not merely to ring the physician with rules to restrain his power. It was to return to the very basis of medical practice, to ask whether respect for patient autonomy (in the sense of using medical technology to further the patient's life plan) was not an essential constituent of excellent medicine and hence an appropriate objective for the physician's power. Pellegrino and Thomasma (1981, 1988) similarly sought to derive medical ethics from the fundamental nature of medicine itself, not from the simplistic importation into medicine of rules that have been found useful in governing modern civil society.

The discussion of the physician's integrity and character as a necessary feature of a shared-power conception of medical practice is important enough to deserve a separate chapter. At this point it will be helpful to return to the idea of personal medical care to refine our understanding of primary-care medicine.

The Essence of Primary Care

Primary care, neglected and looked down upon by American medicine during the explosion of modern medical research and the rise of in-hospital management, has come back into its own in the past two decades. General practice has effectively disappeared as a career choice and has been replaced with family practice, which requires a three-year residency and board certification. Family-practice residency education stresses behavioral and communication aspects of medicine and views the physician's office as an important site of training along with the hospital ward. Spurred by these developments, both internal medicine and pediatrics began to set up primary-care tracks within their own residency programs. Increased attention to cost containment and cost effectiveness has further tilted the scales toward the side of primary care, as have reports that the United States was producing too few primary-care physicians and too many specialists.

Primary care is the first medical care a patient gets for an illness. Except for general internists, who do not see children, and general pediatricians, who do not see adults, primary-care practitioners exclude no prospective patient on the basis of age, sex, type of medical problem, or involved organ system. As a rule, the primary-care physician gets first crack at diagnosing the patient's presenting problem; seldom is a patient referred by another physician who has already made a diagnosis. Primary care is ideally both comprehensive and continuous: the patient's total health, not just a single episode of illness, is the physician's concern, and the physician expects to care for the patient over an extended period. Primary care is fundamentally ambulatory care. The patient decides whether to come and usually has a minor medical problem, if any at all. Hence primary care deals with a group of patients much less passive and vulnerable than the acutely ill individuals confined to bed and made to wear hospital gowns. As part of the definition of *comprehensive*, primary-care practitioners routinely stress preventive medicine and concern for mental and emotional problems as well as physical ones. Teachers of primary care commonly assert that their practice requires a biopsychosocial model such as Engel's (1977) rather than the more traditional biomedical, cell- and organ-centered model.

All these points distinguish primary care from the practice of such specialties as endocrinology, dermatology, and radiology (as well as from emergency medicine, which is first-contact care but makes no claims to comprehensiveness and continuity). They do not, however, suggest that the ethical issues in primary care would be substantially different from those arising in the hospital, the in vitro fertilization clinic, or the neonatal intensive care unit. That the patients are less sick, less scared, and less vulnerable is a difference in degree, not in kind. It seems to be a matter of equal weight if a primary-care physician or a specialist withholds crucial information, engages in risky treatment without consent, violates confidences, or unduly influences patients to enroll in research studies.

Indeed, the new medical ethics proceeded largely by ignoring all such differences. The most exciting cases seemed to involve life-or-death decisions in hospitals, and so the textbooks of the new ethics were full of cases like Karen Quinlan, or the infant with Down's syndrome at Johns Hopkins. Ambulatory and everyday cases found a place in textbooks with a primary-care emphasis only to redress an imbalance, to correct the impression that ethical issues arose exclusively in specialty care, rather than to argue for a primary-care ethics unique to that type of practice.[3] True, family practice could lay claim to what appeared to be a unique ethical issue. Since it defined part of its task as caring for the family as a unit, it had to grapple with possible conflicts of interest among family members: the teenage daughter requesting oral contraceptives and demanding that her parents not be informed is an example commonly cited (Eaddy and Graber 1982). But that issue arose from the family orientation, not the primary-care aspect of family practice.

A more promising tack (assuming that there are some ethically unique features of primary care that deserve separate treatment) is the observation of the central role of the physician-patient relationship in primary care. The typical specialist depends on specialized tools to diagnose and treat

3. Among recent ethics texts, Graber et al. 1985 uses cases drawn from primary-care sources while Christie and Hoffmaster 1986 and Smith and Churchill 1986 tend to argue more for unique aspects of primary-care ethics. My own views on this matter have been heavily influenced by an unpublished paper by Larry Churchill and Alan Cross.

the patient's problem. Take away the surgeon's scalpel or the gastroenter-ologist's endoscope and they are almost totally crippled in the performance of their tasks. It may be argued that the ongoing personal relationship with each patient is the corresponding tool of the trade for the primary-care physician. This physician can decide which symptoms are minor and which are major, when to reassure the patient, when to admit him to the hospital, when to refer him to a specialist, and when to call in a psychologist, not by cutting or peering into the body but by having the personal experience necessary to place what has changed into the context of the patient's life history and immediate environment. To the gastroenterologist, stomach pain may mean peptic ulcer, acute pancreatitis, gall bladder disease, and so forth; but to the primary-care physician, stomach pain may also mean the anniversary of a spouse's death from abdominal cancer.

This observation about the centrality of the physician-patient relation-ship, if correct, begins to point toward some unique ethical features of primary-care medicine. Unfortunately, it is rather vague and ambiguous: to say that the relationship is important sounds more like a platitude than an analysis. It may also be a bit of romantic rhetoric that covers up real problems with modern primary care. There may at one time have existed a small-town, horse-and-buggy or Model-T physician who knew his patients personally and remained in touch with them all their lives; even that is debatable. But the modern primary-care physician is hardly that nostalgic figure. Although the research is not voluminous, some data show that primary-care physicians typically spend much too little time with their patients to get to know them well and perform no better than other spe-cialists in decision-making situations where knowledge of individual pa-tients is at issue.[4]

A group of family physicians at the University of Western Ontario has elaborated a concept of "patient-centered primary care" that is simulta-neously theoretical, therapeutic, and pedagogical (Levenstein et al. 1986). That is, their theoretical statement is accompanied by research showing that patient-centered primary care produces enhanced patient outcomes, in terms of symptom relief, and also by research that illustrates how an effective strategy for training family-practice residents follows from the concept.

For present purposes, the concept of patient-centered primary care can be reduced to one simple idea: *the primary-care physician's approach*

---

4. On the time spent with patients, see Merenstein 1984. On family physicians' inability to anticipate patients' wishes regarding resuscitation, see Bedell and Delbanco 1984.

to the patient's problem is grounded in the way the patient himself defines the problem. If a patient is complaining of shoulder pain, the physician starts to evaluate the patient for shoulder pain and ultimately owes the patient some sort of explanation of why he has shoulder pain and what he is supposed to do about it. The physician, in the course of evaluation, might decide for her own purposes that the correct designation for the problem is *not* shoulder pain. Newly acquired data might suggest that for purposes of both scientific description and correct therapy the problem is better viewed as left lower lobe pneumonia with referred pain from irritation of the diaphragm, or perhaps chronic marital conflict with somatization disorder. If the physician were an orthopedic surgeon and came to either of these conclusions, she might with perfect justification tell the patient, "You've made a mistake. You don't have an orthopedic problem at all. You'll have to see an infectious-disease expert" (or "You should consider seeing a family therapist"). But the primary-care physician can never say, "You've made a mistake in coming to me; you don't have the problem you think you have." The primary-care physician must work within the context of the patient's definition of the problem until either the problem goes away, according to the patient's own report, or the physician succeeds, through a process of open negotiation, to get the patient freely to accept a relabeling of the problem.

The importance of this idea lies in part in its implications for therapy. The Western Ontario research group was able to show that when one looked at symptoms commonly presented to family physicians, acuity of diagnosis and technological sophistication of treatment were not especially good predictors of eventual disappearance of the symptom. What corresponded much better to later symptom relief was the patient's own perception that the physician had agreed with the patient about the nature of the problem and had listened carefully to the patient's explanation of the problem during the initial visit (Bass, Buck, Turner, et al. 1986; Bass, McWhinney, Dempsey et al. 1986). These findings, of course, reinforce the point argued in the previous chapters, that the physician's Aesculapian power is intimately connected with the physician's personality and style of communicating with the patient and cannot easily be sorted out from charismatic and social power.

Patient-centered primary care extends respect for autonomy into an area seldom, if ever, considered by most advocates of the new ethics. It is commonly envisioned that the physician will collect the facts of the case, reach a diagnosis or a set of possible diagnoses, and then propose further diagnostic procedures or therapeutic interventions, from among which the informed patient will then freely select. Patient autonomy is seen to be an issue only at the last stage of this process. Patient-centered primary care, by contrast, forces us to envision a role for patient autonomy throughout this process, since the so-called facts of the case and the diagnostic possibilities considered are no longer under the physician's exclusive control and are necessarily colored both by the way the patient has defined the problem and by the need for explicit negotiation if the physician wishes to relabel the problem. Fried spoke of the goal of medicine as service to the patient's life plan; patient-centered primary care seems to take this seriously: the patient's own characterization of her problem will probably be much more heavily influenced by the bearing the problem has on her life plan than would the formulation arrived at by the physician.

Indeed, how radical a change the patient-centered primary-care concept represents can be illustrated by comparing it to Siegler's (1982b) account of "the physician-patient accommodation." Siegler divides a physician-patient encounter, for purposes of logical analysis, into three "moments": first, a prepatient phase, in which a person decides that he has a medical problem and should seek care from a physician; second, data gathering by the physician to decide precisely what the patient's problem consists of; and third, accommodation, in which the physician and patient (ideally) agree both that the patient will place himself under the physician's care and what that care will consist of.

Siegler, himself a primary-care internist, clearly views his own model as embracing the value of respect for patient autonomy in a powerful way. He also displays full cognizance of the importance of the human relationship within medicine: "Medicine has never been defined solely by its technological capabilities. Rather, the nature of clinical medicine is understood best in the context of an interpersonal accommodation that must be agreed on mutually by both participants" (p. 1901).

It is noteworthy, therefore, that in Siegler's model, patient autonomy is confined to the first phase (in which a patient can choose whether or not to seek medical help) and the third (in which a patient may accept or reject the care, or the care plan, of a particular physician). It does not accept any serious role for patient autonomy in the second phase, in which the physician determines what the problem "really" is and whether it "legitimately" constitutes a medical problem. The negotiation between physician and patient occurs at the last stage; it does not extend to determinating the nature of the problem itself. Siegler considers, but apparently rejects, a suggestion by Mechanic (1978) that every patient is "diseased" in so far as something impelled him to seek medical help.[5] The Western Ontario model, by contrast, imagines a much more substantial role for patient autonomy and physician-patient negotiation in what Siegler would call the "second clinical moment."

It might appear from this focus on primary care that I am leveling a charge of unethical behavior at all specialists and subspecialists in technological fields. But that is not the intent of the discussion. The model of primary care I have presented is not limited by specialty; a primary-care *attitude* need not be confused with primary care as a specialty of practice. The type of physician-patient relationship I have described is accepted by the reflective primary-care physician as her primary diagnostic and therapeutic tool. There is no reason a neurosurgeon or a dermatologist cannot become skilled in relationship building and interpersonal negotiation as a tool of their practice, even though that is not the tool that defines their particular subspecialties.

I suggest that technically oriented subspecialists can be optimally ethical in their contacts with patients in one of two ways. First, they may cultivate what I have called a patient-centered primary-care attitude and approach as a part of their daily practice of their specialties. Alternatively, they may accept the fact that their patients will basically remain strangers to them and that only an ethic of respect for autonomy, rules, and side constraints can properly designate the nature of their relationship. While the former is preferable as a general goal, the latter may in particular circumstances be more honest and realistic.[6]

Toward a Shared-Power Approach

At the conclusion of chapter 3 we looked at some preliminary guidelines for the ethical use of power—owned power, shared power, and aimed power. Preliminary considerations suggested that of these three, shared power might be pivotal.[7] The discussion of various aspects of the physician-

5. As a British physician was reported to have once put it, "There is something wrong with a person who goes to the doctor when there is nothing wrong with him."

6. See chapter 7 below, on the possibility that a different standard may exist for informed consent in primary care as opposed to specialty practice. Dr. Wayne Cooper, a cardiac electrophysiologist, has urged me not to let the specialists off too easily, holding that it is both possible and desirable for specialists to incorporate the important aspects of a primary-care approach into their practices.

7. Presumably this is true for at least two reasons. First, when power is shared, A is less vulnerable than when B has a power monopoly, and B is less tempted to abuse his power. Second, A is more likely to call B to account for how he has used his power, and B is more likely to think, before employing his power, about how he may be called to account in the future.

patient relationship in this chapter has provided additional tools to construct an adequate model of the ethical sharing of power between physician and patient.

First, let us review the power positions of the two participants in this relationship:

1. The physician is likely to hold a near monopoly on Aesculapian power, having the necessary knowledge and skills (which the patient usually lacks) to diagnose and treat diseases.

2. The physician is likely to have a higher level of social power owing to the privileged socioeconomic and educational status of physicians generally.

3. The physician is likely to have a considerable edge in charismatic power. Many physicians are drawn to medical practice, or succeed at it, because they have a natural proclivity for the exercise of this power. Moreover, the sensed powerlessness and vulnerability of someone who is ill reduce any charismatic power, or ability to exercise it, the patient might possess when healthy. (This factor is least consequential in primary-care or ambulatory practice and is most consequential when the patient is acutely and severely ill.)

It is hard for the physician to share social or charismatic power—although the sensed powerlessness of the sick person is a feature of illness the physician can mitigate, and it might be viewed as a sort of sharing of charismatic power when the physician imparts to the patient a heightened sense of mastery or control over the illness.[8] I will discuss in later chapters how the physician can share Aesculapian power by adhering to the obligations of lucidity and autonomy and informing the patient more fully about disease and treatment.[9]

What about the patient's side of the ledger? According to the new medical ethics, the patient gains power only by virtue of being surrounded by boundaries that the physician cannot cross without egregiously violating moral rules. According to the contemporary perception of many physicians—which the new medical ethics has helped shape—the patient gains power primarily as a potential litigant in a tort suit. But both these characterizations of patients' power suggest a hopelessly adversarial relationship in which useful collaboration seems difficult if not impossible. The above

8. The popularity of such books as Siegel 1986 may testify to the possibilities for shared charismatic power.

9. Ironically, the act of sharing power also gives the physician a new sort of Aesculapian power—the power to start and stop the conversation. See chapters 6 and 7.

discussion has suggested, by contrast, two bases of the patient's power within the therapeutic relationship. First, the patient's life plan, and not the physician's life plan or interests, determines the goals of the relationship and the criteria for acceptable or excellent medical practice. The patient's expressed preferences, except in unusual circumstances, are taken as indicative of the patient's life plan and life goals. Second, the patient's way of characterizing the presenting medical problem constitutes the beginning of medical inquiry and places important qualifications on how that inquiry and subsequent treatment will proceed. (This is most true in primary-care medicine and applies with much less force in many specialties.)

Since this way of characterizing the physician-patient relationship will inevitably seem strange from the vantage point of one accustomed to the *power*-less new ethics, some brief comments may be helpful here. As the term *power* has recently seemed more typical of medical sociology or medical anthropology than of ethics, it might seem that there is nothing ethical or philosophical about this account at all, and hence that it must be irrelevant to the physician's moral obligations. I have tried to summarize the ways in which the sorts of power suggested above—particularly on the patient's side—follow logically from a particular *philosophical* conception of the nature of medical practice. The full philosophical argument in support of that conception is obviously beyond the scope of this chapter but may be found in other works on the subject.[10] True, the types of power attributed to the physician derive largely from literary and social-science analyses. They arise less from the essential nature of medical practice and more from the fact that that practice has to be carried out by human beings in a particular social and cultural context. Given that medical practice is a social enterprise, however, it is still the case that any ethical theory ignores those realities at its peril.

Additional support comes from the balance created by the ascription of power to both parties. When the newly formed American Medical Association promulgated its first code of ethics in 1847, it included lists of physicians' obligations to patients and of patients' obligations to physicians. When writers of the new ethics have looked at this code of ethics at all, it has generally been to dismiss the list of patients' obligations as quaintly self-serving. Martin Benjamin (1985), though, has contended that at least a few obligations of patients to physicians can be fully justified. (One example he gives is the patient's duty to report truthfully both his symptoms

10. See Brody 1987d, which in turn draws on Pellegrino and Thomasma 1981. See also White 1988.

and whether he has complied with prescribed treatment.) The new ethics has some difficulty in accommodating this view. My discussion, on the other hand, shows that where power exists, some obligations for the ethical use of that power are to be expected. This is particularly true where the patient's power includes the power to define the nature of the medical problem.

We can also see now why Fried's list of four physician obligations has stood up well in the light of more recent criticism of the new medical ethics. Putting it alongside our three guidelines for the ethical use of power, we can see that Fried in effect anticipated many of these ways of approaching and reinterpreting the issues. We might say that the obligation of lucidity is consistent with the view that the physician's use of power must be owned and candidly acknowledged. The obligation of autonomy allows the sharing of power by increasing patient participation. The obligation of fidelity, understood properly, promotes the owning of power, and also the aiming of power toward ends that are truly the patient's or in the patient's interest. Finally, the obligation of humanity promotes a realistic assessment of continued disparities in power between physician and patient and a search for factors that might reduce or mitigate this disparity. Moreover, characterizing the physician as the servant of the patient's life plan portrays a possibly ironic power reversal: it reminds the physician that the patient retains important aspects of power within the relationship even while in the throes of serious illness.[11]

To summarize, I can now suggest some general guidelines for the ethical employment of power within the physician-patient relationship:

1. The physician should employ all her power to try to effect a good outcome for the patient. *Good outcome* is determined by (a) the patient's

---

11. This irony might suggest that the depiction of the physician as servant is an unrealistic or manipulative denial of the physician's true power. In fact, it is an inherent feature of any power relationship in which the more powerful party maintains and exercises power by influencing those less powerful. This relationship cannot be sustained without implicitly recognizing the power of the "influencees," who could effectively remove all the power simply by failing to be influenced. I am indebted for a reminder of this point to Lawrence Van Egeren's unpublished paper on the Type A personality. McCullough (1989) has called attention to the vast power of medical language to transform a person's life, particularly by labeling him as suffering from a chronic or terminal disease. Again, this points to the patient-centered primary-care model as an important corrective to the abuse of medical power. If the patient's own life story and account of what his problem is necessarily define the way in which the physician must approach the case, then it is less likely that the physician can impose a totally foreign label on the patient's experience. In effect (if not in practice), the patient could always respond, "What you say is all very interesting, Doc, but what does it have to do with my problem?"

life plan, (b) the patient's definition of the presenting problem, and (c) a coherent conception of excellence and quality in the practice of medicine.[12]

2. The physician should try whenever practicable to share her Aesculapian power by informing the patient, in so far as the patient wishes, about the nature of the disease and the treatment.

3. The physician should be alert to the sense of powerlessness often accompanying illness and prepared to respond to it in several ways: (a) by sharing knowledge; (b) by identifying specific psychological sequelae of illness and including their management in the treatment plan, as part of her exercise of Aesculapian power; (c) by explicitly reminding the patient of the power he still possesses and how essential that power is for treatment; (d) by reassuring the patient that her own Aesculapian, charismatic, and social power are employed to secure for him a positive therapeutic outcome.

4. The physician should support and encourage the patient's own exercise of power so long as it is consistent with a good therapeutic outcome and with the patient's long-term goals and interests. When there appears to be a conflict between the patient's use of power and those ends, the physician should employ frank negotiation and persuasion, rather than deception and manipulation, to redirect the patient's power toward the best outcome.

5. Especially in primary care, the physician should regard the physician-patient relationship as a primary therapeutic tool. Her means of seeking a good medical outcome should be designed not merely to resolve the problem of the moment but also to cement and reinforce a mode of relating to the patient that encourages his full and active participation over time.

Much of the rest of this book will be a further elaboration of these guidelines. In the next chapter, however, I will look first at a major tension within medical practice—one that, if not recognized, may obscure some important issues of the use of power.

12. Roger Sider, reviewing an early draft of this chapter, has suggested that effecting a good outcome for the patient entails knowing what counts as a good and healthy life, not just knowing the patient's life plan. This suggestion follows the general line of argument in MacIntyre 1981; but it is a suggestion that I am unable to pursue (or to dissent from) within the scope of this book.

CHAPTER 5

CARE

VERSUS

WORK

I aim to demonstrate in this book that attending to power as a central ethical feature of medicine calls attention to aspects of medical practice that tend to be obscured by the more usual autonomy/paternalism/beneficence approach, and that those aspects are helpful in examining moral problems in health care. In this chapter I will consider a central ethical tension in medicine which has rarely been discussed explicitly in the medical ethics literature but which demands consideration as soon as one looks at the physician-patient encounter in terms of relative power.[1] That tension is between care and work—between the individualized demands of compassion and sympathy and the impersonalized, routine demands of the efficient workplace.

Physicians have frequently commented on popular television doctor shows like "Marcus Welby, M.D." by saying, "Now, if I only had to treat one patient each week, I could be just as compassionate, just as caring, and just as knowledgeable as Marcus Welby." They are suggesting, in effect, that the heroic television doctor can be the sort of doctor he is only if he practices medicine as an avocation and not as a profession.[2]

This observation (whatever self-serving elements it may possess for physicians) seems in keeping with our general cultural image of caring. If the parable of the good samaritan epitomizes the traditional view of care and

---

1. This tension was called to my attention through Richard Zaner's suggestive book, *Ethics and the Clinical Encounter* (1988), although Zaner developed it much less than I would have wished.

2. Indeed, the key difference between the older, heroic doctor shows and the more cynical and more realistic "St. Elsewhere" of the 1980s is the latter's depiction of the stresses of overwork and medical routine.

compassion, then caring and compassion *require a willingness to stop whatever you are doing in order to help.* This suggests that you cannot truly be caring and compassionate if your response to the sight of a needy person is to keep doing what you normally do—even if what you normally do is provide medical "care."

We can now see the direct linkage between power and the care-versus-work tension in medicine. The physician possesses the Aesculapian, charismatic, and social power if she meets a patient while out shopping or if she makes a house call. But in our society, the more usual encounter is in a hospital or an office—the physician's workplace. Immediately upon entering somebody else's workplace you sense an additional power disparity (in the physician's case, an outgrowth of combined Aesculapian and social power) because this is familiar ground to the worker and mysterious ground to you. Instinctively you revert to a more childlike state, as if fearing a scolding if you touch the wrong piece of equipment or press the wrong button. And included in this sense of relative powerlessness is the awareness that what is a matter of unusual concern to you—else you would not have deviated from *your* usual work schedule to show up at the doctor's office—is a matter of work routine to the physician. One part of you (still childlike) hopes that the physician will smile at you and treat you as unique. Another part warns that the physician sees twenty cases like yours each day and that inevitably you are just another face in the crowd.

This sense of relative powerlessness is present in the physician's office but magnified in the hospital. Aleksandr Solzhenitsyn notes this in his pithy description of being admitted to an oncology unit: "In a few hours Rusanov had lost his whole status in life, his honors, and his plans for the future, and had become 168 pounds of warm white flesh that did not know what would happen to it tomorrow" (Solzhenitsyn 1968, p. 12). To most visitors the very architecture of a hospital seems designed to remind them at every turn that they do not belong there, that they cannot possibly find their way around without assistance, and therefore that the staff must be some superior species of being. The overhead speakers utter strangely coded messages which the hospital's denizens show their power by understanding (or, even more awe-inspiring, by ignoring completely). And if this is true of the hospital lobby, consider the impact of an intensive care unit with its thicket of beeping and blinking monitors, screens, wires, and tubes. The average person entering these precincts cannot be blamed for mentally updating Dante and reading "Abandon all power, ye who enter here" over the doorway.

Both in the office and in the hospital, those in power—the physicians, nurses, and other staff—busily try to get their work done. Patients quickly pick up the usually unspoken message that they will get the best "care" precisely to the extent that they facilitate and do not impede the flow of the workplace. In the hospital, the physician visits on daily rounds when *she* wants to. (No matter that the patient is drowsy then and would be more alert later, or that concerned family will be there later but cannot be present then.) Medications and meal trays appear when the nurse or the aide has time, not when the patient would most like them. The patient who complains too much or questions these routines is quickly branded "difficult" and may receive even less sensitive care as a result. These observations do not go to show that nurses and physicians are inhuman; they go to show that they are human. Superficial mechanisms designed to enhance patient autonomy are likely to appear forced and inadequate to both patient and physician if the basic nature of the workplace and the patient's foreignness within it do not change.

In the hospital, it may, ironically, be the interns who are most guilty of using what little power they possess against the patients instead of for them. The intern must often eat and sleep as well as work within the hospital; patients who do anything untoward or unexpected present a threat to the intern's all-too-limited power to control his environment. The novel *The House of God* depicts an intern resuscitating a hopelessly ill patient in the middle of the night, thinking, " 'I wish she would die so I could just go to sleep,' and I was shocked when I realized that I'd just wished a human being dead so I could go to sleep" (Shem 1978, p. 135). It is a thought that many physicians who interned in an acute-care specialty will guiltily recall having shared.

This discussion would suggest that there is a direct conflict between the routine and power of the workplace and the goal of patient autonomy. But my earlier discussion of the power of the physician as a two-edged sword suggests that no such simplistic dichotomy will do justice to the matter. Certainly the workplace mentality erodes patient power and choice whereas more insistence on patient autonomy and patient rights will enhance patient power and choice. Many aspects of the usual workplace routine are unjustifiable, and much can be done to enhance patient autonomy in the usual hospital or office setting. But having said this, we have to confront the fact that many elements of the workplace routine are directly in the patients' interests and that there may be a fine line between those practices and the unnecessary practices that limit patient choice merely out of habit or vanity.

This point is hardly unique to medicine. I summon a plumber to my house to fix my sink. It is my house and my money; clearly I have a right to watch his every move and to demand that he explain to me precisely what he is doing. But *should* I behave in that fashion? At some point it is contrary to my interests to insist on my rights. If I severely disrupt the work routine of this plumber I will receive poorer-quality work as a result. Put the opposite way, up to some point it is clearly in my interest to let the plumber go about his task in whatever way he wishes, is used to, and feels most comfortable with. When he deduces from my inattention that he can deliberately create extra damage and then charge me extra money to fix it, that point has clearly been crossed; but it might be hard to specify in advance exactly where that point lies.

The same observations apply in medicine. The physician is, after all, a sort of skilled craftsman who will probably do good work when he is comfortable and feels in control and may do poor work under stress or where the work conditions are unfamiliar and disturbing. Other things being equal, it is in the patient's interest to allow the physician to do the work in her usual and accustomed way, even when some wishes or goals of the patient are poorly served by that way of doing the task.[3] Other things are probably equal when (for example) a surgeon feels most secure using a special brand of suture in a particular operation and the patient prefers not to use that brand because the manufacturer has business dealings with a foreign country of whose politics the patient disapproves. Other things are most probably *not* equal when a well-informed woman with localized breast cancer prefers a simple lumpectomy followed by hormonal therapy and the physician feels comfortable only performing a modified radical mastectomy. In between these two extremes may lie some difficult judgment calls. Indeed, it is conceivable that an informed and assertive patient may come to value the work done by a certain physician although that physician is made uncomfortable by an open, negotiated relationship with patients and much prefers a paternalistic, authoritarian mode of relating. The patient may weigh the pros and cons of sticking with this physician versus transferring care elsewhere and may end up autonomously deciding to accept a largely paternalistic mode of treatment in this situation.

The obvious rejoinder is that it is too bad when patients must make choices of this sort. Medical training, plus the management of medical

---

3. That patients may already have figured this out is reflected in the data reported by Lidz, Meisel, Osterweis, et al. (1983), that the patient's role of full and equal participation in all care decisions, viewed as ideal in the ethical and legal literature on informed consent, is actually desired by a mere 10 percent of patients. For further discussion, see chapter 6.

systems and institutions, ought to be able to find ways to make respect for patient choice and patient autonomy and the provision of numerous options for care an integral part of the workplace of the health-care provider. But that rejoinder is precisely the sort of conclusion that emerges from a power-oriented analysis, with the avowed objective of a shared-power relationship. It is a conclusion that emerges very slowly, if at all, from the more usual language of autonomy, beneficence, and rights, since that language tends to hold that patients have a right to personal care and autonomous choice and that no features of the workplace routine can morally take priority over that right. Rights language says, in effect, "Are you going to be a worker or a carer? Take your pick." The language of power recognizes the inescapable tension between care and work in medicine.

The Importance of the Tension: Case Examples

Discussion of ethical problems in terms of the tension between care and work brings to light ethically relevant features that would not have arisen had the more traditional language or concepts been used. To illustrate, I shall reexamine three cases typical of those that turn up in medical-ethics courses in the United States, with specific emphasis on the care-work tensions evident in each: the Johns Hopkins case, the Dax Cowart case, and the "Debbie" case.

Richard Zaner, in *Ethics and the Clinical Encounter* (1988), describes a single case in considerable detail to illustrate his main points, which I take to be that the resolution of an ethical problem is to be found in the circumstances of the case and in the conversation and negotiation among the parties directly involved. Zaner's effort provides a warning for what follows in this chapter. He stresses the value of power language and care-work language; but few cases in the literature are known in enough detail to be open to this mode of analysis. I can imagine Zaner is saying that the existing literature is based on the assumption that the application of general ethical principles like autonomy and beneficence is the most useful way to resolve ethical issues, and that the same literature has guaranteed that this assumption can never be challenged effectively. The existing literature presents as cases highly compressed, abstracted, and largely nonnarrative vignettes. Given such "cases" it is impossible to find the material for the kind of answer Zaner envisages; the quick-and-dirty application of general principles is all we can hope for. In effect, what a phenomenologist like Zaner takes to be a case and what classic books like Robert Veatch's (1977) and Beauchamp and Childress's (1983, 1989) take to be a case are totally different. In the three cases about to be discussed we may lack the relevant factual details to discover what a care-versus-work mode of inquiry could add.

I find Zaner unclear on a point that I take to be critical—whether discussion in terms of power and the care-work tension is supposed to *supplant* or *supplement* discussion in the more usual terms of autonomy, beneficence, rights, justice, and so forth. Zaner seems to imply that these general ethical principles can be wholly replaced. I would urge instead an approach that retains such principles as useful for clustering cases and discussing the similarities and differences among them in terms of morally relevant characteristics. I am trying to show that we lose sight of morally relevant features of cases if we use only those general principles and that the language of power can expand and extend that inquiry process. With that goal in mind, let's see what we can learn from some standard cases.

THE JOHNS HOPKINS CASE. A child was born with Down's syndrome and duodenal atresia (blocking of the small intestine preventing oral feeding). Ordinarily the duodenal atresia would be corrected by a simple and safe surgical procedure. But because of the coexisting Down's syndrome and the likelihood of mental retardation, the parents refused the surgery and the pediatrician honored their wishes. The infant was designated "nothing by mouth," wheeled to a distant corner of the nursery, and allowed to die over a two-week period.

This classic case is interesting for many reasons; one is its transition from controversial to uncontroversial status in a little more than ten years. Presumably the case, especially as a videotape dramatization,[4] was widely used in medical-ethics teaching because it represented a genuine controversy. Many were prepared to defend the proposition that if parents did not wish to rear a child with Down's syndrome, it was acceptable to take advantage of a coexisting life-threatening (though easily correctable) defect and to allow the infant to die. The dominant moral position put forth in the neonatology literature between 1973 and 1976 supported this position by depicting the physician first as a provider of information and later as a source of emotional support, but not as someone who may override informed parental choice (Duff and Campbell 1976). By 1983, the President's Commission for the Study of Ethical Problems in Medicine could state flatly that parental refusal of surgery for duodenal atresia in a Down's infant

4. The videotape *Who Shall Live?* was produced by the Kennedy Institute of Ethics at Georgetown University, Washington, D.C., in 1972. For an extended discussion see Gustafson 1973.

unequivocally justified a court order overruling the parents; and few since have challenged this judgment.

There are many reasons for the change. The emergence of the "best interest of the child" as the dominant ethical standard to be applied to such cases is surely one, even though that so-called standard has numerous conceptual and practical flaws (Brody 1988a). Probably more important have been the emergence of an increasingly strong lobby on behalf of the handicapped and their parents and the increasing number of childless couples willing to adopt a Down's child. These changes have been accompanied by a better appreciation, both inside and outside medicine, of the differences between Down's syndrome and more serious forms of retardation.

In 1982, parents refused surgery for a Down's child in Bloomington, Indiana, and the consequences were felt in the state and ultimately in the United States Supreme Court as well as in the White House and Congress.[5] About ten years earlier, in the Johns Hopkins case, basically the same thing happened, with no such consequences; at least for a time the matter was strictly an in-house concern. What accounts for the difference? Clearly social attitude played a role. Were there any other factors?

One of the striking features of the Johns Hopkins case, in retrospect, is the extent to which the withholding of food from the infant and its eventual death were absorbed into the daily work routine of the nursery. One of the parents was a nurse; generally this is mentioned as showing that the parents had accurate information about the long-term prognosis of Down's children. But an equally important point is that this person knew the workplace and would be regarded by the nurses in the unit as a colleague. Not to follow the parental wishes in this case would have been to refuse to do a favor for a coworker, which could be seen as a grave threat to the stability and smooth functioning of the workplace.

The videotape dramatization shows the attending physician announcing to the staff that a decision has been made and that the baby will not have surgery and will not be fed. This seems to have been standard workplace procedure. There is no question of seeking input from nurses or house staff, let alone convening an ethics committee: that is simply not how such things were supposed to be done. Moreover, the existence in the nursery of a patient receiving such a low level of treatment and remaining out of sight and out of mind is consistent with the running and the physical layout of the nursery. This was not, it appears, a high-tech, intensive-care nursery

---

5. The case itself is described in Pless 1983. The subsequent developments are well summarized in Rhoden and Arras 1985.

full of acutely ill infants receiving aggressive life support. Nor was it so full that there was no deserted, out-of-the-way corner into which this infant's isolette could be wheeled. In sum, every feature of the Johns Hopkins case was consistent with business as usual in the nursery.

What of the needs or impulses of the staff to provide care? Are these people heartless automatons? Two kinds of caring are exhibited in the case. The attending physician clearly sees his role as understanding and supporting the parents' choice. They are articulate, and they express their desires in terms of important family values (for example, the impact of the care this child would require on a sibling). A less caring physician (the doctor might say to himself) would brush aside parental wishes as irrelevant and insist on performing the surgery because it was medically indicated, without considering the impact on the lives of the people most affected. Furthermore, those among the nursing staff who see the infant, too, as an object for care are able to retain their values. That the infant, it is reported, took two weeks to die suggests that it received fluids, and that it died more from starvation than from dehydration. Evidently, at least some of the nurses held it and gave it small amounts of water. In this way, while bowing to the inevitability of the infant's death, the nurses could express their natural impulse to relieve its suffering—despite the official order, "nothing by mouth." To the physicians, proper care for this infant meant carrying out parental wishes and saving the family from the burden of raising a retarded child. To the nurses, caring for a baby meant holding it and giving it whatever fluids it could absorb. The workplace setting allowed each group to carry out its agenda without open confrontation.

A third, more subtle variety of caring also came through. Some of the house staff, it appears, felt uneasy about the disposition of the case and later began the process of publicizing it that led to the making of the videotape. But this type of caring, too, could occur without challenging the smooth routine of work. To have qualms, to go home and worry about whether you did the right thing, is a sign of a caring house officer; the callous ones leave their work at the hospital and simply do what they are told without looking back. But it is not the sign of a good house officer, caring or otherwise, to object to the plan of treatment announced by the attending—at least not at that time and place. Still less would any sort of whistle blowing have been seen as a responsibility of the house staff.

In sum, the case transpired as it did, and no one effectively objected to the infant's death, because there was no felt tension between care and work; nor was the work of the nursery substantially disrupted by the incident. Something like this would almost never occur in a nursery today, partly because of a change of social attitudes and partly because the pattern of work in a nursery has also changed in important ways (Kopelman, Irons, and Kopelman 1988; Todres, Guillemin, Grodin, and Batten 1988). Another reason is that the adoption of various ethical principles as applicable to such cases has changed many health workers' conceptions of what it means to care for an infant of this sort. If, as some data suggest, the problem in the modern nursery is much more likely to be overtreatment than under-treatment, it is because of this change in the work pattern. Neonatologists commonly charge that overtreatment results from outside pressures, specifically the new federal law and guidelines regarding medical care of handicapped infants; but that analyses fail to bear out this claim (Nelson 1988) suggests that other forces closer to the nursery are at work. Whether these forces are a change in the conception of the staffer's task based on emerging technologies or ethical overcorrection for the older abuses of the Johns Hopkins type, or both, may be hard to sort out. It is important to note, however, that infants of the Johns Hopkins type—that is, infants with mental retardation plus an incidental congenital anomaly incompatible with life—are quite rare in newborn intensive-care units, whereas low-birthweight infants subject to natural and iatrogenic (physician-induced) complications are quite common (Jonsen 1982; Strong 1983b). An overcorrection that tries to compensate for a handful of cases like the one at Johns Hopkins by stressing maximal treatment even where benefit is doubtful will therefore end up subjecting a large number of infants to nonbeneficial treatment.

THE DAX COWART CASE. In 1973, Donald Cowart received severe burns in a gas explosion in Texas, in which his father was killed. He eventually requested that his treatment be discontinued and that he be allowed to die. He was subjected to daily immersions in a whirlpool to prevent skin infection, which he found excruciatingly painful. As he knew that at the completion of this treatment he would be left blind and without the use of his hands, he judged the outcome not to be worth the pain. The physicians at the University of Texas Medical Branch continued treatment against his wishes, relying on the consent of Cowart's mother and the family attorney. Cowart, who later changed his name to Dax, eventually completed legal training and has spoken publicly on numerous occasions about the injustice of his forced treatment.

This case, of the three discussed here, is known in the most detail. The viewpoints of most of the actors in the drama at the time the medical decisions were being made were recorded on videotape and in print, and we also have that crucial element that distinguishes a true narrative from a case vignette, a record of what happens next.[6] The story of Dax is typically presented as a paradigm instance of paternalistic interference with patient autonomy, and the debate then proceeds about whether Dax, in his burned, blind, crippled, and pain-wracked state, is capable of sufficient autonomous choice to make it mandatory to respect his wish to die by stopping treatment.

At least one commentator (Platt 1975) called attention early to evidence of a care-versus-work conflict in the case, as documented on the first teaching videotape made of Dax's psychiatric assessment. The scenes of the patient being immersed in a whirlpool tank and then rebandaged, a procedure that he reported as exquisitely painful, depict strikingly callous disregard among the unit staff for Dax's experience. A radio blares in the background, machinery whirs, and the place seems more like an automobile repair shop than a sanctuary for suffering humanity. Moans or statements of pain bring forth no response from the attendants who are methodically applying the dressings; a shriek elicits a muttered, reluctant apology. Since Dax's pain must have been due in large part to inadequate doses of narcotics, I suspect that the tone of allowing work to dominate care and drive out almost all perception of the patient as an individual might well have been set by the attending physicians, with the lower-ranking staff simply following the dominant pattern.

It was apparently possible for the staff to ignore Dax's experience of pain; such neglect probably was felt by many other patients and was part of the work routine. What was unique to Dax and could not long be ignored was his persistent request to be discharged and to be allowed to die, uttered in terms that suggested rational thought. Dax was pleading with them to put aside their work and pay attention to him and what he was saying about himself. In Dax's terms, care would have required this attention to his individual needs and to the reasons behind them; but this burn center was in the business of skin grafting, debriding, and preventing infection and appeared incapable of interpreting care in this fashion.

The center could, however, determine that a patient was becoming a barrier to the smooth work routine; and, as almost always occurs within

6. The case of Donald Cowart, as it occurred in the hospital, was captured in *Please Let Me Die*, a teaching video from the psychiatry program at the University of Texas Medical Branch, Galveston (*Videotape Library of Psychiatric Disorders*, vol. 29, May 1974). See also White and Engelhardt 1975; Platt 1975. Later developments as well as much richer background information are depicted in *Dax's Case*, a film prepared by Concern for Dying, 1984. For further commentary, see Kliever 1989.

medical and other institutions with a major power differential between the workers and the clients, the fault was attributed to the patient. In Parsonian terms, Dax must be deviant to be creating such a fuss (Parsons 1978); the goal was to label the deviance in such a way that it became somebody else's job to deal with it, leaving the burn team free to continue whirlpooling and bandaging. This was readily accomplished by labeling the deviance as psychiatric in origin and deciding that the psychiatrist was the person responsible for fixing it.

So the psychiatrist, Robert White, came to interview Dax, who presented him with the same plea—stop the work routine long enough to listen to me and see what care for me and my needs would actually entail. To a greater extent than the burn treatment team, White did this; he refused to go along with the initial theory that Dax was just depressed and that a pharmacological behavioral "fix" was all that was needed. White at least gave Dax credit for being rational. But he was not willing to go the next step, which would have been to say that the institution, not the patient, had a problem: it was imposing on this patient a pattern of care that was good for almost all patients *but not for him*. It was then exacerbating the problem by refusing to acknowledge it and calling the patient crazy instead. For White to take this stance would have been to side with patient rights and patient autonomy, and it would also have been to bring work to a halt. He refused, implicitly, to do this. Instead, he adopted a course that could be construed as making Dax's behavior the subject of his own work routine while allowing the burn team to go on with their work routine. Instead of stopping work long enough to listen to the patient, both White and the burn team went on with the work, at two separate levels.

White's part of the work routine consisted of what would be called psychotherapy by his defenders and manipulation by his detractors. It consisted of reinterpreting Dax's wishes in terms of White's frame of reference—not as a wish to stop treatment and be allowed to die but as a wish to regain control. It then proceeded to a carefully tuned procedure of seeming to give Dax the control White believed he sought while keeping all real control in medical hands. Eventually Dax gave in and allowed treatment to continue. This could have occurred for one of several reasons: (1) White was right about what Dax really wanted; (2) White was wrong, but Dax found the pseudo-control too tempting a halfway gain to pass up; (3) Dax simply got tired of fighting against the odds; (4) Dax realized that he was so close to the end of treatment that it was not worth his while to keep struggling.

At the time the burn treatment team faced their decision, they had few resources within the hospital to assist them in resolving an *ethical* issue; hence they can be forgiven if they elected to construe the matter as a psychiatric one. Today it is becoming much more common for hospitals to form ethics committees to assist in cases like Dax's.[7] The committee membership typically reflects the various professions at work in hospitals. It is likely that had such a committee existed in Dax's time and place, the burn physicians, the psychiatrists, and the nurses and physical therapists would all have had representatives on it.

This analysis in terms of care versus work helps to show a particular promise as well as a particular risk of the ethics committee mechanism. If awareness of the care-work tension is explicitly a part of the charge and training of each committee, then the committee may be especially alert to factors of work routine and how they might influence both the decisions made and the way patients and families are perceived by staff. It is quite possible, for example, that a representative committee would know without being told what are the dominant work routines in each hospital unit and in what ways those routines predictably clash with certain patient interests and wishes. (By contrast, an individual ethics consultant, who may be familiar with the daily work routine of only a few units, may have great difficulty discovering such factors in operation.) But if the committee is trained or charged in a different fashion, it may routinely fall into the trap of always sympathizing with the hospital workers and seeing the patient and the patient's request through the workers' eyes. The risk that the committee might simply serve as a rubber stamp for institutional interests has been pointed out several times, but I mean here specifically the interests created by comfortable work routines, not the financial interests that are usually intended when this risk is discussed. If this negative scenario were played out fully, the patient whose need for individualized care disrupted the dominant work pattern of the unit would never get a fair hearing before the ethics committee. Clearly this issue has great importance for how ethics committees are trained and how they see their function.

THE "DEBBIE" CASE. In 1988, the *Journal of the American Medical Association* published a brief case report (the author's name was withheld by request) recounting the mercy killing of a young woman terminally ill and in pain from ovarian cancer by an on-call gynecology resident, who injects her with an overdose of morphine. Although this brief case vignette is much more recent than the preceding two, it seems destined to come in

---

7. On the concept, and the potential problems, of ethics committees, see Cranford and Doudera 1984; Kanoti and Vinicky 1987; Lo 1987.

for an equal amount of discussion.[8] It is extremely sketchy, leaving questions about whether the case itself is real or fictional and, if real, just how many years ago it happened. The action described—a sleepy on-call resident administers an overdose of morphine to end the misery of a terminally ill cancer patient—has been widely condemned for failing to adhere to the sort of guidelines or safeguards that even strong advocates of an active euthanasia policy would insist on.

The structure of the vignette forces the care-work tension onto the reader at the onset. The resident is awakened by a nurse who reports that the patient cannot sleep. The patient is not the resident's: the inadequate regimen of pain relief is the work of a private attending physician (who is no doubt snoring contentedly in his own bed at this moment). In effect, the resident has been awakened to clean up some other doctor's mess. Under the circumstances, the question is not, "What is the optimal care for this patient?" or "How can I begin the process of talking with this patient to see what she really wants?" but rather, "What can I do to solve the problem quickly and get back to bed with the least likelihood that I will be called again later by these same nurses for this same patient?" You don't have to be a medical psychologist to see that the circumstances are not conducive to thoughtful reflection over a matter as grave as active euthanasia. Here is the House of God's "I wish the patient would die so that I could get some sleep" with a vengeance.

Thus, one observed tension between care and work goes to support the condemnation of this resident's action. But although this condemnation was almost universal, the lessons drawn from the case vignette were argued hotly in the later exchange of letters and editorials in the journal. One point of view was that active euthanasia is immoral, pure and simple: physicians must never be involved in killing their patients under any circumstances, and the journal's editor was to be condemned for publishing a piece like this, which could be construed as endorsing active euthanasia (Gaylin et al. 1988). A divergent point of view was that although this particular action was to be condemned, the problem of active euthanasia was much more complicated, and the main lesson was the need for more humane relief of symptoms for dying patients, not a blanket condemnation of active euthanasia in principle (Vaux 1988; Lundberg 1988). (That is, if active euthanasia is to be prohibited, it can only be because humane and efficacious relief of pain and other symptoms of terminal illness is readily

8. For case "report" itself see "It's over, Debbie" 1988; for further discussion see chapter 3, note 5.

available; if medicine cannot or will not relieve those symptoms, it is hypocritical to condemn active euthanasia.) Which of these points of view is more supportable requires a subtler analysis of some of the care-versus-work issues underlying the "Debbie" case.

We might first note that the physicians denouncing active euthanasia in response to the case would presumably endorse many instances of passive euthanasia or withdrawal of life-prolonging treatment. Their across-the-board condemnation of active euthanasia therefore ignores two complications. First, it may be hard to say in a particular instance whether the patient's death is the result of active or passive means—as in the case of withdrawing food or fluids. Second, even if an unequivocal distinction could be drawn, it is by no means clear that the active-passive distinction is in itself morally controlling or even morally relevant; other features of the case may outweigh the active-passive issue in moral terms (Menzel 1979; Rachels 1986). Besides these complications, the opponents of active euthanasia ignored the practical experience with active euthanasia that has been accumulated over recent years in the Netherlands (Pence 1988). Although the Dutch experience may not by itself constitute a reason to endorse active euthanasia, it remains true that available data do not support the notion that a policy of active euthanasia, frequently resorted to, has produced the sort of moral disaster the opponents' theory would predict.[9]

If both analytic and practical considerations argue against a blanket condemnation of all instances of active euthanasia, why did the opponents (among them some of the most illustrious names in contemporary biomedical ethics) react as strongly as they did? It is my guess that they were responding primarily to the power dimension of the active-euthanasia debate, as discussed briefly in chapter 3. Their response to the "Debbie" case was based as much on their fear of how the public would view them as on their desire to clarify the issues for their fellow physicians. They seem to have assumed that the public reaction would be one of terror at the thought that a trusted physician might someday administer a fatal dose in

9. At this writing the truth about the active-euthanasia policies in the Netherlands remains uncertain. The bulk of published material supports the notion that euthanasia is generally being restricted to cases of voluntary request and that the occasional lapse is punished swiftly. (A physician who purportedly euthanized several senile residents of a nursing home was reported to have been sentenced to prison.) Most published articles attacking the policy speak vaguely of possible abuses but give no hard evidence. Personal reports I have received from American and British visitors to the Netherlands, and from Dutch physicians involved and uninvolved in the euthanasia movement, vary widely in their assessment. The range of opinions is captured in Fenigsen 1989 and Rigter 1989 and a subsequent exchange of letters in the *Hastings Center Report* (November-December 1989).

the name of kindness. The only proper reaction was a self-righteous de-
nunciation of any such act as outside the pale of medical morality.

Public reaction is in truth quite different. First, recent opinion polls
show a majority of respondents approving of active euthanasia in certain
circumstances.[10] Second, the widespread public dread is not of the mur-
derous physician but of the overzealous one: a prolonged and lingering
death tied to machines and tubes seems to hold greater terror for the average
person than Debbie's sleepy and misguided resident. Letters to the editor
from several nonphysicians were published in the same issue of the journal
in which the opposing letters and commentaries appeared; none of those
correspondents condemned active euthanasia, and all expressed concern
about inhumanely prolonging life in the terminally ill. The public, indeed,
seemed quite concerned that the power of medicine would be used against
them rather than for them as they lay dying; but it was the chemotherapy
infusion and the intensive care unit, not the syringe of morphine, that they
had in mind. If the goal of the opponents of active euthanasia was to relieve
public fears about medicine, their supposed reassurance landed wide of
the mark.

All these observations about the opposing viewpoint can be made readily
without drawing on the care-work tension. But further discussion of that
tension on a deeper level supports this line of thought. Consider again the
workplace within which that resident found himself on that night. He was
not called because a dying patient had been in a state of severe, unremitting
pain for forty-eight hours. He was called because the patient was unable
to sleep. (The presumption was that a sleeping pill, not pain medication,
was needed. Indeed, under those circumstances, his getting up to see the
patient at all instead of simply giving the nurses a phone order for a sedative
was to the resident's credit—and perhaps further evidence that the case
was either fictitious or else occurred many years ago.) When he arrived at
the nursing unit, he was not greeted by any sort of frantic plea for the
resolution of what was, after all, an intolerable and professionally unjustifiable situation. He was greeted matter-of-factly, as if a patient unable to
sleep and hence awake to bother the night nurses was a problem. But a
dying cancer patient in great pain who was receiving totally inadequate
analgesic therapy was all part of a day's work there.

We would ideally have wanted this resident to assess the situation and

10. Typical is a poll of 1,982 adult Americans conducted by the Roper Organization in
1988, in which 58 percent of respondents favored allowing physicians to end the life of
terminally ill patients at the patients' request.

then tell this patient, "You do not have to be in this much pain. We will be taking steps immediately to get it under control. If need be we will sedate you to the point of coma; but we will get rid of the pain one way or another." And a resident who had trained in a good inpatient hospice unit or a good pain clinic would have had this patient free of pain within two hours. But even a brief review of the workplace shows that this approach would be as out of place in this particular hospital ward at this particular time as a bar mitzvah at the Vatican. It is quite likely that the resident lacked the training to manage the patient's problem properly (it is questionable that the dose of morphine he says he used was adequate even for analgesia, and it would hardly constitute a predictably fatal dose). Even had he known how, instituting that rational management plan would most likely have been met with incredulity if not outright opposition from nurses, the pharmacy, and the attending physician the next morning.

We can now have a little more sympathy for (without approving of) the thinking of that resident as he walked into the room that night. He knew that the patient was dying and in terrible pain, and that the only possible thing medicine could do for her was to end that state of affairs by one means or another. He also knew that the usual work routines of the gynecology unit were totally unequal to the task of giving this patient what she needed. So he concluded that only by doing something totally out of the ordinary—indeed (I hope), unprecedented in his short career—could he possibly give the patient what she needed and desired. He chose wrongly. But we can now see that the basic ethical value in cases like this is not the approval or disapproval of active or passive methods of intervention but rather the duty of the physician to use the powers of medical science to secure for the patient a death as comfortable and dignified as possible, defined in the patient's own terms. To precisely the extent that pain control, psychological support, and the like have been made readily available and have been fine-tuned in their efficacy, will active euthanasia appear an unnecessary or indeed a less humane alternative. But when the workplace of medicine has neglected those skills and procedures, then we can expect active euthanasia to look ever more attractive to both patients and physicians. To say that what defines the core of medical morality is that, first and foremost, doctors must never kill, and then to add as an afterthought that of course doctors must find ways to soothe and comfort the dying without killing them, is a high-minded but inadequate rendition of the obligations of medicine toward the terminally ill patient. It places devotion to abstract principle ahead of real care of the patient, since real care demands attention to the nuances of individual cases. By contrast, the ideal state of medical practice in this regard would be when active euthanasia is shunned by all physicians because to perform it would be to admit gross clinical incompetence, there existing so many better treatments for dying patients of all types and under all circumstances. In this ideal state of medicine a moral prohibition of active euthanasia would hardly be necessary.[11]

I propose as an agenda for the remainder of this book to develop a conception of the physician-patient relationship, construed both as one-on-one and as a broadly social relationship, which seeks the sharing of power as a means toward my criteria for the responsible use of power in medicine: owned power, aimed power, and shared power. The tension between care and work presents one of the most common ways in which health professionals do two things simultaneously: first, refuse to share power with the patient (since the professional and not the patient controls the workplace); and second, remain unaware that the power has been monopolized or that power is even an issue (since the work routine is as much part of the background environment, and hence hidden from critical reflection, as water is to a fish). There is, therefore, a value in adding questions about the care-work tension to any checklist of questions to ask when conducting a medical-ethics inquiry or work-up. Unless one begins explicitly to inquire, "What work routines typify this particular medical-care setting or team of professionals? In what ways might that work routine conflict with the individualized care needs of this patient? To what extent are the involved professionals consciously aware of this potential for conflict?" then it is highly likely that many important ethical problems—along with the possible routes to their resolutions—will remain hidden from view.

11. This, in effect, was the thinly veiled charge against the Dutch medical profession in the British Medical Association's *Euthanasia Report* (April 1988). Briefly, the BMA claimed that it takes hard work to listen carefully to a dying patient to find out the precise sources of his anguish and devise a humane response; to kill the patient is much simpler.

CHAPTER 6

INFORMED

CONSENT:

DEFINITION

AND

MODELS

I nformed consent in medical practice has been a ticklish test case for the new medical ethics. Superficially, it sounds like a success story. It was only in 1957 that the term *informed consent* was coined.[1] Today, almost all physicians recognize the need to obtain informed consent for various procedures, and the term is ingrained in medicine's daily vocabulary.

But this superficial appearance belies a deeper set of problems. Informed consent became a subject for legal involvement in medical practice, through negligence law, before it became the subject for detailed ethical analysis.[2] This meant that practicing physicians were first introduced to the concept as a legal intrusion on medicine, and not (as the ethicists would have had it) a natural component of a physician-patient relationship that respects patient autonomy.[3] Thus, when physicians disclose information to patients and request their consent, they do so with an attitude of giving in to intrusive foreign influences on proper medical practice, and not of performing a vital and central function of medical practice. Not surprisingly, under these circumstances empirical research reveals many gaps in informed-

1. The term appeared first in an amicus curiae brief filed on behalf of the American College of Surgeons in the case of *Salgo v. Leland Stanford University*. For further discussion see Katz (1984); Faden and Beauchamp (1986).

2. This contrasts, say, with the issue of withholding nutrition and hydration from terminally ill patients. That matter did not come before courts until authoritative ethical analyses, such as the President's Commission report (1983), had already appeared; and the courts tended to rely on those ethical analyses in drawing their conclusions.

3. See the discussion of Fried's (1974) "rights in personal care," by which the concept of informed consent would arise naturally from the rights of autonomy and lucidity, in chapter 4.

consent practices by physicians and many practical barriers toward fulfill-
ment of the promise of the concept.

A Definition of Informed Consent

A thick volume by Ruth Faden and Tom Beauchamp, *A History and Theory
of Informed Consent* (1986), draws on two decades of work on this subject
by both legal and philosophical thinkers and in the contexts of medical
practice, medical research, and social-science research. The authors' analysis
of the concept illustrates both the significant results achieved by the "new"
medical ethics and the gaps and weaknesses that are related at least partly
to the reluctance to deal with power as an essential concept.

Faden and Beauchamp follow the trend of the "new" ethics in locating
informed consent under the general umbrella of respect for patient autonomy; the purpose of consent is respect for patient autonomy, not good
outcomes. Therefore, they devote much effort to analyzing, first, what
autonomy consists of in medicine. Noting that one could speak of either
persons or actions as being autonomous—each case requiring somewhat
different criteria—they argue that autonomy of action, and not autonomy
of the person, is relevant to informed consent. (That is, a person suffering
from substantial incapacities of thinking and decision making might yet
make a single reasonable, informed decision; they would regard the person
as nonautonomous but the action as autonomous.)

They then consider three necessary conditions for autonomy of action:
the action must be intentional; the action must be done with understanding;
and the actor must be uncontrolled by coercive influences, whether internal
or external. An action is either intentional or it is not. But both *understanding*
and *uncontrolled* (or *uncoerced*) represent relative values on a continuum:
one seldom if ever has either no understanding or full understanding, and
one seldom if ever has either total freedom from any coercive influence or
total lack of freedom. One might be inclined to suggest that autonomy, as
a moral ideal, requires full or optimal understanding and freedom from
coercion. But here Faden and Beauchamp nod in the direction of practicality
and propose that the condition of most interest is not full or optimal
autonomy but *substantial* autonomy. Actions are autonomous so long as
they are performed under conditions of *substantial* understanding and *substantial* absence of control or coercion. The implication is that their definition allows the majority of human actions and choices to be viewed as
autonomous. If we adopted the requirement of full understanding and full
freedom or voluntariness, then an autonomous action would be a rare event
in human experience and of little interest to practical morality.

Although they wish to link informed consent conceptually with auton-omy, Faden and Beauchamp do not wish to make the two terms coextensive. Hence, to define informed consent, they add a fourth condition to the three necessary conditions for autonomy. A patient gives informed consent if and only if (1) he acts intentionally; (2) he has substantial understanding of the act and its consequences; (3) he is substantially free from coercive control; and (4) he authorizes the physician to provide the treatment in question (p. 278).

From their discussion, Faden and Beauchamp seem to believe that "au-thorizing" requires formal or explicit authorization; they pay little heed to the possibility of implied or assumed authorization. Their view seems to be similar to that taken in a book by Beauchamp and McCullough (1984), who held that informed consent is almost totally absent from primary-care practice because no *explicit* disclosure and authorization occur in most primary-care encounters. These authors concluded that primary care is thus basically paternalistic. They discounted the possibility that implied consent could be an equally good form of consent in a primary-care setting, and Faden and Beauchamp seem to pursue that line of thought.

Ignoring some of the realities of primary-care medicine might be taken as a warning sign that Faden and Beauchamp have gotten off the track somewhere in their analysis. But in fact they do not regard this point as of any importance to their enterprise. For they proceed to make the rather astonishing claim *that their task is to describe what informed consent ought to consist of in theory, and that it is largely irrelevant whether anything corre-sponding to that concept takes place in practice* (1986, pp. 274–80). I take this to mean that they think they have derived their definition of informed consent from all the appropriate first principles of philosophical ethics, theory of the person, theory of action and causation, and so on. If they then look at medical practice and find nothing there that fits their definition, their conclusion will not be that their definition is flawed; they will conclude instead that "real" informed consent simply does not exist in medicine. Of course, they fail to explain why their theory and definition would then be of any interest to someone interested in medicine or in medical ethics.

This avowedly theoretical and nonpractical agenda might explain a fur-ther puzzle in Faden and Beauchamp's approach: their labeling of two "senses" of informed consent. For them, informed consent in sense$_1$ is the moral concept (in either medical practice or research) and occurs when the above four conditions are met. Informed consent in sense$_2$ is consent as defined by a legal or administrative policy. What they wish primarily to say here, it seems, is that one can obtain informed consent in sense$_2$

but fail to obtain informed consent in sense$_1$, such as when a physician gets a patient to sign a piece of paper but does not check to be sure the patient understands what is written on it. Alternatively, a physician may obtain consent in sense$_1$ but not in sense$_2$, such as when the patient is fully informed and makes a voluntary choice but the physician fails to record the details in the medical record. The problem is to see why one would wish to regard the moral and the legal as two alternative *senses* of informed consent. If one's agenda is purely theoretical, it is handy to have two senses of informed consent, deriving one strictly from ethical and philosophical principles and the other strictly from legal precedent, common law, constitutional protections, and so on. One could then engage in interesting theoretical analyses to see where the two senses overlap and where they do not. But someone concerned with medical practice and its improvement would likely wish to commit herself to the moral sense of informed consent and then view legal and administrative rules not as a coequal "sense" but as practical means and mechanism to insure that informed consent (in its moral sense) is carried out by physicians. The question would then be an empirical one of the practical consequences of different legal and administrative mechanisms and requirements.

To sum up, there are pluses and minuses to Faden and Beauchamp's analysis, arguably the most sophisticated to have yet emerged from the new medical ethics. The pluses involve the definition itself, which calls attention to what they generally take to be most crucial in assessing whether a patient has given informed consent. They worry about whether the patient understands the proposed medical intervention, its consequences, and the existence and consequences of any practical alternatives to it. They worry about whether the patient knows what he is doing—that when he says he wants something, he truly wants *that* thing and not something else that he has confused with it. They worry about whether the patient is being unduly influenced or controlled by other people (ourselves included) or by internal forces like fear, addiction, depression, or metabolic imbalances. And they worry about whether the patient sees this process as part of *participating in a decision* and not just as polite conversation or pro forma ritual.

The further pluses include the distinctions between substantial autonomy and full autonomy and between autonomy of the person and autonomy of action. Relating informed consent to autonomy of action, for instance, may help isolate informed consent as one discrete element in the physician-patient relationship; it may be argued that the physician-patient relationship overall is relatively more concerned with the autonomy of the person whereas informed consent is more narrowly focused on the autonomy of individual actions and decisions.

But a fair assessment also includes the minuses, which have to do primarily with the overall theoretical strategy and the identification of two coequal senses of informed consent. If I begin my critique from the standpoint of the power taboo phenomenon, then Faden and Beauchamp seem to have little interest in exploring the complexities of power relationships in medical practice that a deeper analysis of informed consent as a *practical* concept might uncover. This charge may seem unfair, for they review in some depth several empirical research studies of informed consent and patient and physician reactions to it (as I will do below). But the point may be that the new medical ethics, with its taboo regarding power, is happy to mention social-science research so long as it is carefully bracketed and does not intrude directly into the arena of philosophical analysis. It is not mention of empirical fact that is missing; it is the idea that the results of one's philosophical analysis need to be checked against empirical fact before they can be accepted as philosophically adequate.

I propose to try an alternative strategy: starting with the empirical observations, developing models that attempt to respond to the facts, and then testing the models against a combination of philosophical and empirical considerations. For all further purposes in this chapter, however, the definition of informed consent as developed above will be perfectly suitable.

Empirical Facts and Possible Models

The new medical ethics customarily begins discussion of informed consent with the theory of patient autonomy and its practical implications for the rights of patients to be informed and to decide on their own medical treatment. But medical ethicists need not today feel obligated to use the same starting point. They have been advocating respect for patient autonomy for more than a decade, at the same time that courts have been finding various ways to come down hard on physicians who inadequately disclose known risks of medical treatment or possible alternatives to the recommended treatment. Moreover, with a renewed interest in empirical research on doctor-patient communication and on matters related to medical ethics, we have additional data on what is happening in medical practice in response to these legal and ethical exhortations. (Some of the most important research was commissioned by the President's Commission on biomedical ethics as part of their preparation for a detailed report [1982] on informed consent.) Instead of asking from what moral principles the pious exhortations arise, we can start by asking what the pious exhortations have done for the practice of medicine. Although the details are important and the method of research is crucial to determining whether the research helps with ethical thinking, it will suffice for present purposes to sketch out the most important trends in the research results fairly broadly.[4]

Practicing physicians at all levels of training appear to show little understanding of what informed consent is all about. The law locates informed consent as part of the basic right of self-determination, and medical ethics locates informed consent within the ideal model of the physician-patient relationship. But physicians see informed consent as a legal practice, not as part of doing medicine; and they fail to see any basic link between jumping through the perceived legal hoops and doing anything valuable for the patient or for patient self-determination. When physicians disclose information, the underlying motive is often to avoid legal trouble and seldom to improve the quality of patient care (Lidz et al. 1983).[5]

Some physicians take an almost perverse pleasure in pointing out that it is just as easy to manipulate patients with full disclosure as with incomplete disclosure, so long as one subtly emphasizes the right points (Lidz et al. 1983). What arouses concern is not a comment like this but the tone in which it is offered. The physician does not appear to say, "I know that ethics requires respect for patient self-determination, but—alas!—I remain a weak sinner, and treat patients paternalistically." The tone instead is, "You and I both know that practicing good medicine means doing what we think best for our patients. Then those lawyers came along and insisted that we do silly things that don't help our patients but fit the lawyers' concept of patients' rights. But the joke is on them, for it turns out that we can play their silly game, disclosing mounds of information, and *still* make sure that we end up doing what we know is best."

Physician disclosure of therapeutic information is driven by a precon-

4. For a concise summary of much of the relevant empirical data, see Faden and Beauchamp 1986: 98–99 and associated footnotes.

5. I would supplement this research finding with a personal observation gleaned from attending medical conferences, grand rounds, and journal clubs during this period. Physicians may be impatient with presentations that are labeled "doctor-patient communication" or "patient education," possibly preferring to discuss the latest calcium channel blocker or third-generation cephalosporin; but they at least acknowledge those topics as pertinent to better caring for patients and better serving patients' needs. By contrast, a conference on informed consent (which should ideally be presented by a lawyer) is seen as an unpleasant but necessary intrusion, something like a disaster-preparedness drill. What is almost totally missing from the mind of the average clinician (I would allege) is that one could be talking about basically the same thing in addressing any one of those three topics.

ceived protocol and not by any active process of assessing the patient's need or desire for information. Asked to guess how much information patients want, physicians routinely guess wrong—usually on the low side (Strull et al. 1984). When patients explicitly call attention to their informational needs by refusing some treatment that the physician has recommended, the physician may respond by repeating in rote fashion all the information previously given (perhaps in a louder voice), or may simply shrug her shoulders and allow the patient to do without the treatment. But what is virtually never done when treatment has been refused is to ask the patient *why* he refused and then to tailor the subsequent disclosure of information to the patient's specific concerns (Appelbaum and Roth 1983). In other words (and at some risk of overgeneralizing), talking *to* the patient about medical facts may be much more common than it used to be, but talking *with* patients about medical facts remains rare.

If this sounds like a resounding rejection of the new medical ethics on the part of physicians, the patients have registered their own dissent. Thinking in medical ethics tends to view disclosure and participation in decision making as a logically linked, two-step process: the first is necessary for the second, and the second is the main reason justifying the first. But what philosophers have joined, patients have cheerfully put asunder. Patients claim that they want more information from physicians about their disease and their treatment (Strull et al. 1984) and even say that they would pay more for it if necessary (although a follow-up study to see if they would put their money where their attitude questionnaire is has not to my knowledge been carried out). But when asked why they want the information, they do not answer as the philosophers say they should. Patients, it seems, want information so that they can feel that they are being treated like people and not like slabs of meat being shunted between points in the health-care system. They want information so that they can better comply with their physician's recommendations. They want information so that they might register a veto (admittedly rarely) if the physician's choice seems especially ill-conceived—here the philosophers are starting to get a bit warm. But in one detailed study, only about 10 percent of patients said that they wanted information because they wished to participate substantially in their medical-care decisions (Lidz et al. 1983).

Of course, this empirical finding might simply be the flip side of the two findings mentioned above. Patients tend to want to be good patients and to do what their physicians seem to expect. If physicians, despite the "new" exhortations, expect and value patient passivity in decision making, then patients are likely to be passive. But the cart-horse problem aside, these findings are still important if a goal of the philosophers is to produce any actual medical reform. When patients demand something of the health-care system as their right, in the United States they are likely to get what they seek. We have seen this in such varied areas as heart and liver transplants covered by insurance, fathers' being allowed in the delivery room and in the operating room during Cesarean section, and walk-in convenience clinics open during evening and weekend hours. When the philosophers but not the patients demand something, change is likely to be much slower; and the patients are clearly not demanding participation.

In sum, the empirical data will not allow us to view informed consent—as it has developed under the "new" medical ethics, hand in hand with medical negligence law—as a resounding success. According to these studies, fifteen years of exhortation seems to have done far less than might have been done to secure patient autonomy a more privileged place in the value system of both doctor and patient. There is an important proviso to these depressing findings: the studies we have reviewed generally reflect hospital practice and outpatient subspecialty practice and indicate little about primary-care medicine. But as of now, there is no data to make us think that the picture is much better for primary care, and there are some reasons to suspect that the situation there is even worse.[6]

At this point we are faced with two issues: a theoretically satisfying definition of informed consent, and empirical data showing that that definition has not been translated successfully into practice. We may now look at some alternative strategies for addressing this disparity. Toward this end I present three models, which would need fleshing out before they could be seen as strategies for practical implementation.

Paternalistic model. The facts show that informed consent is a farce. Return to a model of frank physician beneficence and give up the idea that patient participation is meaningful.

Legalistic model. Continue to use tort law, specifically the law of negligence, as the primary means of enforcing physician cooperation. Emphasize complete disclosure of all potential risks that the patient might need to know to make an informed decision. Judge the adequacy of disclosure in the light of later events, especially in cases of adverse outcome.

Conversation model. View informed consent primarily as a sort of conversation between physician and patient designed to involve the patient in

6. For example, see Merenstein 1982 on the short amount of time spent by family physicians with the average patient—certainly limiting opportunities for serious approaches to informed consent.

medical decisions in an informed way to the extent that the patient wishes. The physician's duty is to lay the groundwork for, facilitate, and promote this sort of conversation. The process and not the precise facts disclosed or withheld is what should be judged. Since it is harder to give objective criteria to judge a process of this sort, education of physicians, not negligence law, will have to play the major role in securing reform.

The paternalistic model is a logically possible way to resolve the disparity between theory and practice, and possibly a majority of physicians would favor it, although many would not. I, of course, cannot accept it, since I wish my critique of the "new" medical ethics to be a step forward, not a cover-up for reactionary retreat.

The legalistic model is somewhat peculiar. Legal scholars and philosophers who have sympathetically followed the reasoning of the high courts that have put forth subjective standards for adequacy of disclosure might deny that it correctly reflects the current law of informed consent. They might argue that it reflects physician ignorance and paranoia about the law rather than what the law is really telling physicians to do. I will offer two points in defense of my formulation of the model and later will show, I hope, why the model has some utility as a counterpoint to the third model.

First, no matter what the law says, this model describes how many physicians have understood the legal pressure they face. These are not necessarily physicians who wish to return to paternalism but physicians who wish to promote greater patient participation yet are unsure what they are required to do and where they should put their emphasis and energy. The physicians may be legally uninformed, but this model at any rate describes the practical impact that legal developments have had on physicians' behavior.

Second, some aspects of the model are true to a large extent. So long as tort law remains the avenue by which disputed cases come before a public tribunal, the most obvious feature of a case will be the harm suffered by the patient, and reasoning will start with the harm and work backward to the actual consent process that was used. In this setting it is very hard to judge a consent process on its own merits without either party having foreknowledge of what is going to happen down the road: in short, it is hard to judge the consent process from the viewpoint of the physician who has to design and implement it. Moreover, as degree of participation allowed in relation to degree of participation desired is a "soft" concept, and the number of facts disclosed (or at least written down) seems by contrast a "hard" concept, there is a strong tendency under tort law for the duty to obtain informed consent to degenerate into a duty to disclose information. No matter what else the law might or might not say about informed consent, I think that these implications are undeniable.[7]

Finally, there is the conversation model, which at first glance seems totally foreign to medical ethics and its current vocabulary. It is derived almost wholly from the work of Jay Katz (1984), who has looked in detail at informed consent as an ethical and legal concept. But Katz has also looked hard at the psychology of the physician-patient encounter and has identified all the barriers that have traditionally impeded a dialogue designed to secure for the patient the role of active and informed decision maker. These barriers are rooted in the psyche of both physician and patient and in the culture within which the encounter occurs. For Katz, the purpose of calling attention to all these barriers is not to promote the return to paternalism or to justify continued reliance on a legalistic model; it is to show precisely in what direction the movement for reform must proceed and what energy it would require. In Katz's view, the tradition that states that good medical care excludes patient involvement is thousands of years old; the movement that calls for increased participation of patients in their medical decisions dates effectively from 1957. But Katz has no trouble determining that the thousand-year-old tradition is wrong and the new movement is right; and neither is he under any delusions about how hard it will be to oppose the tradition.

I argue that Katz's model is the best, in large part because Katz's psychological insights forced him to take the power aspects of the physician-patient relationship seriously. Of all three models, conversation provides the best metaphor for describing what a realistic shared-power approach to medical decisions might look like. But first we have to convince ourselves that the conversation model can be used as a tool for analysis and can distinguish better from worse physician-patient encounters—in short, that "conversation model" is not simply another way of saying "anything goes."

The typical rhetoric of the "new" medical ethics, power-shy as it is, often denies any intent toward medical reform. The "new" medical ethicist got invited into medical schools and hospitals by proclaiming, "I'm not here to tell you what's right or wrong; I'm here to help you analyze the issues." That rhetoric was useful but simple-minded, and I doubt whether any so-called ethicist either believes it or says it today. But it should be especially clear from what has been said so far that *any model that takes*

7. For a rare example of an attorney agreeing with physicians that the current tort law is not a proper guide to the practice of informed consent, see Green 1988.

the definition of informed consent seriously is a strategy for the reform of medical practice. The empirical data have indicated an intolerable degree of incoherence between the concept of informed consent and the practice of physicians, even where physicians use the term *informed consent* to describe what they are doing. The legalistic model is the least reformist, because it basically advocates more of the same, but even it assumes that more of the same will eventually yield significant behavior changes. Therefore, when comments about the extent of reform needed or envisioned are made below, we should not assume that the discussion has departed from the realm of medical ethics.

Disclosure of Remote Risk: A Test Case

Definitions like that of Faden and Beauchamp, presented in the first section of this chapter, clearly do important analytic work. They allow us to approach purported instances of informed consent or purported cases of violation of patients' rights and determine precisely which of the most important elements are present or absent. To the analytic philosopher, the conversation model appears unable to carry off this sort of task. The "rules," if any could be given, for what is a conversation and what is not, when one begins and when it ends, whether subsequent conversation is the start of a new one or the continuation of an old one, and—perhaps most important—what counts as a good or rational or effective conversation, seem much too vague to guide us when in exploring something like informed consent. A metaphor, to be useful, should clarify and not obfuscate; and it would seem that a conversation model or metaphor must flunk this basic test.

As I wish to use the conversation metaphor later to point the way to useful and practical reforms, I must defend its analytic utility. I will try to apply Jay Katz's model to an issue I do not think is thoroughly dealt with in his book: the extent of the physician's duty, if any, to disclose serious but very low-probability risks. If the conversation model helps us toward new insights into this application, I will take it that I have illustrated its potential utility.

A typical example of the problem of remote risk is the duty of the radiologist who proposes to perform urography (intravenous pyelogram or IVP) to disclose to the patient that the diagnostic procedure carries an estimated one-in–40,000 risk of death. To most previous commentators, especially those tending toward the legalistic model, a low-probability risk of death or other catastrophic consequence is exactly the sort of thing that ought to be included in any *adequate* disclosure of information to the patient. On the other hand, to physicians, a duty to disclose this slim risk has generally appeared to be the height of insanity. One radiologist was led to propose that all his fellow specialists refuse to disclose this risk and if necessary cite standard of care as the defense if this refusal were ever challenged in court rather than cave in to what he viewed as unrealistic legal pressures (Allen 1976). It seemed to Allen that one can talk about patients' rights at great length, but ultimately professionals will have to decide what is a rational and sensible practice of their craft and what is not. He felt comfortable in declaring that a duty to disclose this risk was absurd on its face and thus could form no part of rational professional practice.

The most common response to arguments like Allen's is to assume that they reflect the paternalistic model and dismiss them. Indeed, the arguments traditionally offered in defense of this position fall comfortably within the paternalistic model. The oldest chestnut is that patients will be scared off by such frank disclosure and refuse to undergo tests and treatments that are clearly to their benefit. This argument has tended to fall by the wayside, since empirical studies and prolonged experience fail to provide any validation for it.

A slightly more cogent argument is a sort of catch–22, which asserts that no *reasonable* patient who needs an IVP would change her mind simply because she was told about a one-in–40,000 risk of dying. Either we could predict in advance that this remote risk will be inconsequential for the decision—in which case why feel any duty to disclose it?—or else we could predict that the patient would change her mind—in which case she is being unreasonable and hence cannot serve as a model for the duties we owe patients generally. First, this argument tends to assume that every patient for whom an IVP has been ordered really needs it. Sadly, experience with other test procedures and operations in the United States suggests that rather less than 100 percent of cases fit that criterion. The one-in–40,000 risk may not by itself change the patient's mind; but it might serve to remind the patient that the supposed benefits of urography had not been well explained and that it would be wise to ask many more questions before proceeding. Second, if no reasonable person will be talked out of needed urography by disclosure of a remote risk, why not let reasonable people make reasonable decisions by giving them the requisite data?

Subsidiary arguments relate to the time and expense of full disclosure for all procedures and all patients. But these arguments, again, seem only to reinforce the paternalistic origins of these views. Few physicians begrudge

the time and expense attached to some new surgical procedure so long as
the new procedure is thought to produce better outcomes. It seems inherent
in quibbling over time and expense to assume that enhanced consent
procedures will *not* lead to any improvement in outcome—which is the
same as saying that patient autonomy does not count as a good outcome.

To summarize, almost all the arguments customarily raised against disclosure of remote risks sound like more of the old paternalism, which is
hardly worth the time to refute. But this labeling ignores the possibility
that some *nonpaternalistic* arguments might be offered to show, at least in
a limited way, that disclosing remote risks is professionally inappropriate.
Whether such arguments are possible requires that the debate be joined
and carried out in some depth; and since medical paternalists no longer
seem interesting enough to debate with, the attempt has seldom been made.

It is precisely at this point that the conversation model offers a fresh
look, giving us a chance to get out of the paternalism-antipaternalism rut.
That model would have us ask the question, In what way would mention
of remote risks occur within the context of physician-patient conversation
of the sort that is designed to allow the patient an opportunity to participate
in decisions? In what way, if any, is a conversation that includes discussion
of remote risks superior to a conversation that excludes it?

To begin to answer those questions, we have to specify a bit more closely
what sorts of behavior the conversation model entails. Here I will sketch
what I take to be the primary implications of this model, again drawing
heavily from Katz but interpreting the model with an eye toward the more
common setting of primary-care medicine instead of assuming that the
conversation occurs with a specialist or subspecialist:

1. The conversation takes place in the context of a relationship where
it has previously been made clear to the patient that the physician welcomes
both additional questions and active patient participation in decisions. No
messages or signals have been sent that being a "good patient" entails being
quiet and passive.

2. The conversation, insofar as disclosure of information is concerned,
goes something like this: "I recommend that you have an IVP. This is an
X ray of the kidneys that is done with a dye injected into one of your veins.
I think it could benefit you in the following way. [Here the physician
describes the patient's diagnosis or diagnostic possibilities and how IVP will
aid in choosing the best management of the illness; included would be
some mention of the consequences of not doing an IVP.] The main risk

associated with the IVP is if you happened to be allergic to the injected dye. There are a few other risks that are quite remote in your case. Would you like to ask me any more questions about this?"

3. Once the physician has volunteered the most pertinent data based on her assessment of what the patient needs or wants to know in order to make a sound decision, she takes the patient's lack of further questions as an indication that the patient's need for information has been met.

4. If the patient asks for additional information, the physician continues the conversation until the patient indicates that his questions have all been answered. If the patient asks for details about the remote risks, the physician responds with a lengthier discussion of them.

5. The physician is free to frame the information disclosed in a manner that she feels will best help the patient make a reasonable choice. She might say, for example, "I think you may be putting too much weight on that particular risk. In my experience it almost never happens." The physician does not, however, withhold any requested information or dismiss the patient's own weighing of the risks and benefits once it is clear that the patient has heard the facts. (Admittedly, there is a fine line, easily crossed, between framing the information in a helpful way and manipulating the patient's choice by selective disclosure. But this problem is implicit in the physician-patient relationship as I have described it; it will be discussed further in chapter 8.)

I take these five points to be a reasonable description of how a primary-care physician, motivated to mold her behavior to the conversation model, might recommend and obtain consent for an IVP. The question now is whether this conversation would be *better* if the physician volunteered specific mention of the remote risk of death. Recall that the issue is not that of withholding the information or of lying; if the patient indicates a desire to know more about the remote risks, the physician is obligated to answer all those questions.

We are now in a better position to see a possible justification for the argument, rejected above as paternalistic, that rational professional practice would exclude volunteering such information—namely, how would one expect that topic to come up in any *reasonable* conversation? This justification, while admitting that we cannot specify in advance necessary and sufficient conditions for a reasonable or complete conversation, assumes that once the conversation has occurred we can review it and critique it in accordance with some widely shared (if often implicit) criteria. At one extreme of reasonableness will be a conversation that proceeds crisply from initial premises to final conclusion, with each sentence following logically from the previous one. At the other extreme will be a rambling discourse that bumbles from one irrelevancy to another. The attempted justification alleges that a one-in–40,000 risk of death is sufficiently tangential to all the main themes of the discussion so that the mention of it would push this conversation closer to the "rambling" end of the spectrum.

This justification may be part of the strategy of the reductio ad absurdum replies to informed consent that have occasionally appeared in letters to the editors of medical journals, especially in the mid–1970s. Physicians fancying themselves witty have prepared detailed consent forms for riding on a bus or an airplane, apparently hoping to show that if a legalistic laundry list of risks sounds ridiculous in other commonplace activities, it must be ridiculous for medicine too. In a similar vein, the person trying to show that a mention of the remote risk of death is tangential and not central to a reasonable patient conversation about IVP might note, "If you feel obligated to throw in the risk of death from IVP, why don't you also mention the remote risk of death from driving to the X-ray lab? If you calculate them out, the probabilities may well be roughly equivalent."

Of course, these consent forms for buses and planes have a ready rejoinder—that the average person *already knows* about the remote risks associated with bus, plane, and auto travel but cannot be expected to know about the sorts of remote risks attached to medical procedures. If one is already committed to a legalistic model of informed consent, that rejoinder seems sufficient to require exhaustive disclosure. But within the conversation model, one remains skeptical. First, is it really true that the average person does not know that a remote risk of death is part of many medical procedures? Periodic surveys of the news media suggest that this idea has been regularly presented to the general public, especially since such deaths have sensational news value. Furthermore, it is still the case that the presence of serious but low-probability risks *as a general notion* has already been included in our model conversation. How much *more* specific does one have to be to have gotten the point across before one can be accused of going off on an unreasonable conversational tangent?

In sum, a variety of explanations could be given as to why a reasonable conversation would exclude explicit mention of this remote risk, unless the patient requested the information. None, however, is likely to be completely convincing. And so the discussion should proceed to the next logical point: if the physician is obligated to disclose this risk explicitly, how should she bring the matter into the conversation? We can now envision several different ways, but each gives rise to problems.

1. "I feel that I have to tell you that there's a one-in–40,000 chance of dying from the IVP, although really the risk is so remote that I wouldn't worry at all about it if I were you." This formulation conveys the fact accurately enough, but it also conveys a strong message that negates the importance of the fact. This seems self-defeating if the object is to let the patient decide how much weight to place on that fact. The more subtle message is that the physician feels silly about mentioning the precise risk but feels she has to mention it anyway. If this is not for the patient's good, then whose good is being served? Is the physician fearful of a lawsuit? Is the physician following institutional orders of some sort? Why are considerations that have nothing to do with the patient's welfare intruding on this discussion?

2. "Also, before you make up your mind, remember that there's a one-in–40,000 risk of dying as a result of the IVP." Here again the fact is disclosed adequately, but a very different message is being sent. Now it sounds as if the physician thinks the patient ought to take this risk seriously into account. It is now the physician who seems to be saying that a one-in–40,000 risk is a grave matter.

3. "There's a one-in–40,000 chance of dying as a result of the IVP." This formulation seems, on its face, totally neutral. But its effect is likely to be very much like that of (2) and not neutral at all. The physician no doubt could have said a lot of things about the IVP and its risks and benefits. But the fact that she deliberately chose this piece of information as worthy of inclusion in a necessarily brief conversation seems to label it as being weighty.

4. "There's a one-in–40,000 chance of dying as a result of the IVP. Most people probably would see this risk as being so remote that it would not affect their decision. A few people, for good reasons of their own, would see this risk as a serious matter and would take it into account. Now, which way you prefer to view the matter is a decision only you can make." This phrasing seems superior to the others. At any rate, the general statement, "In your situation, some people would do X, while others would do Y," is often suggested by skilled interviewers as the best way to give the patient the widest possible permission to make a free choice. Where the choice is really something of a toss-up, this approach makes good sense. But the risk here is, after all, remote. The mere fact that the physician has devoted four sentences to it instead of one seems to be another example of making it seem far more weighty than she thinks it deserves to be. Furthermore, we have gained additional objectivity and given the patient permission for freer rein, but at a cost of adopting a much less personal

tone. The physician is now in the position of laying out alternatives and (it seems) disavowing responsibility for which one the patient chooses. That the physician wants the patient to make a wise decision, and that she wants to aid the process as best she can, seems to have dropped out of the message.

I could suggest other locutions, but by now the main point should be clear. Instead of merely asserting that the remote risk would be tangential in a reasonable conversation, we are now in a better position to say precisely why; and the point would never have been made had we not had the conversation metaphor to guide us. *In a reasonable and realistic medical conversation, we cannot disclose this remote risk without at the same time conveying additional messages that are both unintended and confusing.* It therefore seems that we have done our duty by relating the general existence of remote risks; and that unless the patient asks, explicit inclusion of those risks makes the conversation less useful, not more so, from the patient's perspective.

The conversation model has thus far appeared to support the idea that the physician need not voluntarily disclose remote risks, in opposition to what seems to be the majority view within the "new" medical ethics. But the limitations of this conclusion have to be noted. We have been imagining a primary-care setting in which the primary-care physician discusses an IVP for a patient with whom she has created a relationship over a period of time. The unreasonableness of remote-risk disclosure derives from several features of this setting. First, the goal is to help the patient make the best decision, not to provide the patient with maximal knowledge.[8] Second, the level of personal contact and the history of the relationship predispose to the "hidden messages" argued for above; if one is in a more technological or specialized environment where one *expects* to be treated impersonally, then an impersonal disclosure of a fact will *not* produce these same unintended messages. And third, the primary-care physician recommends such a wide range of interventions for so many different sorts of problems that she cannot possibly maintain a detailed knowledge of the remote risks of each. Everything I have said about the conversation ignores the basic

8. This statement may seem absurd on its face, as additional knowledge is usually seen as a necessary precondition for rational, active participation. For an example of how these factors can be separated, see Greenfield, Kaplan, and Ware 1985. In that study, one group of chronically ill clinic patients received a sort of assertiveness training and the second received additional teaching about their disease. Videotape analysis showed the first group participating much more actively and effectively in a subsequent interview with the physician, whereas the second group scored higher on a knowledge test about the facts of the disease.

fact that few primary-care physicians would know the one-in–40,000 figure unless they had just been reading up on the subject. But the standard office conversation requires that the data to be presented are known to the physician; a break in the conversation to look something up, or rescheduling for a further visit at a later date, leads again to the problem of signaling unintended messages about the importance of the fact.

But none of this is true of the specialist's office, where in all likelihood a few procedures are repeated frequently each day. And none of this is true about a written disclosure form, which can dispassionately lay out all facts, roughly in order of importance to the average patient, without sending any unintended or confusing messages (assuming that the form is written in readable language). The patient can read the first paragraph of the form and then skip the rest if he wishes; he cannot as easily tune out the primary physician's spoken word if she elects to disclose all risks exhaustively. And so the same argument that excludes disclosure of remote risks from rea-sonable primary-care conversations tends to *require* the disclosure of such risks in more specialized settings, especially where the logistics are made easier by access to printed or videotaped disclosure packages.[9] According to the conversation model, it is one thing to have a verbal discussion with a patient about a decision he has to make, and quite a different matter to hand the patient a printed form or set him down to watch a videotape; the criteria for adequate disclosure may vary among these settings.

Finally, we can compare the conversation analysis of disclosure of remote risks to a recent court decision on the physician's lack of duty to disclose such a risk. In *Precourt* v. *Frederick,*[10] the Massachusetts Supreme Court found in favor of an ophthalmologist who, before treating a patient with corticosteroid drugs following surgery to repair a retinal detachment, failed to inform the patient that aseptic necrosis of the hip joint was a possible side effect of high-dose steroid medication. (The patient not only remained blind after surgery but suffered from the joint disorder and eventually had to have hip replacement surgery.) The risk of aseptic necrosis was consid-ered to be remote; one expert testified that in a literature review of thousands of journal articles he was unable to find a single case report of aseptic necrosis of the hip following corticosteroid use in ophthalmologic surgery of this type. However, aseptic necrosis is a known, if rare, side effect of corticosteroids in other contexts. Attorneys sympathetic to physicians found

9. For an opposing viewpoint, see Coles et al. 1987, arguing that ophthalmologists should not be required to disclose the more remote risks of cataract surgery.

10. 395 Mass. 689 (1985); for a detailed analysis, see Curran 1986.

this decision to be a refreshing reversal of the tendency in earlier cases to rule that the duty to disclose risks was virtually limitless (Curran 1986).

What reasoning did the court employ to reach its decision? The decision seemed to hinge primarily on two points. The first, already suggested, was the non-occurrence of this particular side effect in ophthalmological practice. The second was the observation that corticosteroid treatment is a customary (and indeed essential) sequel to surgical correction of a detached retina. Given some chance that the surgery could restore eyesight, the court felt that no reasonable person would refuse the combined surgical-plus-drug regimen out of fear of aseptic necrosis of the hip.

Now, by referring back to the conversation model, we can see justification for lack of a duty to disclose this risk (or rather, lack of a duty to be informed about it, since it is highly unlikely that it ever crossed the mind of this ophthalmologist to mention it) along the same lines we used to refute a duty to disclose the risk of death from IVP—that it would divert a previously sensible conversation onto a direction that is likely to prove confusing or less useful for the patient. But this sort of justification is different from the two reasons offered by the Massachusetts court. (Their first reason seems to take conversation issues into account.) Still, one would be tempted to ask why the physician's specialty makes any difference. If aseptic necrosis is a known toxic effect of corticosteroids, it would seem that all specialties that employ corticosteroids, at least in high doses for a relatively long time, would have an equal duty to disclose the risk to patients. There is nothing special about ophthalmologic surgery that would render patients immune to the side effects of drugs that have been reported elsewhere. And so, at a minimum, the court's first argument seems poorly framed.

The second argument ought to be rejected because it is a throwback to the paternalistic model. Why decide what a reasonable person would do instead of assuming that the person is reasonable, telling him the facts, and letting him decide? Taken to its logical conclusion, this argument overturns the basis for informed consent. I might welcome a court decision that puts limits on the physician's duty to disclose because it sees that physicians need not engage in extreme or excessively burdensome activities in order to promote patient autonomy. But I would not welcome a court decision that pulls the rug out from under respect for patient autonomy simply as a means to limit the physician's duty to disclose.

To summarize, the duty to disclose serious but low-probability risks exists, but it is more limited to specific medical contexts than previous analyses have suggested. The "test case" of remote risks has shown that the conversation model can be a useful tool for analyzing informed-consent practices. Indeed, it offers more cogent arguments than does a recent, widely cited court decision. We can proceed, then, to use the conversation model as a framework for a more detailed discussion of informed consent in primary care.

CHAPTER 7

INFORMED

CONSENT:

SHARED

POWER AND

TRANSPARENCY

We have looked at three models of informed consent that represent possible solutions to the practical barriers discovered by empirical research. The conversation model has some attractive features and has also been shown to offer useful analyses of problems like the duty to disclose remote risks. We can now take the discussion further—recalling the earlier observation that any ethical model for informed consent is likely to be implicitly a reform program for aspects of medical practice—and ask how the conversation model aids in identifying the optimal responsible use of the physician's power on the patient's behalf. I have already discussed the issue of shared power in the physician-patient relationship generally; now I will apply this more specifically to informed consent.

First, consider the uses of power that can interfere with the patient gaining adequate knowledge and participating actively in the decision. The most obvious seem to be outgrowths of the physician's charismatic and social power. They take the form of the various signals sent to patients, both by the physician's behavior and by expectations people have about physicians—that questions or prolonged discussion are unwelcome and are signs of "bad" patient behavior. A commonplace example is the physician saying,"By the way, do you have any questions?" with his hand on the doorknob ready to walk out of the examining room. The verbal message, and perhaps the message the physician consciously intends, encourages participation; the much stronger nonverbal message signals clearly how unwelcome any bid for participation would be.

Admittedly these uses of power are generally not intentional; but they have cemented incorrect biases in the minds of physicians. By offering patients no real choice except to be passive recipients of advice, physicians have convinced themselves that patients prefer it that way and really have no desire or need for more information or participation. Of course, patients themselves may have come to believe this for equally illegitimate reasons: we have no way of knowing the extent to which the striking research finding that only 10 percent of patients desire full participation in medical decisions arises from the fact that most patients have never experienced full participation and don't know what they are missing.[1]

This use of power, effectively to cut off questions and participation while explicitly denying that one is doing any such thing, is a clear target for any useful reform in medical practice. It is a good target because it is (the Chief of Medicine notwithstanding) in no way essential for the patient's healing. No doubt this use of power streamlines the physician's tasks and makes it possible to get through a larger number of patients in an afternoon; but a physician who needs to employ this technique to get through the day is seeing too many patients to give each the care he deserves—the tension between care and work has slipped too far toward the work side.

There is another form of physician power that threatens to interfere with the patient learning all he might need to know. It is the power to end the conversation; or, more fully, the power to decide when enough has been said on a particular medical subject. If the physician mentions, "I want to recommend this antibiotic for your sinus infection, even though it has some possible side effects," and the patient asks, "What sorts of side effects do you mean?" the physician will say some things and then, at some point, decide unilaterally that enough has been said. True, the patient does have the right to say, "Tell me more"; but the power differential growing out of the physician's relative monopoly on technical medical knowledge makes this unlikely. If the patient does try to exercise his own power in this fashion, he is much more likely to irritate the physician than he is to learn any really useful information. The patient, it is true, could exercise power in other related ways. He could, for instance, go to the library and look up the side effects of the drug in the *Physician's Desk Reference*, and then use his newfound knowledge as a basis upon which to open the next interview with the physician. But in at least some medical encounters there will be no opportunity for these alternative means and the physician's power to end the conversation will be decisive.[2]

1. When patients are specifically trained to become more assertive and involved in their own medical care, they tend to demonstrate a high level of satisfaction, besides showing some improvement in their ability to live with their diseases (Greenfield, Kaplan, and Ware 1985).

2. One might wonder why I have focused on the power to end discussion of a particular topic instead of the more-often-addressed power to frame the way that the information is

Two things are worth noting about the power to end the conversation. The first is that Jay Katz, for all his insight in devising the conversation model, seems not to have been aware of this power or its implications. He argues as if the conversation approach puts physician and patient on an equal power footing, at least in theory. But my analysis suggests that this power disparity is irreducible, even though this in no way makes informed consent impossible. The second point is that we know a fair amount about the psychology of physician decision making in many medical contexts, but we know virtually nothing about how the primary-care physician decides when enough has been said in reply to a patient's question. The conversation model would suggest that this is a vital research question.

Addressing this power problem further leads us to see an important advantage the conversation model has over the legalistic model as a vehicle for medical reform. Imagine the physician saying, "Now that I'm aware of this irreducible power problem, I want to make sure that it doesn't get in the way of promoting optimal patient autonomy. So how am I to decide when I have said enough on a particular subject?" The legalistic answer would appear to be, "You haven't said enough until you have covered all possible negative consequences the patient may later suffer and, if he suffers them, feel aggrieved that he was not warned of them in advance." But this answer is unrealistic (and thus leads to a legitimate part of the physicians' resentment of what they see as unwarranted legal intrusion into medical practice). It assumes that these possible negative consequences are finite and that the well-trained physician has them at her fingertips in advance; if so, failure to disclose them is either a willful decision to withhold information or else a sign of negligent ignorance of crucial medical facts. In actuality, the range of possible negative consequences is much more extensive than most lawyers seem to think, and the ability of even the best-trained physician to think of them in advance of their occurring is quite limited.

Here, *Precourt* v. *Frederick* (see chapter 6) may be an instructive example.

presented. (This latter power has led some physicians to claim that they can follow the letter of the law on informed consent and still manipulate patients to make exactly the decisions that the physician himself favors.) To be sure, the power to frame information is open to abuse by paternalistically minded physicians. I have chosen to focus on the power to end the conversation precisely because even physicians who disavow paternalism still must choose to end the conversation at some point. The power to end the conversation remains with the physician no matter how much one bows in the direction of patient autonomy. Moreover, the two manifestations of physician power are arguably identical: the power to frame the conversation and the power to end the conversation can be used responsibly, to help the patient focus on what is most important, or irresponsibly, to deny choice.

The toxic effect resulted from the use of a drug instrumental in securing a successful outcome to the surgery. But when the ophthalmologist solicited the patient's informed consent for the surgery to repair a detached retina, it must have been hard to anticipate and list all the risks of the surgery *plus* those of the drug *plus* those of any other drugs and treatments that are also adjuncts to the surgery. If the corticosteroid had induced a stomach ulcer (another commonly listed side effect) best treated with the antiulcer drug ranitidine and the patient had suffered a toxic reaction to that drug, would the physician be negligent for having warned the patient of the possibility of an ulcer but not the possible toxicities of ranitidine?

I do not want to overextend this line of argument. When physicians can anticipate possible risks, they should be disclosed, and that holds true for single therapies or for related packages of therapies. My point is that the legalistic thinkers seem to take medicine for a more cut-and-dried, predictable practice than it is.

The problems with the unrealism of the legalistic answer to this physician's question lead in turn to what may be the most important reason why even nonpaternalistic physicians have so much trouble seeing informed consent as part of medical practice instead of an artificial graft. The problem is that according to the legalistic model of informed consent, the physician never knows when she is finished. Most medical tasks that are widely accepted as part of the body of skills the good physician should possess have agreed-upon endpoints. When I have prescribed the right number of doses of an effective antibiotic and proved that the urine is sterile by a follow-up culture, I have finished treating a bladder infection. When I have asked the patient about mood, somatic symptoms, obsessive thoughts, sleep patterns, and activity patterns; offered reassurance as to the normality of their reactions and feelings; and scheduled an appropriately timed return visit, I have finished a counseling session for normal reaction to grief. But because the list of possible risks of any complex medical intervention is endless, the physician can never finish full disclosure according to the legalistic model—or, what amounts to the same thing, she can never know for sure that she has finished. The nonpaternalistic but sensible physician can only conclude that she is being asked to perform a task unlike anything else in medical practice when she is asked to obtain informed consent.

How are things different under the conversation model? That model is, in one way, equally perplexing, but in another way much more reassuring and informative. The perplexing part comes if the physician requests a recipe to assure that disclosure and discussion will be adequate in all cases and that no second-guessing will be possible. The conversation model does not pretend that it can provide any such algorithm. Neither can the legalistic model, but it seems to demand one. (Because it assumes that any well-trained physician can readily foretell all the risks of any procedure, it suggests that if a doctor doesn't have such an algorithm at her fingertips, she must be negligently ignorant of medicine.) The conversation model, on the other hand, shows why no algorithm is possible: we all know what a conversation is, and with a little thought we can come to realize that nobody can give rules for how to have a good conversation in advance, even though we could more or less agree on whether the conversation was a good one in retrospect.

The reassuring part of the conversation model comes from the common-sense aspects of how conversations are judged. If the task is full disclosure, nothing in either medical training or life experience prepares the physician to know when that task has been carried out. If the task is to have a conversation that will promote and facilitate patient involvement in the medical decision to the extent that the patient wishes, then the physician has a much better sense, even in the absence of rules or algorithms, of what she is being asked to do. If she takes the idea of patient autonomy seriously, then at times she will cut a discussion short because she judges that all that is necessary has been done. But she will be just as likely to draw the conversation out further by quizzing the patient on whether he truly has sufficient information on various points, or whether he has reflected carefully on what he has been told. Both the way the conversation is going at the time and what she has learned in the context of the evolving relationship with the patient will guide her in deciding when it is time to continue and when time to close. Some of these judgments will later, in hindsight, seem erroneous; but that is the nature of a complex human relationship. At least in primary-care medicine, the ongoing relationship will often provide later opportunities to correct earlier mistaken judgments before any irreparable harm is done.

Some Objections

I have up to this point been defending the conversation model of informed consent as the best route to the reform in medical practice that would assure a shared-power relationship. We now need to consider some possible objections to the argument:

1. The conversation model is a cover-up for a blatant return to paternalism; it fails to protect essential patient rights.

2. The conversation model inadequately responds to important empirical data showing that patients generally desire full disclosure.

3. The conversation model assumes a preexisting ideal relationship and says nothing about either how to start up such a relationship from scratch or what to do in settings where it is unrealistic.

The first objection is most likely to come from defenders of the legalistic model, who still fear physician paternalism as an omnipresent danger to the rights and interests of patients. They remain distrustful of any power discrepancy between physician and patient. Since the conversation model (as I have argued above, in contrast to Katz's view) retains an irreducible power disparity, it seems no different from the old paternalism.

The idea of defending the patient from the possible misuse of power by taking power away from the physician is unsatisfactory because it forgets the nature of the rights we wish to protect in the first place. As Fried has said, these are basically "rights in personal care"; they make sense within the context of a physician-patient relationship that treats the patient respectfully and tries to use medical knowledge and skill to promote the patient's life plan. Any manipulation of medicine that effectively destroys personal care, hampering the physician in the task of finding out the patient's life plan and of seeing what medicine can do to further it, thereby undermines any rights worth protecting. So long as the declawing of the physician is restricted to charismatic and social power, personal care is to a large degree preserved. But the argument above was designed to show that the legalistic model attempts to eliminate a variety of physician power that is Aesculapian in its origin and cannot easily be separated from the physician's essential power to heal.

In chapter 4, we saw the fallacy of any approach that proposes by rules and regulations to make the clinical relationship doctor-proof. Inevitably, since the physician must retain some power to be able to heal, the ethical practice of medicine will continue to rely on the good intentions and good character of the physician (see chapter 16). Many spin-offs from the conversation model will appear blatantly paternalistic so long as we assume that the physician is either unconcerned about paternalism or else chooses to be actively paternalistic. But if we assume that the underlying intent is to avoid paternalism, to allow the patient to participate as fully as he wishes, and over time to identify and remove systematically any barriers to full participation, then a much different picture of the conversation model emerges.

Consider in this connection the statement of the physician who claims that no matter how full his disclosure, he can always manage to manipulate the conversation to get the patient to decide exactly as he (the physician) wants. To the legalist, this will seem the ultimate fate of the conversation model—giving up frank paternalism and replacing it with more subtle manipulation. But the only physician who would make such a statement without shame is one who has not adopted the basic concepts of the conversation model as guiding principles and who does not really believe in either disclosure or participation. We would have to assume that a physician truly committed to the conversation model would both be aware of the dangers of manipulation and actively try to avoid it.

I would ask the defenders of the legalistic model precisely how the power equality between physician and patient that they seek could be achieved in practice. This practical strategy must go beyond the punishment of a physician's failure to disclose adequate information; it must prospectively assure that each patient gets all the information he needs and gets to participate fully in every encounter. Would the ideal be that each visit to the primary-care physician's office be made in the company of a skilled lawyer? But even a lawyer knowledgeable in health matters would run into the same disparity of Aesculapian power—the power of the physician to declare that enough has been said on a particular topic. Does this then mean that the patient must be accompanied by another physician? But if one physician cannot be trusted, why should two be better? The point is not to reduce this to absurdity. Mechanisms such as the establishment of a patient advocate or ombudsman undoubtedly help promote a shared-power situation, and indeed the value of taking a trusted friend with you to the doctor's office is something the conversation model would endorse in many circumstances. (The question then turns to ways in which a three-way conversation could cover ground that a two-way conversation couldn't.) The point is that even highly intrusive and impractical schemes fail to eliminate the power disparity between physician and patient.

In a nutshell, my response to the first objection is this: The patient ideally has a right to a relationship that assures that he will be treated with respect and that medical knowledge will be used to further his own life plans and values. Both to show respect and to find out how medicine can be applied to his specific life issues, a particular sort of sustained, reasonable conversation is necessary. If legal forces and regulations end up encouraging that sort of conversation, so much the better. But experience suggests that the legalistic model, at least as it is usually perceived or understood, has done no such thing but has instead put additional barriers in the way of reasonable, sustained conversation. Hence the legalistic model fails to protect the patient's essential rights.

The second objection is suggested by the striking research finding that patients do not place much value on participation in decision making but that nevertheless they seek much fuller disclosure of information than physicians are wont to provide. As one set of investigators concluded, physicians habitually overestimate the extent to which patients want to be involved in decisions and underestimate the extent to which patients seek out information about disease and treatment. Indeed, some patients asked for information about precisely the sort of remote risks that seem rather off the subject in a meaningful, decision-oriented conversation. It could be argued, therefore, that the conversation model, which provides a rationale for less full disclosure than that demanded by the legalistic model, is a move away from what patients really want.

I think that the problem, that the conversation model might institutionalize underdisclosure if widely adopted, demands serious discussion. Several points, however, tend to mitigate it. First, the conversation model necessarily focuses on the primary-care relationship, but few studies have been conducted in that setting. The physician who takes the model seriously will return to the issue of education and information at each visit and will view disclosure as something occurring over time, not completed at one sitting. We do not know much about how well patients feel their needs have been met when exposed to a relationship of this sort. Second, the conversation model tends to be self-correcting. If a physician misjudges the patient's wants, the conversation as it unfolds ought to reveal that fact, so long as the atmosphere created is one of open acceptance of the patient's agenda. Third, if patients indeed want detailed disclosure of remote risks (which for practical reasons is difficult to achieve in primary care, no matter how extensive the conversation), this tends to argue for providing printed forms and other educational aids as a backup to conversation, not abandoning the conversation concept.

The third objection is not really an objection but instead a call for expansion of the model. A full description of how to facilitate and promote conversation of the sort I have been talking about in all medical settings— with new patients, with well-established patients, in subspecialties, in emergency rooms, with children and adolescents, with retarded patients, and so forth—would be a course in how to practice medicine. Much of this teaching in fact occurs in the modern medical school, where supervised interviewing of patients has gained a place of importance in the curriculum (although providing information to the patient and involving her in the process still lag far behind eliciting information as a curricular goal). Still more of it takes place in primary-care residencies, where behavioral scientists increasingly teach alongside clinicians. These communication skills are hardly ever linked explicitly with "informed consent"; the teaching is called "patient interviewing" or "doctor-patient relationship" or "patient education." It is this trend, largely, that leads me to conclude that the reform of medical practice implicit in the conversation model is a realistic goal, for at least some of its essential elements are already being accepted into medical practice under other labels.

The conversation model helps the reform process first by helping identify which behavioral skills it requires (an aspect of medical ethics that its teachers, until recently, often neglected, preferring to address ethics purely in cognitive terms). These skills, however, remain fragmented until the conversation model provides a set of objectives for their application. For example, consider how the model modifies the ideal first visit of a new patient to a primary-care physician. In addition to the standard medical history of past illnesses, life habits, and risk factors, questions like the following suggest themselves: What have your relationships with your previous doctors been like? What did you most like and most dislike about those relationships? What did you especially hope to get out of coming here for your care? What is the ideal amount of information you'd like about illnesses and treatment? How much do you want to be involved in making decisions about your own care? (It should be noted that the "first visit" in a primary-care setting often extends over three or more actual office appointments, lest it be thought that there would never be time for these sorts of questions.)

This intake interviewing and data gathering would ideally provide the physician with four general types of knowledge about the patient: biomedical problems, including risk factors and preventive issues; the family, occupational, and community environment within which the patient lives, with some early hypotheses about how that environment may affect the patient's health; a cultural-anthropological assessment, which includes some understanding of the patient's medical worldview and how he tends to explain illnesses and treatments within the context of his cultural belief system; and the answers to questions like those listed above, which is part of what has been labeled the "values history" (Doukas and McCullough 1988). For the physician to gather this rich collection of data, the "conversation" has necessarily to have been going on for some time, and implicitly both physician and patient have evolved a set of rules and guidelines for how that conversation should proceed—what is essential, what is tangential, and what is off-limits.

The physician may now begin to set out further guidelines for continued conversation based on her assessment and integration of all the data. Let us imagine that this patient has some risk factors for coronary disease that have to do with life-style issues; but his own preferred belief systems about disease causation tend to discount the importance of those factors. If the patient's value history suggests a strong desire to participate, the physician may try to enlist the patient's active involvement in addressing the disparity between the patient and physician belief systems. If the value history reveals a passive or uninvolved patient, the physician may elect to steer the conversation toward discussion of whether that passive stance really meets the patient's medical needs and whether it is open to change. Alternatively, the physician may *temporarily* go along with the patient's approach and ask, for example, that he bring his wife along on the next visit so that the physician can explore with her changes in meal preparation and daily routine that will reduce her husband's risk of coronary disease.[3]

Conversation that proceeds along these lines therefore provides a mechanism to nourish and sustain the shared-power physician-patient relationship. It embodies the shared-power concept in that conversation is by nature a mutually participatory activity, even though one or the other party may dominate at a given time. The physician retains, irreducibly, a significant power advantage in the form of the Aesculapian power to stop the conversation by declaring that enough has been said on a specific topic. But if we adhere to the primary-care perspective of the physician-patient relationship, the patient has a compensatory power advantage: although the physician may take the conversation off on many different medically dictated tangents, the conversation must in the end return to address directly the patient's own perception of his problems. The patient's way of understanding his problems and what they are doing to his life thus sets the agenda for the proper practice of primary-care medicine and must guide whatever conversation occurs.

The goal, of course, is not to equalize power for its own sake: medicine is not arm wrestling. The goal is to use both powers—physician's and patient's—in tandem to produce, as efficiently as possible, the best and most skilled application of medical knowledge to the patient's problems to secure an outcome that best aids the patient in living out his life plan. I stress efficiency because my focus is on primary care. No matter what

---

3. The choice to allow the patient to remain passive is only temporary, assuming that the relationship is long-standing. Depending on how the patient and wife react during their joint visit, for example, the physician may gain a much clearer picture about the origins of this apparent passivity and how it could be changed. Or, as often happens, the physician will realize that what he thought was passivity is actually a more complex set of coping mechanisms that works well for this family and needs to be respected.

changes occur in the financing and organization of medical care in the future, it is likely that primary care will remain high-volume medicine. But neither should the emphasis on efficiency be seen as a doctor-centered concern. Patients also have many tasks to get done in their daily lives, and good medical care and good health are only one of the myriad things that they value. Patients seek convenient access to primary care and quick resolution of their medical problem. Primary-care conversation is a constant trade-off between completeness and efficiency. The committed primary-care physician is dedicated to the ideal that he can provide the best medical care when he best understands all facets of the patient and his environment. But complete knowledge of the patient and his environment, just like the "complete history and physical" so prized by the academic internist, is a myth, for theoretical as well as practical reasons. At any step along the way, there are gains from slowing down the conversation for greater comprehensiveness and gains from hurrying up to complete the task at hand. The craft of primary care demands an ability to weigh those competing gains rapidly as the conversation proceeds. Although it may be tempting to view the irreducible tension between comprehensiveness and efficiency as the rock on which the conversation model must break up in the end, it is more realistic to see the tension as defining the very nature of primary care, so that any model of primary-care medicine must work within its constraints. It is therefore a component of the tension between care and work, which must be accepted and accommodated rather than resolved or eliminated.

The biggest future challenge for adherents of the conversation model will be to suggest practical feedback and assessment strategies to help the physician and patient assure themselves that the conversation is on track and meeting the patient's needs. Medical conversation is not just any old sort of conversation; it has a specified agenda, goals, and limits. It will not do to assume a physician-patient encounter was a success just because neither party walked out on the other or called the other names. An important goal of the conversation model, at least in primary-care settings, is to improve the efficiency of conversation by giving the patient an important role and allowing the physician to interpret the patient's silence or acquiescence as an indicator that enough has been said and that the patient's needs have been met. The model bogs down if we assume that it is always the physician's responsibility to assure optimal patient participation. No reasonable conversation can proceed if it must constantly be interrupted with remarks such as, "Are you *sure* you have enough information to make up your mind? Are you nodding your head because you've participated to the extent that you want, or because you think I'll get angry if you ask more questions?" At some point this sort of conversation becomes a cross-examination rather than mutual participation—and, more important, it signals disrespect for patient autonomy rather than the reverse.[4]

For the conversation model to succeed, patients will have to become more active in the medical dialogue than they have generally been in the past. When they want more information or want to discuss matters in more depth, they are going to have to say so and not expect the physician to read their minds. Research indicates that patients can be taught this fairly easily and that once they have, positive health benefits result (Greenfield, Kaplan, and Ware, 1985). But in the face of a centuries-old tradition of patient passivity, we cannot assume that this transition will occur automatically or smoothly.

This gives us another reason to focus on primary care, since that is the place in medicine where new forms of conversation and communication can be tried out with the fewest life-and-death decisions at stake, with the patient having his capacity for autonomy least compromised by serious illness, and with the most opportunity for early mistakes to come to light and be corrected. Another question worthy of extended research is whether greater patient participation in primary-care decisions will carry over into more complex medical decisions in other settings. It is tempting to assume that if the patient is involved early in decisions on whether to treat a respiratory infection with antibiotics, and in decisions on whether to try drugs for borderline hypertension or stick with exercise and a low-salt diet, he will eventually be better prepared to participate fully in decisions about respirators and dialysis in the intensive care unit. But this assumption cannot be adopted without empirical justification. One advantage of the conversation model is that it may prompt research into those aspects of

---

4. This point, by the way, reveals a hidden contradiction within the legalistic model. That model makes two assumptions: first, that patients are capable of autonomous choices; and second, that physician paternalism must be squelched to allow the patient room to exercise autonomy. The contradiction arises only at the point that one demands especially intrusive and forceful measures to contain all types of physician paternalism—not just out-and-out coercion and deception but even the more subtle forms of manipulation and undue influence. At some point this becomes a statement that patient autonomy is so fragile and weak that measures much more stringent that those required for actions and decisions outside of medicine are needed to protect it. But that in turn denies the first assumption, that patients are in fact capable of a reasonable level of autonomous choice. In this connection, it is important to see that respect for patient autonomy may actually impose duties on patients within the physician-patient relationship—among them, the duty to participate in various conversations. I am indebted for this argument to Michael J. Meyer (unpublished paper presented at the Society for Health and Human Values, October 1989, Washington, D.C.).

the clinical encounter that have the most to do with promoting an ethical relationship of shared power.

From Conversation to Transparency

Consider yet another objection to the conversation model:

4. Although informed consent ought not be solely a legal concept, it is nevertheless true that legal protection will be required to safeguard patient rights from the occasional serious abuses. But the conversation model is too vague and subjective to allow it to serve as a test or standard in a court of law. Therefore, although it may be a helpful heuristic to encourage reform within medicine, it cannot replace the legalistic model.

This objection cannot be turned aside as readily as the other three. Whereas ethics can concern itself with the usual or even the optimal case, the law must worry about the worst possible cases and provide some legal protection or recourse. But if something like "We had a conversation" is to be allowed to form the physician's defense in a court case, then patients would seem to be without any substantial legal recourse. Somehow the law must be able to formulate a standard of informed consent that will guide jury deliberation in a clear way, perhaps letting the physician off the hook if a good-faith effort was made but holding the physician accountable if the patient's need or desire for disclosure was ignored or overridden. And yet we have seen the arguments to show that so long as the legalistic model is allowed to function as the dominant court test (or the physicians' perception of the court test they are likely to face), then true reform of medical practice will be next to impossible.

I propose that it is possible to develop the conversation model in a direction that would allow it to function as a legal standard of informed consent for purposes of tort law.[5] Although this proposed legal standard would not offer a cut-and-dried checklist to see whether adequate informed consent was obtained in a contested case, it would nevertheless serve as a useful guide to judges and juries in making an unavoidably subjective judgment. This standard might be called the *transparency standard*.

The transparency standard would hold that valid consent to treatment has been obtained when (1) the physician has rendered the decision process, by which the recommended intervention was arrived at, transparent to the patient; (2) the patient, on the basis of the disclosed rationale and the

5. This section of this chapter is based on Brody 1989d. As I have no legal training, I have relied heavily on conversations with Margaret Wallace and her reactions to earlier drafts of the material.

associated facts, has been allowed to ask questions and has received satisfactory answers; (3) The patient then authorizes (by action or by acquiescence) the recommended intervention or an alternative one.[6] The idea of transparency requires that the physician make it a habit to *think out loud* about the recommended interventions in language accessible to the patient. Physicians who routinely do this and take pains to make this an expected part of each encounter with a patient could then feel reasonably secure from legal difficulties due to inadequate consent.

The question of which risks the physician is obligated to disclose to the patient in order to get valid consent would be answered by the transparency standard: "Precisely those risks that the physician weighed seriously before deciding what intervention to recommend." Two things should be noted about this reply. First, it may seem quite vague for purposes of a legal decision; and yet it is not any more vague than the alternative two answers suggested by now-prevalent legal standards: "Those risks that physicians generally reveal to their patients in the relevant community of practice" and "Those risks that a reasonable person in the patient's situation would want to know before deciding." Second, it may seem that even the most careless and neglectful physician has an ironclad defense: he can state that even though the risk was obvious and grave, he simply failed to take it into account when he recommended treatment. But this defense would put the physician in a serious bind, because he could be judged negligent for *not* having considered that risk, assuming that the standard of care for his specialty required him to do so. The physician could get himself off the hook on informed consent only to impale himself more deeply on the charge of negligence.[7] Because the transparency standard requires that the physician reveal clearly his process of thinking, he can more readily be held accountable for a failure to think properly.

Getting out of the informed-consent frying pan into the negligence fire might not seem to physicians to be a useful change in the legal standards. Yet I would argue that it accomplishes a major goal of getting the issues into their proper places—no small feat if we want physicians to derive a clear and useful message from the tort system. It places under the title of

6. Here I disagree with the definition offered by Faden and Beauchamp (see chapter 6) that requires explicit authorization. I suggest that explicit authorization is seldom a feature of the average encounter in primary care.

7. A shrewd attorney for the plaintiff in such a case would of course take full advantage of this feature by charging the physician with negligent failure to adhere to the standard of care at the same time that a charge was made of failing to obtain the patient's informed consent.

informed consent whether the physician made his thinking clear to the patient, and under negligence whether that thinking was good or bad. This seems to get things the right way around instead of trying to use the doctrine of informed consent to police bad medical decisions.

What about those situations in medicine where physicians *don't* think? This comment is not necessarily a criticism of physicians, since it is an unavoidable (though perhaps unpalatable) truth that a good deal of medical practice is routine, and physicians match treatments with illnesses fairly automatically. The transparency standard suggests two answers here. One is that under that standard physicians would be more likely to think carefully about these situations instead of treating them as routine. Few physicians wish their patients to view them as unthinking automatons, and if they got into the habit of sharing their rationales for treatment openly with every patient, they would feel less satisfied with these previously unquestioned responses.[8] The second, a bit more to the immediate point, is that one can make routine decisions every bit as transparent as complex ones. The physician can say, "I see a lot of people with this particular problem, and when I do, I always treat it this way. Do you have any questions about that?" The patient then has the option of accepting the routine nature of the treatment as a sign that the risks are quite modest and the benefits highly probable, or else he can ask questions to discover whether the physician has considered carefully enough the features of his own case that may make it unique. But in either instance the patient knows exactly what is on the physician's mind and can respond accordingly.

The greatest challenge to the transparency standard comes not in primary-care practice, where interventions that have major risks or for which major alternatives exist are likely to be the exception and therefore will automatically call for more careful thought and discussion. Instead, the problem occurs in specialty practices where physicians routinely do fairly risky procedures, and the physician thinking out loud about whether to recommend a procedure may not mention the risks because they have become so much a part of his daily practice. As the old joke goes, the surgeon who tells the patient, "Don't get all excited about this operation; I do ten of them every week," may elicit the reply, "Well, *I* don't have ten of them done on *me* every week." This problem suggests that the trans-

8. It is perhaps worth noting here that some physicians choose to devote time to teaching medical students and residents out of self-interested rather than altruistic motives: to have an informed learner constantly asking questions about one's diagnoses and management choices is a clear impetus toward a better-informed and more self-conscious style of medical practice.

parency standard would have to be applied differently in that setting, as indeed has already been mentioned for the conversation model. Where the risks and alternatives for a given procedure are specifiable in advance and where the physician does a fairly small number of such procedures over and over, there seems no excuse not to have written handouts, videotapes, or similar educational aids to be sure that these are known to the patient.[9] Again, the point is to make clear to the patient what has gone into the physician's thinking, and having standard forms for standard (albeit risky) procedures properly indicates to the patient what is being proposed. It lets the patient see what the physician considers to be routine and compare it with what he himself views as routine, and it lets him see that the treatment, though risky, is at least not experimental or untested. Thus the transparency model would hold physicians who repeatedly do a small number of somewhat risky interventions to a different and more exacting standard.[10]

I have noted that a major problem with the legalistic model is that it sends physicians a message that is at odds with the best medical care. The transparency standard, by contrast, reinforces the conversation model in especially useful ways. It encourages the sharing of not only the physician's conclusions and recommendations but also the processes that led to them. This allows the patient to be an active participant in the decision-making process and creates an expectation that the patient may wish to participate in this way. (As a rule, one does not make the effort to explain one's thinking to somebody else unless one expects that person to carry on the thinking process or at least critique it thoughtfully.) It encourages not merely the disclosure of facts but the putting of those facts into a meaningful context. By making both the thinking process and the context more plain, it facilitates thoughtful and useful questioning from the patient. By forcing the physician to be explicit about the starting assumptions as well as the final recommendations, it may signal to the patient when the physician has failed to grasp the patient's view of his own problem. For example, if the patient is convinced that he has a life-threatening illness, and the physician's reasoning is based on assumptions that are appropriate only

9. At this point I would disagree with Coles et al. 1987, who suggest an approach similar to the one I propose for ophthalmological surgery. I think that they are correct in principle but that their model would be better applied to primary care rather than to ophthalmology.

10. This might seem to be favoritism on the side of primary care. It relates more closely, however, to the fact that the specialist is more likely to be a stranger to the patient, and so conversation, to be meet its purpose, needs these educational aids. By contrast, the primary-care physician would be held accountable for adequacy of conversation over time in a way that the specialist is not.

for minor, chronic problems, then the patient will immediately note the discrepancy and either challenge the physician's assumption or ask for further clarification.

It seems, then, that a shared power conception of the physician-patient relationship can best be served by adopting the conversation model for purposes of medical education and translating that model into a workable transparency standard for purposes of legal review and accountability. These conclusions follow both from empirical data suggesting that the present-day doctrine of informed consent has simply not had the desired effect on physicians' behavior, and from analyses of standard theories of informed consent, which reveal a tendency to paper over irreducible power disparities between physician and patient instead of squarely facing their implications.

An article purporting to defend "benevolent deception" in primary care described a case of a teenager requesting help from a physician in relation to her sexual activities. If the parents demanded to know the details of treatment, the physician, it was argued, would be justified in providing only partial or deceptive information (Lincourt and Sanchez 1984). Against this analysis, one might well argue that these authors have suffered from a fundamental confusion between two ethical issues, lying and confidentiality. The problem of lying or telling the truth comes up when the party to whom one would reveal (or not reveal) the truth has some strong moral claim to that information. By contrast, confidentiality arises as an issue precisely when the other party has no moral right (or a questionable right) to the information that would be disclosed. The teenager's case is one of preserving confidentiality, not lying, and hence it has limited if any relevance to the question of benevolent deception.

Although I am in sympathy with this rejoinder, I also find it significant that these authors would have lumped together two different ethical issues that, according to the conventional wisdom, ought to be strictly distinguished. Indeed, there is a clear reason to consider truthful disclosure and confidentiality as closely related issues: both have to do with the physician's power to control information.[1]

There are, in the view of today's medical ethics, two major ways a physician might abuse the power to control information about a patient.

---

1. Christie and Hoffmaster (1986) entitle a chapter in their book on ethical issues in family medicine "Control of Information," but they address only truth-telling issues without mentioning confidentiality.

One is when the physician discloses the information to someone from whom the patient wished it kept private. The second is when the physician fails to disclose that information to the patient himself. This juxtaposes virtually the oldest and the newest pronouncements in Western medical ethics. The duty to maintain patient confidentiality has a venerable pedigree going back to the Hippocratic oath and before. The duty to disclose even "bad news" to the patient, is quite recent. For most of the history of Western medicine, and according to the vast majority of its practitioners,[2] the real abuse of the physician's power was not failure to disclose; it was the disclosure of any information that the patient would find emotionally distressing or that might distract him from the task of following the prescribed regimen and returning to health. The traditional image of the physician portrayed the strict control of both types of information—keeping private matters from others, and keeping distressing news from the patient—as a fundamental skill, almost a defining skill, of medical practice. Authors as far removed in time as Plato and Oliver Wendell Holmes used precisely the same analogy to describe the physician's skill: truth and falsehood should be doled out to patients with the same care, precision, and foresight called for by the administration of medications.[3]

By maintaining confidentiality and by keeping unpleasant news from the patient, the traditional physician established himself as a powerful figure, both socially and in his own estimation. This core reason for the two practices may have contributed to the general absence of detailed ethical commentary on truth telling and confidentiality throughout much of medical history. Such behavior was something the apprentice learned from the master, not something the master himself had to justify to a critical audience. Moreover, when justifications were offered for these professional practices, they tended to be utilitarian, calling attention to the benign consequences of the use of power, not to the power itself. By maintaining confidences, the physician established the trust of the patient and therefore facilitated the full disclosure of symptoms and habits without which ac-

2. An excellent historical overview is Reiser 1980. One important dissenting view was lodged by John Gregory in the eighteenth century; see McCullough 1978. For other important dissents, see Hooker 1849; Cabot 1903.

3. "Again, a high value must be set upon truthfulness. If we were right in saying that gods have no use for falsehood and that it is useful to mankind only in the way of a medicine, obviously a medicine should be handled by no one but a physician" (Plato, *The Republic*, III.388; 1945, p. 78. "Your patient has no more right to all the truth you know than he has to all the medicine in your saddle-bags. . . . He should get just so much as is good for him" (Holmes 1883, p. 338).

curate diagnosis and management could not occur. By withholding distressing news, the physician prevented the deleterious health effects of shock, depression, and other negative emotions on the patient's already weakened system.

I know of no historical commentator who has offered a combined ethical discourse on confidentiality and truth telling. But such a discourse would include the following points:

1. Information is a potent force that can produce both benefit and harm to the patient.

2. In a state of full health, most adults can manage information for themselves, keeping some things private and finding out the truth about those matters that most concern them.

3. In illness, a person loses this ability to handle information. Needing help with the most private functions, he discloses what he normally keeps hidden. Psychologically distraught, he becomes incapacitated by news of even mild setbacks or dangers.[4]

4. Therefore, upon calling in the physician, the patient effectively hands the control of personal information over to him in trust. The physician in turn is judged by how effectively he uses his power to produce a good outcome for the patient. The power over information is therefore mingled with all other aspects of Aesculapian authority, like the power to use instruments and medications, and is judged according to the same standards.

Here the physician who withholds or manipulates information in a highly paternalistic fashion does something praiseworthy, not morally corrupt. Clearly, however, these conditions, which prevailed in Western medicine roughly from Hippocratic times until the dawn of the twentieth century, no longer hold. Besides the social changes regarding respect for autonomy and distrust of authority, more and more people consult their physicians in a state of relative good health. And even when a serious or fatal illness occurs, people become patients relatively early in its course and before they are in extremis either physically or psychologically.

In reaction to this "old" paternalism, the "new" medical ethics proposes firm principles. The patient must be told the truth about her own condition, except in those circumstances where she might autonomously refuse certain

---

4. It is worth comparing this outline argument to the modified version of the Grand Inquisitor's argument in chapter 2, as both rely on the weakness and vulnerability of the sick to justify medical paternalism.

types of information; and confidentiality should be honored except in those unusual cases where the threat of harm to another person, or to the patient, is so great as to justify overriding this rule. Certainly these principles embodying the basic moral value of respect for individual autonomy serve as a counterbalance to the paternalistic tendencies that have shaped the history of medical practice. The question in this chapter is whether these firm principles adequately address the irreducible power issues in the physician-patient relationship. As we previously discovered with informed consent, simply advocating respect for autonomy does not eliminate important aspects of the physician's power; and appeals to autonomy may not provide the whole answer on how that power may be used most responsibly.

I suggest that the power relationship between physician and patient, as regards control of information, must be modified from the old formula to meet present necessities. For confidentiality, this requires that the traditional practices be largely maintained while updating them to fit the changed circumstances of medical practice. For truth telling, it requires that the traditional lying to patients be stopped, all the while retaining a sensitivity to the physiological power of negative emotions.

Confidentiality

The arguments for dismissing patient confidentiality as a "decrepit concept" (Siegler 1982a) are powerful. The Hippocratic physician worked alone and visited the patient in the patient's own home; all the medical records he needed he carried inside his head. Today's physician works in groups and teams, which cannot function unless information about each patient is readily available to any member at all times. When a patient is hospitalized, it is not unusual for fifty to sixty people to have good reasons both to walk into the patient's room and to have access to the medical chart. The law requires that instances of communicable disease, suspected child abuse, gunshot wounds, and other conditions be disclosed to public agencies. Patients voluntarily (more or less) sign a variety of permissions that allow insurance companies and others access to portions of the medical record. Moreover, this record itself is hardly of the physician's making. The physician signs the hospital record and effectively guarantees its accuracy, but she herself may have generated less than one-fourth of the record. It is safe to say that no physician in the United States today reads every word in her patients' charts. For those parts of the chart that contain important facts recorded by nurses, social workers, and other ancillary staff, this omission is unfortunate. But many parts of the chart contain information satisfying administrative or bureaucratic needs instead of patient-care requirements.

The physician lacks the power to control completely this monstrous body of information. Does this mean, then, that medical confidentiality is obsolete and that any moral appeals must be instead addressed to, say, medical records clerks or insurance administrators? Answering this question requires, first, an analysis of why confidentiality is important to patients and, second, an analysis of what power the physician actually possesses to control information in ways that are relevant to the patients' wishes and interests.

To the first point, there is an obvious reply and a more subtle reply. Clearly, direct harm can result when certain information about individuals is made known to others. The recent AIDS crisis has driven this point home with a vengeance. When loss of insurance, loss of job, and loss of one's home have all followed the inappropriate disclosure of an individual's seropositive status, avoidance of harm has to be seen as a significant moral factor when addressing issues of confidentiality (Dickens 1988).

This obvious reply is important but also limited. Philosophers have noted that it may as easily undermine confidentiality as support it. After all, in some cases one may be able to avoid harm to the individual precisely by releasing private information, as in the case of making known someone's plan to commit suicide to those who are in a position to thwart it. Moreover, in many instances in which we would consider disclosure of private information morally offensive, no clear harm would result, nor would it have been expected to result. The physician who details his patients' intimate secrets as cocktail party chitchat acts in a morally outrageous fashion, independently of whether any harm comes to the patients themselves as a result of his disclosures.

The more subtle reply has to do with how control of information affects the maintenance of different sorts of relationships. It is helpful to begin by depicting one's relationships with others as a series of concentric circles around the central point which represents the self. Along the smallest circle are the most intimate and long-standing relationships. Along the next largest circle are relationships with close friends. More distant friends and acquaintances occupy circles farther out, until we get to the largest and most distant circle, comprising those with whom we have only instrumental relationships, like the clerk at the supermarket (Beauchamp and Childress 1983; Brody 1989c).

The point of this model is that we control these relationships to a large extent by controlling the amount of private information to which these parties have access. We will ordinarily tell our most intimate associates nearly all our thoughts and feelings (though never all of them). We will disclose virtually none of them to those along the outermost circle. We can shift people from one circle to another by changing information disclosure: we can make a casual acquaintance more of a close friend by revealing more, and we can cool off a very close friendship by making a habit of revealing less. Indeed, what it means to be an intimate associate or a close friend is largely bound up with the amount and type of information that is exchanged.

Therefore, when one takes from people the right to control who has access to that sort of information, one robs them of the power to control personal relationships. In effect, if I can disclose the most private information about you to the supermarket clerk, I can place that clerk on a par with your most intimate family members. This radical disempowerment explains why the violation of confidentiality is such a basic moral indignity.

Now, among the various circles of human relationships, the physician-patient one occupies a contradictory position. Though it may be friendly, as a rule the patient does not regard his physician as a close and intimate friend; the relationship, from the patient's side at least, is largely an instrumental one, aimed at furthering and protecting his health. But it happens—unlike in most other instrumental relationships—that in order to secure the offered benefit, the patient is forced to disclose to his physician matters that he would ordinarily disclose only to his most intimate acquaintances. This unavoidably gives the physician a good deal of power over the patient and his relationships.

It now seems important to ask, in the event that the patient finds himself disempowered with regard to these relationships and losing control over private information, whether this loss of power and control occurred through some preventable or willful act of the physician or is simply a sad consequence of our modern, technological society. This question should be taken seriously on both sides, for we live in a world in which technology and complexity have challenged our abilities to control relationships and information. For example, so long as I choose the convenience of paying for purchases by credit card instead of by cash, I am going to leave a wide trail, on paper and in computer data banks, of what I purchase, where I spend my time, and where I travel, and a great many people are going to have access to that information, both appropriately and by surreptitious means. Yet in spite of the world in which we live, many people manage to retain the necessary degree of control to have rewarding relationships with family and friends, and others may choose whether to respect that control or act against it. So it will do neither to expect miracles from the physician, as if he could single-handedly simplify modern life, nor to speak as if modern life takes the physician off the hook completely.

The concept of shared power goes partway toward defining a set of realistic physician duties regarding patient confidentiality. The first step in appropriately sharing power to disclose information with the patient is making clear to him the nature and extent of the problem. Some data suggest that the average patient thinks that privacy in medical settings is guarded more carefully than is realistic, and indeed more carefully than physicians think they must (Weiss 1982). The physician would appear to have a duty to tell the patient how information is handled in both office and hospital settings, who generally has access to the records, and how hard or easy it is for others to obtain the information.

This discussion about information handling in medical settings should accomplish two things. First, it should help avert overly facile promises by the physician such as "Anything you say to me will be held in the strictest confidence." Possibilities for information leakage exist in almost all modern care systems, and it is only fair that the patient should know that. Second, it may give rise to specific negotiations about what should be included in the written record. In an example that is becoming commonplace, the physician may advise the patient at risk for HIV infection to be tested anonymously through the local health department instead of ordering the test through a standard laboratory and having the information become part of the chart.[5]

Next, the patient may be asked some questions about his own wishes regarding control of information. "Are there particular people or organizations to whom you especially want me to disclose, or not to disclose, information about your medical care? Do these wishes for disclosure or nondisclosure cover all medical information or only information on specific topics?" These data may be entered in the record in the same way (for example) that one might record a patient's wishes regarding a proxy decision-maker or other advance directives.

These general wishes cannot substitute, of course, for explicit patient

5. However, excluding information about HIV status or HIV risk factors from the medical record may seriously compromise patient care when somebody other than the primary physician must make a decision about a new onset of illness. Several states have recently passed laws providing strict penalties for anyone, including health-care personnel, who discloses confidential information about the patient's HIV status. This legal protection may go a long way toward gaining patient acceptance of having this information recorded in the medical record.

consent to reveal specific pieces of information at a later date. The point of this preliminary discussion is twofold. First, it signals to the patient how seriously the physician takes the matter and may start the patient thinking harder about issues he had previously not considered. Second, it can serve as a guide in those circumstances where the physician must decide whether to disclose information when it would be inconvenient or impossible to consult the patient first. It should be explained to the patient that this information will be used as a general guide only and that no one on the treatment team will reveal information without explicit consent.

A further implication of shared power is a duty to disclose to the patient when confidentiality has been breached in the pursuit of a more pressing moral duty. When the physician discloses information as required by law (such as reporting suspected child abuse) or to protect threatened, identifiable third parties from substantial harm (such as disclosure to the unwitting sexual partner of an HIV-seropositive patient), it is generally held that disclosure is morally justified. The harm of disclosing private information behind the patient's back, however, need not be added to the harm of disclosing that information against the patient's wishes or interests. Candid discussion with the patient of the need to disclose the information in question seems required, and in some cases it may allow the maintenance of a trusting physician-patient relationship that otherwise would have been demolished by the disclosure.

This third point raises the difficult issue of when breaching confidentiality is justifiable. On this score, an autonomy-benefit analysis and a power analysis seem to give almost identical answers. Specifically, the autonomy-benefit analysis would require the following conditions to be met: (1) The harm to be avoided is great, there is a high likelihood that the breach of confidentiality will avoid the harm, and there seems to be no other practical way to avoid the harm. (2) Whenever possible, the patient is given the opportunity first to disclose the information voluntarily (or to prevent the harm in some other manner). The patient is informed that the physician will find it necessary to breach confidentiality if the patient does not take this opportunity. The decision to breach confidentiality follows open discussion with the patient on these points.

The first condition assures that the benefit side of the scale is morally weighty. The second condition assures that maximum respect for autonomy has been shown even if breach of confidentiality is the eventual course of action.

The power analysis, following the three rules for responsible use of power listed in chapter 3, would proceed as follows:

1. Shared power requires that the patient be given the opportunity to prevent the harm or disclose the information and that the patient have a chance to try to talk the physician out of the breach of confidentiality (perhaps by showing that there is an alternative way to avoid the harm that does not require breaching confidentiality or by demonstrating that the harm is not as great as the physician believed).

2. Owned power requires that the patient be informed that the physician intends to breach confidentiality (or has done so, in cases where circumstances preclude prior consultation with the patient).

3. Aimed power requires that the exercise of power have its intended effect—that is, that the harm be actually avoided and that it be substantial enough to warrant this use of power.

Both sets of rules place the need for open discussion of the moral dilemma with the patient in a somewhat new light. Not only does respect for autonomy, or respect for persons, require that one be informed when other parties intend to override one's basic rights. But also creative and unanticipated resolutions of the dilemma may arise from frank discussion and negotiation. Factors of which the physician was unaware, or to which the physician had given too much or too little weight, may be clarified.

Truthful Disclosure

Two major studies of truthful disclosure of the diagnosis of cancer (Oken 1961; Novack et al. 1979) are commonly cited as milestones in the transition between the old and the new medical ethics. In 1961, Oken found more than 90 percent of physicians unwilling to tell a patient the truth about his having cancer; in 1979, Novack, using almost the identical questionnaire, found more than 90 percent willing to disclose the diagnosis. On the surface, this seems like a triumph for the principle of patient autonomy within less than twenty years.

Further analysis suggests some problems with the rosy picture of autonomy triumphant over paternalism. First, many things about cancer and its treatment changed in the interval between the studies. Most important, cancer changed from a disease seen by the general public as an invariable death sentence to one against which many effective treatments could be marshaled. Second, the administration of those treatments in most settings required informed consent—as we saw in previous chapters, possibly less because of respect for patient autonomy and more because of perceived legal and administrative pressures.

Moreover, the twin studies indicate that one thing did not change between 1961 and 1979—the dogmatism and inflexibility demonstrated by the physicians. In each study the physicians responded that their own clinical judgment told them which policy on disclosure of information was correct; and they stated that they did not anticipate altering that policy on the basis of any new information in the future. There is more to this point than the irony of falling back on "clinical judgment" to defend a practice that has, according to empirical evidence, been turned inside out within twenty years. There is also the suggestion that physicians are ill prepared to attend to individual patients and individual treatment situations in deciding what to do, but are prone rather to fall back on a comfortable formula. And that would seem to bode poorly for sensitive and compassionate care of patients based on individual needs.[6]

Further evidence that the new medical ethic of truthful disclosure may have more problems than it first appeared to have comes from more recent studies. Novack and colleagues (1989), in a separate study of physician behavior, found that doctors advocated deception in a number of circumstances in medical practice, especially deception directed at persons other than the patient, when it seemed a convenient way out of a jam. The justification proposed for most such uses of deception was purely consequentialist and gave short shrift to concerns about autonomy and rights. Reich (1989) has claimed that an exclusive focus on the patient's right to know the truth about his condition falls far short of appreciating the important issues of suffering and compassion in serious and terminal illness.[7] He argues that "the clinician's anguish over constantly and directly exposing himself or herself to the pains and torments of the dying" (p. 105), in addition to the patient's own possible anguish and fear of death, cannot be brushed aside as interesting psychological factors of no great ethical weight. Reich instead argues for an approach that recognizes the physician's possible suffering and provides a compassionate response to it, as a precondition for the physician's being able to provide, compassionately and truthfully, the sort of support that the dying patient needs.

Is there something missing from the standard analysis of truthful disclosure? Consider the following two cases:

6. Examples of criticisms of physicians who adhere to the moral duty to disclose truthful information but display striking disregard for the feelings and wishes of the patient in doing so can be found in Springarn 1978; Cousins 1980.

7. See chapter 16 for a more detailed discussion of Reich's analysis of suffering and compassion in medicine.

A physician orders diagnostic tests for a seriously ill patient and discovers the presence of cancer. He elects to withhold this information and tells the patient instead, "There are a few abnormalities in the tests, but everything should come out just fine. Tomorrow I'll be starting you on a new course of treatment that should correct what's wrong."

A physician examines a patient and diagnoses a common, easily curable illness. In the back of his mind, however, he is aware that there is a slight chance this could be an early sign of cancer. He elects to withhold this information and says to the patient, "I'm sure things will turn out all right if you take these pills and get lots of rest as I advised. But, on the off chance you are not over this in about five days, please call me back so we can check into it some more."

I will assume that the considered judgment of most readers would hold that the first physician acted wrongly and the second physician acted correctly—so long, of course, as there are no important unknown features, such as a prior request from the first patient not to be told "bad news." The standard analysis would defend these judgments by noting the relationship between truth and autonomy. To make her own choices, a person must know where she is situated and what her options are. To withhold the information essential for those tasks is to undermine her autonomy, to treat her as a means only rather than as an end in herself. Respect for the autonomy of others therefore entails that they have a right to truthful information. In ordinary human relationships, this right may be recognized simply by not lying or deceiving. But in fiduciary relationships like the physician-patient relationship, the corresponding duty is more exacting. As the physician may come to know things that the patient cannot discover for herself but which may nevertheless be very important to the patient's free choice, the physician has a special obligation to disclose information of importance and not merely not to lie about it (Beauchamp and Childress 1983; Brody 1989c).

But this standard account has difficulty explaining the different moral judgments that attach to the two cases. It might be said that a patient has a right to know a diagnosis but no right to know a hunch or a suspicion. But all that separates a diagnosis from a hunch is a degree of probability, not a difference in kind; and besides, clients commonly consult experts to learn their hunches or suspicions without demanding certainty. Or it might be said that a diagnosis of cancer poses several important choices for an individual, whereas the physician's suspicion of a slight probability of cancer raises no choices of practical import; therefore, autonomy is at stake in the first case but not in the second. But why shouldn't the existence of a slight possibility of cancer be of importance to at least some patients? How can the physician know in advance that the matter would not be of practical importance to this particular patient? Why would not the concept of transparency (as discussed in the previous chapter) mandate disclosure of this slight probability, since it crossed the physician's mind? After all, no one is proposing that the physician scream and flail his arms about as if the sky were falling; he merely is expected to state calmly that there may be some slight possibility of a cancer. Can that information honestly be said to be frightening or even incapacitating to a citizen of our modern world?[8]

It therefore seems that grounding the duty of truthful disclosure solely in respect for patient autonomy may entail a stronger disclosure duty than common sense would accept. For this and for other reasons, some have proposed that truthful disclosure must be seen as equally grounded in the principles of autonomy and beneficence (Gadow 1981; Beauchamp and McCullough 1984). The practice of medical deception throughout most of the history of Western medicine presumably occurred through the dominance of the benefit principle: physicians judged that harsh truths harmed patients and soothing lies helped them. If physicians now have changed their tune and tell the truth most of the time, it may be because they have come to respect patient autonomy, or it may be because they have recalculated the risk-benefit ratio and have decided that the truth may be more beneficial, or lies more harmful, than had previously appeared.

The reintroduction of the benefit principle leads to a discussion of the physician's power to help or to harm the patient by giving or withholding information. This in turn shows the incompleteness of Reich's (1989) analysis of why truthful disclosure remains a difficult ethical problem for the

---

8. Would the transparency standard described in chapter 7 require disclosure of the possibility of cancer in the second case, since the matter crossed the mind of the physician? Presumably, if the basic rule of transparency is "think out loud," this disclosure should be made; and yet this seems unreasonable, as it would require that the physician blurt out all sorts of unpleasant and basically useless information. But before rejecting the transparency standard, it is important to recall that that standard was introduced within the context of a conversation model, for which the ultimate test was, "What information would be exchanged in a reasonable conversation?" It seems quite plausible that the information about the remote risk of cancer would not come up in a reasonable conversation about the patient's visit; the same reasoning applies here as to the disclosure of remote risks (chapter 6). Moreover, our hypothetical physician has not exactly failed to disclose his concerns: he has included a warning about calling back if symptoms do not improve. The patient who had a higher-than-average need for information could always ask at this point, "If they don't get better, what would that mean?"

physician. It is not simply because the physician hesitates to share the patient's suffering once the patient learns his true state of affairs, but also because the physician is trying to weigh exactly what to say and what to withhold and the extent to which any information can relieve suffering as well as how it can cause suffering. The outcome the physician fears is not just that the patient will collapse psychologically from a dread diagnosis. She may also fear remorse and self-doubt at seeing the patient's anguished response to what she has chosen to say.

The point here is analogous to a consideration raised previously in discussing informed consent. Patient autonomy may be a comforting verbal formula to convince us that the power has been taken away from the physician and given back to the patient. But it fails to recognize the power that irreducibly remains with the physician. No physician ever tells a patient "everything"; and for no medical diagnosis is there one single truth that gives the physician objective and unequivocal guidance concerning what words ought to be said to the patient. No matter how frank or how full the disclosure, the physician selects both how much is said and how it is said. How the patient will use what is said to make decisions; what the patient has previously said he wants to hear; what the likely emotional impact will be; what emotional reactions the physician is prepared to handle; and how much time the physician has, all must play a part in the choice that the physician finally makes. For these reasons, respect for patient autonomy alone may give the physician very incomplete moral guidance. Instead, it is worth asking what counts as a responsible use of this considerable power to disclose information.

At this point, a review of the biological origins of that power may be helpful. The biopsychosocial model previously alluded to (Engel 1977) holds that psychological states can, under appropriate circumstances, affect health outcomes. A specific example of this is the placebo effect—a change in the patient's condition that results from the symbolic dimensions of a healing intervention rather than from its specific pharmacological or physiological properties. A unifying concept that can explain many aspects of the placebo effect, and psychological or symbolic healing more generally, is to link the change in the patient's health status to the altered meaning that the illness experience comes to have for that patient. In turn, meaning may be broken down into several components: the explanation the patient has for the illness and how well it fits into the patient's preexisting worldview; the sense of care and concern shown by others toward the patient; and the patient's own sense of mastery or control over the illness and its symptoms (Brody 1980, 1986, 1988b).

It follows from this that the physician has the power to improve the patient's health status to the extent that she can alter the meaning that the patient attributes to the illness experience in a positive way (in addition to the power to utilize other therapies that act through somatic routes).[9] But this is not always an easy task. Sometimes the choice of a few words, or mere body language, may make the difference between a patient who feels cared for and a patient who feels abandoned; or between a patient who feels competent to control symptoms and one who feels victimized. As a general rule, if physicians are most effectively to understand the meaning an illness has for the patient so as to be able to alter it positively, they must be attuned to the role that the illness plays in the unfolding story of the patient's life (Brody 1987d; Kleinman 1988). In turn, this observation links the meaning model of placebo effect and symbolic healing to the patient-centered conception of primary care summarized in chapter 4. If physicians are going to enter into the required negotiation with patients to be sure that they understand the presenting problem in the patient's own terms, they will have to listen carefully to the patient's story of the illness. This then gives the physician enhanced power to attach a more benign and less frightening meaning to the illness experience in terms that the patient will recognize as being relevant to him and his circumstances.

It may be difficult enough to try to balance autonomy and beneficence in deciding what to disclose to a particular patient and how to do so. But this analysis suggest that the balancing act may be even more delicate. All three "rules" for the responsible use of power may apply here. The physician must first of all recognize precisely what power she does and does not possess to help or to harm the patient through information disclosure (owned power). She must try to use the power she does have to maximize the benefit and to minimize the harm (aimed power).[10] Finally, she must strive to make the patient as much as possible an active participant in the process of disclosing information, encouraging the patient to ask questions and to react to the information given (shared power).

9. Here it is important to remember that most medical treatments work simultaneously at the somatic and the psychological-symbolic levels. Unless the physician is treating an unconscious or unaware patient, most medical interventions will affect the physical and chemical characteristics of the patient's body and will also *mean something* to the patient. In this sense the placebo effect accompanies almost all medical therapies and is not restricted to so-called inert therapies; see Brody 1980, 1986.

10. There is no reason in this analysis not to include enhanced patient autonomy as one of the benefits of information disclosure. This again assumes, in the terminology of Nozick (1974), that one is willing to view autonomy as an end constraint rather than as a side constraint.

The guideline of shared power is not simply, as it might first appear, a nod in the direction of respect for autonomy. Rather, it is a necessary condition for assessing the way that power has been used and its consequences for the patient. The balancing act among all the moral values and guidelines pertinent to truthful disclosure is so complex that it is virtually impossible for the physician to predict what will be *best* to say to the patient (including how much to say and how to say it). Instead, the physician who wishes to do the best possible job of disclosing information will need to follow many cues that arise in the course of the interview, making numerous midcourse corrections as she goes along. The patient who feels comfortable participating actively and candidly in the process will provide the most, and the most useful, cues. The passive patient who believes that it is his appointed role to sit silently and absorb whatever the physician says does not give the physician the same opportunity to fine-tune the disclosure as it proceeds.

We can now return to the two brief cases noted near the beginning of this section to assess why one nondisclosure of cancer is defensible and the other is not. In the first case, the classic paternalistic nondisclosure of "bad news," the physician correctly perceives the power that the diagnosis has over the patient and tries to use that power to produce a good outcome by withholding what would cause emotional distress. But he achieves this apparently good result only at the cost of ignoring many important aspects of the patient's situation. As Gadow (1981) noted, truth is a two-edged weapon. It can scare, depress, demoralize, and confuse. But it can also relieve (by turning vague, unmanageable fears into approachable certainties). It can aid in making a wide variety of decisions (whether to get a second opinion, what to tell one's family and friends, how to manage one's finances, what attitude to adopt in living the rest of one's life). It can help make the patient a coparticipant in a possibly arduous course of treatment instead of a victim of toxic effects. The physician, in this case, does more than violate the patient's right to autonomy by withholding the diagnosis; he makes a judgment (almost certainly on insufficient data) about the relative values of the benefits and the burdens of telling the truth. Moreover, because his nondisclosure has the consequence of closing off further dialogue, the physician is likely never to receive the cues he would need to redirect his disclosure efforts in a more positive direction. His power will inevitably in this case be well intended but poorly aimed.

Moreover, this physician seems to have thought very little about contingencies. What if the patient asks for more details about the "few abnormalities in the tests?" What if the patient asks for more details about the treatment and its risks? What is the physician going to say to other family members—will he leave the entire family unaware of the danger this person faces, or will he involve them in a conspiracy of silence that is likely to strain family bonds? If any of these contingencies results in the patient later finding out that he indeed has cancer, then the patient will still get all the harm of the disclosure plus the harm of knowing that the truth had been withheld from him when he had a right to expect it. The implications for trust and emotional support within the physician-patient relationship are obvious.

What about the second case? There the assessment of disclosure of the remote chance of cancer mirrors our previous discussion of the disclosure of remote risks in informed consent. The physician has calculated that the chances of the patient being *empowered* by the information is extremely low. Moreover, there may be considerable emotional distress from the physician's frankly saying "I think it is unlikely, but it is possible that these symptoms are an early sign of some sort of cancer." The emotional distress may be considerable. Knowing about the physician's moderate concern will not help the patient make any important decisions and could sway the patient to make some unwise ones. For example, the good primary-care physician knows that a head-to-toe search for a hidden tumor in a patient with no clear symptoms pointing to that diagnosis is more likely to produce false positives than it is to turn up a curable disease that would have become incurable had it been discovered later.[11] But the disclosure of this remote risk to a fearful patient might lead him to request just such a fruitless search.

Further, the physician has also solicited a cue from the patient by noting that he wants the patient to call back if things do not turn out as planned. This will allow the more concerned or fearful patient to ask, "What sorts of things should I look for?" or "If things didn't get better soon, what other things would you be concerned about?" The physician can then share more information about remote risks with the patient, continuing as long as the patient indicates a desire to hear more. Usually the patient will feel reassured that the symptoms point to a benign diagnosis; to dishearten this patient by forcing on him the remote risk of cancer would seem to serve no useful or humane purpose.

All that we know about the placebo effect and the therapeutic impact

11. I do not mean here to suggest that such screening for occult cancer as mammography and cervical Pap smears is not of value. I am referring instead to the patient who has vague or nonlocalized symptoms of the sort that may be associated with cancer less than 5 or 10 percent of the time and hence are almost always associated with some benign diagnosis.

of the physician-patient encounter (Novack 1987; Thomas 1987) would suggest that the more positive, reassuring approach is likely to improve the patient's medical outcome, whereas arousing anxiety or uncertainty may retard a good outcome. The physician who would then feel obligated to mention the remote chance of cancer even if unasked appears to have a peculiarly legalistic view of his role. He fails to own the power that he possesses by acting as if he were a sort of reference book to which the patient comes to look up answers. And he aims his power very poorly by forgetting that information that assists the physician's mental process would be taken totally out of context if it were mentioned to the patient in this sort of medical interview.

In short, physicians most effectively empower patients neither by reflexively disclosing nor by reflexively withholding any particular sort of information. They empower patients by creating an atmosphere that encourages participation and dialogue; by following carefully the cues provided by the patient as the dialogue unfolds; and ultimately by aiding the patient in placing the new information in the context of the patient's life experience and life story in the most meaningful, encouraging, and health-promoting way.

Thc primary-care focus gives us an interesting vantage point from which to view the apparent love affair of medical ethics with life-and-death cases. Indeed, we might begin to entertain the uncharitable assumption that the readiness to focus on these exciting cases—what has been labeled "neon ethics"—might serve to conceal a selective blindness, precisely the sort of thing that we would expect ethical analysis to reveal rather than to aid in covering up. In this chapter I will discuss what I take to be a key example of this blindness: the rescue fantasy.[1] I will show how the rescue fantasy links a series of cases that otherwise seem dissimilar and then review it in light of my proposed rules for the responsible use of power.

One recent advance in the methodology of medical ethics has been an increased appreciation of how one organizes or arrays sets of exemplary cases. According to the more traditional analytic view, or "engineering model," doing medical ethics meant knowing a set of ethical principles and knowing how to apply them to particular cases; the study of the cases themselves was an illustrative but secondary exercise. Increasingly this model is being rejected in favor of models that focus on how we pick out the morally relevant details of a case and—closely related—how we sift

---

1. I am unsure of the precise origins of this term. Albert Jonsen has referred in several places to a "rule of rescue" or an "age of rescue" to describe the perceived imperative to utilize available technology to save identifiable lives; see, for instance, Jonsen 1986a. In psychology, the term *rescue fantasy* has been used to refer to an inappropriate assumption of power by the therapist, who may believe that only he can "fix" the client's problems; this delays the better therapeutic outcome in which the client comes to accept responsibility for making changes in his own life.

through sets of cases in search of morally relevant analogies and disanalogies.

It follows from this that when we arrive at a new insight in medical ethics, it may change the way in which we group cases or issues: we may see a relevant similarity where previously we saw only divergence. I would argue that the power perspective can be shown to be insightful in this way. Consider, for example, the following five cases:

1. A woman terminally ill with leukemia and carrying a possibly viable but very premature fetus undergoes a court-ordered cesarean section, against her own wishes and those of her family and physicians, to save the fetus. The woman's death is hastened and perhaps rendered more painful by the surgery, and the infant lives only a few hours (This is the Angela Carter case: Annas 1988b).

2. A pregnant woman sustains serious head injuries and is declared to have suffered brain death. The body is maintained on a ventilator for many weeks, until the fetus becomes viable and can safely be delivered by cesarean section (Dillon et al. 1982; Field et al. 1988).

3. A proposal is made that in cases where cardiopulmonary resuscitation is predictably futile a do-not-resuscitate order not require patient consent, although the patient and/or family should be notified (Tomlinson and Brody 1988). A strong objection is registered by a distinguished ethics panel on the grounds that the proposal undermines respect for patient autonomy (Farber 1988). This is stated in spite of the generally accepted dictum that a physician has no obligation to offer any patient futile therapy. The ethics panel appears not to realize that in stating their objection, they are in effect separating cardiopulmonary resuscitation from all other types of medical treatment.

4. An infant with congenital liver disease, who has previously undergone three liver transplants followed by rejection of the organ in each case, is transplanted with a fourth liver. Meanwhile other infants are dying of liver disease because of inability to pay or because of the great scarcity of infant-size donor organs.

5. Patients A and B both require heart transplants and are awaiting suitable donor organs. A heart becomes available that would be a good tissue match for either. A will die within a week if he does not get his transplant; but after transplant his prognosis for functional life is limited to perhaps five years owing to other disease complications. B will survive four to six weeks without a new heart; but once he receives his transplant, he is expected to gain twenty to thirty years of functional life. Because of

the uncertainty as to when another heart with a good match will become available, it is quite possible that if B does not get this heart, he will die before another is found. Based on existing allocation policy, the transplantation program allots this heart to A.

Ordinarily these cases would be placed in different categories. The first case would be seen as a problem in patient autonomy, here of a conflict between maternal and fetal therapeutic interests. In the second case no such conflict can be argued, since the pregnant woman, being dead, can no longer have any rights or interests; and so the rights or interests of other parties—the fetus, if it can be said to have rights or interests, or the surviving next of kin—should be controlling. The third case would be seen as a classic dispute between patient autonomy and physician paternalism, raising the question of whether refusing to administer futile therapy when the patient requests it could be classed as true paternalism. The fourth and fifth cases would be seen as problems in the allocation of scarce resources (distributive justice).

I suggest that in spite of these genuine differences, there is indeed a common thread among the cases that becomes apparent once one adopts the power vocabulary. I submit that in each of the above situations, *if* an incorrect decision has been reached, it arises at least in part from the involved physicians having fallen under the spell of the rescue fantasy. Indeed, in the first case (as legal commentator George Annas charged) the fantasy proved to be contagious; the court, as a result of deciding to hold the hearing in the hospital instead of in a courtroom, contracted the fantasy and ordered a procedure that most of the involved physicians were not seeking. I will support this contention by explaining the nature of the rescue fantasy, indicating how and why patients reinforce this fantasy among physicians, and noting ways in which it may lead to unsound ethical reasoning.

The rescue fantasy is a power trip: it envisions the physician having the power to snatch the patient from the jaws of death. Probably most students are possessed by it to some degree upon entering medical school and it is part of the popular folklore about physicians. In days of old, at least, it was implicitly used by medical school professors to spur the students on to greater efforts: unless you listen carefully to my lecture about the hexose monophosphate shunt (said the biochemist in so many words), someday you will kill a patient.

The problem, of course, is that most of medical practice is not like that at all. Most patients visiting a primary-care physician either have nothing medically wrong with them, or have something that will go away if left to itself, or have something chronic that can be managed but never cured. Even when patients have a problem that is curable if treated properly and could be disastrous if missed or mishandled, the timing is wrong for the rescue fantasy: The case unfolds slowly, over days or weeks; if the physician misses something or makes an error at the early stage, there are many opportunities to correct mistakes before permanent harm is done. And so the real-life case that fits the rescue fantasy—if I don't act now, and if I don't do the right thing, this patient will lose his life or his health—is almost nonexistent. (Ironically, in real-life medical settings that fit this description, such as emergency trauma centers, the rescues may occur several times a day, but they offer very little satisfaction to the physicians because almost all procedures are reduced to automatic, unthinking protocol.)

It might seem under these circumstances that all practicing physicians would jettison the rescue fantasy as an worn-out piece of baggage from their naive student days; and to a large degree this occurs. But the fantasy, I suggest, hangs on to a surprising degree, for several reasons. First, the folklore is powerful, and the Lazarus imagery compelling.[2] Second, to give up the rescue fantasy would be felt subconsciously as the giving up of a vital part of the physician's self-image—*the sense of the power to control bad outcomes*.[3]

The sense of power to control bad outcomes is a two-edged sword, as all physicians in the United States are now acutely aware. Sherman Mellinkoff (1987) captured this in an anecdote: "The patient wants to know

2. The image of rescue is intimately linked in our folklore with that of the hero, who, it appears, always engages in action, never in restraint. This hero image clearly influences the behavior of those who enter medicine. I am indebted to comments from John R. Stone and Leonard Fleck on the importance of this point. See also Gilligan and Pollak 1988: "In American medicine ideals of heroic achievement have overshadowed the value of nurturance and close personal affiliation. Technological advances have repeatedly been gained at the expense of the doctor-patient relationship" (246).

3. The power of this myth of control is illustrated by a passing reference in a volume on medical ethics by a theologian, whom one might have thought to be as free of the rescue fantasy as possible. Drane (1988) discusses the conflict between autonomy and benefit in cases of life-prolonging treatment: "As the patient moves from an acute and easily cured illness into chronic illness and finally into greatly reduced quality of life and the dying process, beneficence, as medical best interest, weighs less, and autonomy, as patient personal preference, weighs more" (p. 72). What is strange about this passage is the notion that a dying that is unencumbered by the overuse of medical technology cannot be said to be *medically* a good thing; it becomes good only by appeal to the patient's own (nonmedical) values. This in turn seems to equate good medicine with always trying to rescue, no matter how low the chances of success or how severe the burdens imposed.

who his or her physician is. One delightful patient I saw on rounds one day looked at the array of doctors and students advising him and asked with a twinkle in his eye, 'Tell me, which one of you fine lads am I supposed to sue?' " Fear of malpractice litigation is so strong among American physicians that the humor of such a remark is very thin. But the more basic point, for Mellinkoff, is that diffusion of responsibility through impersonal team care deprives the patient of one of the most important comforts and reassurances that medicine can provide. For the patient, this is the image of a powerful physician who is the one person who can save him from the harm that threatens. Namely, it is the rescue fantasy as the patient experiences it. Rescue by a group lacks this sort of flair; it does not meet the deep need of the patient for an all-powerful parent figure. From the physician's perspective, it is a difficult dilemma: I can accept the power to control outcomes and the responsibility that goes with it and thereby open myself to a lawsuit if things turn out badly, or I can deny any such power and thereby deny both to the patient and to myself the fantasy that keeps both of us going in this world of sickness and death. From the patient's perspective, it is simpler: If I cannot find anyone who will take responsibility for how things turn out, then I have no doctor.

I emphasize here that I am trying to depict a level of thought that seldom reaches conscious awareness. Logically, of course, we can distinguish among bad outcomes that arise from a variety of sources: limitations in the present state of medical knowledge; statistically predictable but random and uncontrollable occurrences; errors of judgment or technique that are unfortunate but are only human and form no recurring pattern; and recurring errors of judgment or technique that indicate culpable negligence. But the subconscious, which blurs all such distinctions, forms part of the reality of the physician's and the patient's mental life; it is the backdrop against which information is processed and decisions are made.

What I conclude from all this is that medical situations that fit the description of the rescue fantasy, or can somehow be construed to fit that description, will be treated as a special and important class of medical situation for reasons physicians and patients mutually (if subconsciously) strive to maintain. Accordingly, when well-accepted ethical principles appear routinely to be ignored or misapplied in a category of cases, one might ask whether something like the rescue fantasy is at work.

Consider emergency cardiopulmonary resuscitation, often referred to in hospital parlance as a "code." The dispassionate application of sound ethical principles would argue that where therapy is predictably futile, the physician has no obligation to offer it even when the patient requests or demands it. Yet the entire emotional life of the hospital community pro-claims that cardiopulmonary resuscitation is different. No other medical treatment is announced over the hospital loudspeaker system. Few other medical treatments demand that staff stop whatever they are doing and literally run to the spot. Few other treatments produce the palpable ad-renalin rush in participants and onlookers; indeed, few medical treatments attract onlookers at all, whereas the control of traffic not immediately involved in the code is a common problem in hospital resuscitations.

The rescue fantasy sets up two barriers to accepting the proposal that patient consent not be required for a do-not-resuscitate order when re-suscitation would predictably be futile. First, the rescue fantasy opposes labeling any resuscitation as futile in advance, as that seems to admit lack of control over bad outcomes. "You never know until you try" is more consistent with what the fantasy requires. Second, the fantasy opposes taking a security blanket ("Doctor, I want you to do everything") away from the patient, no matter how illusory the security. "Sure, he's going to die, but you can't just sit there and let him die without at least trying to do something" is again what the fantasy requires. Remaining in the back-ground is the fear that if this proposal were to be accepted, there would be fewer codes, which is bad because codes are exciting and are one of the hospital's main rituals for keeping the rescue fantasy alive.

The rescue fantasy also explains some reactions to the no-code issue that otherwise remain inexplicable despite their widespread occurrence among hospital staff and in expert reports and guidelines. Cardiopulmonary resuscitation was developed and tested in a highly select group of patients: otherwise healthy people with temporary but serious cardiac arrhythmias who would die without resuscitation and who could be restored to a fully functional state with resuscitation in many instances. More by seepage than by design, the procedure came to be standard practice for all hospitalized patients, so that now the presumption is that no one is allowed to die in a hospital in the United States without an attempt at resuscitation. As one physician noted, we seem to have forgotten the difference between those who die because their hearts stop and those whose heart stops because they are dying (Graham 1988).

The requirements for patient or family consent tend to presume that when someone refuses resuscitation, she trades in life for death. From the majority of published ethical analyses and guidelines one would gather that resuscitation was successful at least 70–80 percent of the time. One has to look elsewhere to discover that under the best possible circumstances resuscitation is successful in restoring heartbeat only half the time (and even then less than 20 percent survive long enough to leave the hospital); whereas in more chronically ill patients and those with major organ system failures a 0–10 percent response rate is more common (Moss 1989). This means that resuscitation is less likely to work precisely among those patients in whom cardiac arrest can be predicted and with whom a conversation about the matter can take place beforehand. All the work that has gone into devising detailed do-not-resuscitate policies suggests that important patient interests may be in jeopardy. But how are a patient's interests compromised when he refuses a possibly burdensome intervention that has at most a 10 percent chance of succeeding?

Nurses used to complain with complete justification when physicians would privately state that a patient was not be coded but would refuse to write an order to that effect. The shoe is now on the other foot: physicians may complain that the nurses are after them to decide, "Is this patient a code or a no-code?" whenever a seriously ill or elderly patient is admitted, often before a firm diagnosis has been reached. Ethical deliberations about appropriateness of care that would best be phrased, "What plan of management is optimal for this patient, given her expressed wishes and her interests?" are habitually raised by hospital staff as, "Should this patient be made a no-code?" There exists an almost magical expectation that *code* or *no-code* will convey a plan of patient management and resolve all care dilemmas in advance.

Physicians sometimes accuse nursing staff of practicing near-abandonment of patients who are designated no-code, of going into the room less often and sometimes ignoring basic nursing or comfort measures. While many nurses reject these charges, others admit that they are sometimes on the mark.[4] The same fear affects physician willingness to raise the code issue with patients or family, as if to ask about the appropriateness of a do-not-resuscitate order is tantamount to saying, "We have written you off."

In sum, a logical analysis of the resuscitation issue requires, first, that resuscitation be considered a medical treatment with well-understood indications and contraindications; and second, that decisions on whether to resuscitate be approached within the context of the overall plan of optimal medical management for that patient. But the rescue fantasy undermines attempts to apply this logic. That hospital staff still commonly regard

4. For an example in which an intensive investigation and discussion of this issue occurred in a community hospital, I am indebted to Dr. Jack Stack. The hospital eventually developed a new do-not-resuscitate policy based on its findings.

resuscitation decisions as arcane and perplexing, despite the volumes of analyses and guidelines that have been published on the subject, attests to the liveliness of the rescue fantasy in the hospital culture.

Another author who seems to feel that something like the rescue fantasy is endemic in medicine is attorney Nancy Rhoden (1988). She approvingly cites Jay Katz (1984) on the "magical thinking" that characterizes many physicians and on the fact that physicians view a patient's death as evidence of personal failure. Rhoden attributes to the prevalence of this view in medical circles, and to the courts' rather abject acceptance of this medical status quo, what she takes to be an important anomaly in court decisions regarding treatment refusals on behalf of incompetent patients. Most courts have allowed for treatment withdrawal, and yet the standards they propose—clear and convincing evidence that the patient, if competent, would have chosen nontreatment and death—are almost impossible for the average family or proxy decision-maker to meet. It is as if the courts are saying two contradictory things: first, that treatment withdrawal seems eminently reasonable when the facts of the case are taken into account, and second, that aggressive treatment of all dying patients ought to be the norm and especially weighty reasons must be brought forth before anything less can be permitted. The courts further reveal their ambivalence when families sue health facilities, charging wrongful overtreatment of the patient without appropriate consent. Two such cases (*Bartling* v. *Superior Court* in California, *Estate of Leach* v. *Shapiro* in Ohio) were dismissed on what seem to be extremely flimsy grounds, even though the cases displayed egregious indifference to the wishes of the family and of a competent patient. To Rhoden, this signals that courts wish whenever possible not to mess around with an informal system that makes the physician and not the patient or family the primary decision-maker in terminal-care cases. Although courts may allow petitioning families to refuse treatment, they may claim at the same time that such decisions ought to be made privately by families and physicians in the hospital setting and should not come to court at all. Yet courts will not impose penalties that would have the effect of forcing physicians and hospitals to take the patients' and families' wishes more seriously.[5]

An emergency cesarean section for fetal distress is in many cases the obstetric equivalent of a code. Moreover, whereas resuscitation may be

---

5. Since this chapter was drafted, the legal climate has begun to change. Courts are occasionally willing to hold that patients or families need not pay for life-prolonging medical care that was administered contrary to their clearly expressed wishes.

discouragingly unsuccessful an emergency section will produce a viable and apparently healthy infant most of the time. Thus emergency sections have the potential to support the rescue fantasy even more than do codes. We might then suspect the rescue fantasy at work if society's repugnance at allowing bodily invasion of a competent adult over her strenuous objections is routinely set aside when a court of law deals with cesarean section to save the fetus despite maternal refusal.

One example of case 2 illustrates the power of the rescue fantasy to override even fears of litigation; which are often believed to dominate the thinking of contemporary American physicians. The physicians involved stated that they were unsure of the legality of continued ventilation of the maternal body but elected to "sin bravely" and proceed anyway (Dillon et al. 1982, p. 1091). A feminist commentator has noted that postmortem ventilation of a pregnant cadaver implies a morally troubling view about pregnancy—that being pregnant is a bodily function which does not require the woman's consciousness or choice, and that successful completion of pregnancy ought to be a woman's highest goal and hence becomes a fitting memorial after her death (Murphy 1989).[6] Whether one agrees or disagrees with what was done in case 2, what tends to support Murphy's thesis is that the physicians involved in these cases give no evidence of having considered what their treatments imply for the status of the woman; nor do they reflect on the tragedy of a child's starting its life in this fashion. This seems further proof of the power of the rescue fantasy to distract attention from matters of potential moral importance.

The transplantation cases might be expected to be resolved by standard principles of distributive justice: organs would be allocated by a perfectly random system, so that no person counts as more worthy than any other, or else they would be allocated where the potential benefit is greatest. Whether one accepts Kantian or utilitarian reasoning on this subject, it is unlikely that one would favor a policy of entitling those who stand less chance of benefiting than other potential recipients. And yet in both cases 4 and 5 this seems to have occurred. In case 5 it seems to have been because of immediacy of need, and this fits with the social tendency to save a single identified life in preference to saving many anonymous or statistical lives. The key point here is that in case 5, if patient A dies, his physicians would think that he died "because we turned him down for the

6. It should be mentioned for completeness that Murphy's otherwise useful commentary is marred by sloppy language and reasoning regarding brain death. She refers to "life support" and "somatic life" and argues for a patient's "right to a speedy death," all concepts that fail to apply to a being which is in fact already dead.

heart and gave it instead to somebody who would get more long-term benefit." If patient B dies, he would die "because no good match was available when he needed it." The physicians would have to accept responsibility for A's death in a more direct fashion than B's, and by their own account that death would constitute an instance of refusal to rescue. By the dominant ethos of the physician—especially the surgeon, and especially the transplant surgeon—this is unacceptable, and distributive justice be damned.

Case 4 presents a slightly different application of the rescue fantasy in its more basic manifestation as a refusal to admit that bad outcomes may be outside one's control. Other things being equal, physicians will offer more extended and more aggressive treatment where the condition being treated is in some sense iatrogenic, even if that treatment violates principles of justice and may not truly be in the patient's interests. It is almost as if physicians engage in a ritual attempt to undo their unfortunate results— possibly unbecoming in a profession that prides itself on its scientific objectivity, but a fully human and understandable impulse nonetheless. If the fourth transplant works, the case goes down as a success and the three failures are wiped off the slate—as are the deaths of the three other children who could have gotten those livers.

An Objection

I anticipate an objection from those completely satisfied with the standard ethical vocabulary. They will probably say that all this business about a "rescue fantasy" is of limited, if any, ethical importance—just an entertaining look at some psychological and emotional factors that influence medical thinking and behavior. But when we get to the bottom line the question still is, what ought to be done? And when we analyze cases 1–5 we must employ the language of autonomy, beneficence, justice, and so forth to decide what ought to be done. *Why* physicians sometimes fail to see what ought to be done is beside the point; it is a question for social scientists and not for medical ethicists.

Before I reply to this objection, it is worth repeating a fundamental premise of this book. I do not disagree with the position that ultimately, for the successful analysis of an ethical problem, we will want to bring to bear the standard vocabulary of ethical principles. I do not propose that talk of power or rescue fantasies or whatever will replace talk in terms of those principles. At issue, then, is whether ethics talk extends beyond those principles into so-called emotional issues like the rescue fantasy or if it stops short.

A preliminary reply to the objection is that the discussion so far about the physician's power and how it is perceived by both physician and patient implies strongly that a good deal of the physician-patient relationship is bound up in meanings, symbolism, and perceptions. To try to describe that relationship while leaving out those emotional and psychological factors is to misdescribe, or at least underdescribe, that relationship. In that sense, to call for a return to power vocabulary in medical ethics is to challenge the comfortable line of demarcation that leaves all "objective" ethical considerations on this side of the line and all "messy" emotional factors on the other.

A more specific reply is that the rescue fantasy will creep in even when one thinks one is talking strictly in terms of received ethical principles. This, at least, was Annas's (1988b) contention in case 1. He argued that the certain terminal outcome for Angela Carter was allowed to intrude on the thinking of the court in inappropriate ways. Where the proper issue was that of respecting the wishes and rights of Angela Carter as an adult citizen, even in her dying, the thinking that seduced the court and led to the trampling of her rights was, "If we can no longer rescue her, can't we at least rescue the baby?" The issue officially addressed in this case was maternal autonomy and interests versus the competing interests of a possibly viable fetus. One participant in the case, objecting to Annas's analysis, argued that maternal autonomy was not violated, because in trying to save the fetus the court was simply trying to carry out the patient's previously expressed wishes and values. But in order to assess whether Annas was correct, it seems crucial to ask whether something like the rescue fantasy was operating implicitly.

A similar point could be made about cardiopulmonary resuscitation. When one raises questions about the possible futility of resuscitation or asks why resuscitation should be put in its own special category of medical treatment, the common rejoinder is, "Well, if you don't resuscitate, then the patient is dead, pure and simple. No other medical treatment poses such an immediate and stark choice between certain death and life." This rejoinder claims, by implication, that probability estimates and cost-benefit analyses applicable to any other therapy are somehow inappropriate when applied to resuscitation.

Indeed, something like the rescue fantasy may even infect so "objective" a methodology as quantitative decision analysis. One team of investigators learned from interviews that patients routinely considered certain states of prolonged disability or suffering as states to which death would be preferable. But when they reported these findings in the standard language of their discipline—by means of a utility scale ranging from zero to 100, where 100 represented the value of perfect health and zero the value of the "state worse than death" (death itself ranked a 10 or so)—their colleagues objected that there was something obviously wrong with their data analysis. The colleagues assumed that if perfect health was 100, death must be zero: a "state worse than death" was something their methodology could not handle.

The same assumptions might have been operating in a preliminary attempt to apply decision analysis to resuscitation decisions. On the first such effort, the investigator could not arrive at any data on either low probability of success or poor outcome that made it rational to write a do-not-resuscitate order, because the 100 percent probability of death without resuscitation multiplied by the low utility value assigned to death overwhelmed any figures that were plugged into the other decision options.[7] The investigator could justify a do-not-resuscitate order only when he added a negative utility evaluation for being subjected to the resuscitation procedure itself, independently of its outcome—and that indeed may be how many patients think about resuscitation and what they would use to justify their wishes not to be resuscitated. These examples show the difficulty in getting around the idea that being rescued from death is necessarily the highest good that medicine can achieve, even within the bounds of a mathematical analysis.[8]

A Problem with Aimed Power

The rescue fantasy is a feature of medical thinking that will occasionally distort ethical reasoning and yet will be missed if cases are analyzed only in the more usual terms. It displays once again a central feature of the physician's power that was discussed in chapter 2: the sense of power over disease and death is not something that physicians grasp for their own ends and that patients find threatening; it is something that serves the needs and interests of the patient as much as those of the physician, and patient behavior will in many ways tend to reinforce the sense of power. Thus, where we find a manifestation of power, such as the rescue fantasy, interfering with sound ethical reasoning, it will often not do simply to make physicians or nurses conscious of these factors. It may be necessary to

7. This happened so long as economic factors were excluded from the analysis. When economic factors were included, the analysis shifted over, and it could never be shown to be rational *not* to write a do-not-resuscitate order.

8. I am indebted to David Rovner and Robert McNutt for data and observations referred to in this paragraph.

address patient's feelings, assumptions and behaviors before anything can change.

To begin to view the rescue fantasy more precisely so as to apply to it our proposed guidelines for responsible use of power, it may be helpful to review one medical-ethics manual to see how it differs from other sets of guidelines on terminal-care decisions and the withholding of life-sustaining treatment. In *Clinical Ethics* (1986), Jonsen, Siegler, and Winslade invert the typical way of presenting ethical-decision strategies. Consider by way of contrast the report of a committee of the Hastings Center (1987), which was itself modeled after the very influential report of the President's Commission (1983). It puts forward an impressive list of fundamental values, including the benefit to the patient and the moral integrity of the health professional; but it starts off, like all similar documents, by focusing on the autonomy and the rights of the competent adult patient. From the rights of the competent adult to refuse life-prolonging treatment, the document moves to methods of substituted judgment and advance directives for those patients who have lost competence or whose wishes are not known. After considerable discussion of these ethical intricacies, it moves, almost as an afterthought, to a list of medical-care strategies that might result from the application of those decision rules, including aggressive life-prolonging care, palliative care aimed only at providing comfort, and time-limited trials when the benefits of a proposed treatment are in doubt.

Jonsen, Siegler, and Winslade elect to begin their manual (aimed primarily at house officers in internal medicine) with precisely this list of possible strategies of medical intervention. Discussion of the wishes of the competent patient and the determination of competence for these purposes deliberately occupy second place. To those who view the fundamental issue of medical ethics as patient autonomy versus physician paternalism, this inversion appears a throwback to paternalism, which can only be opposed by enshrining respect for autonomy as primary in the hierarchy of moral values. But Jonsen and colleagues reply quite reasonably that the question, "What does medicine have to offer you in your present predicament?" seems logically prior to the question, "Given those possible interventions, which, if any, do you prefer?" Jonsen, Siegler, and Winslade seem here to grasp firmly the fact of the physician's power monopoly when it comes to saying what the problem is in medical terms and specifying the range of acceptable medical responses to it.[9] This power monopoly cannot be ar-

9. As this volume is written primarily for hospital practice and does not truly reflect a primary-care perspective, it is not surprising that it gives primacy to medical considerations

tificially erased by appeals to respect for patient autonomy, however im-portant autonomy might be at the next logical step in the decision process, when an array of choices can be laid out before the patient.

I submit that the standard reference works on life-and-death decisions begin with the assumption that most ethical problems in this area are shared-power problems of autonomy versus paternalism. Jonsen and his coauthors seem to have made a useful departure from this trend by sug-gesting that the problem of *aimed* power may be more central than is often appreciated. An obvious guideline for the responsible use of power, as stated previously, is that it be aimed properly, which requires in turn that there be a clear and attainable objective, that the means chosen have a reasonable chance of attaining that objective, and that there be a discernible proportionality between means and ends.

At this point I will depart from the published literature and report from personal experience, over a seven-year period, of meeting regularly with third-year medical students on their medicine clerkship to discuss ethical issues of their choice and occasionally consulting on difficult ethical cases.[10] Although the details of the life-and-death cases under discussion differed widely, one general similarity emerged: students rarely asked about the end or goal toward which medical care was directed. My tentative conclu-sion is that this failure to ask what appears to be an obvious question is not related to any lack of thoughtfulness or clinical acumen on the part of the responsible attending physician or senior residents. Instead it seems to be the proverbial forest-and-trees problem when daily rounds inevitably become dominated by discussion of laboratory values, respirator settings, antibiotic and pressor dosages, and the like. Determining and documenting a complete set of medical diagnoses and keeping the patient alive until rounds the next morning can easily become the lone objectives of the medical team.

The unspoken but deeply persuasive rejoinder to the question of the goal of medical care is, "Why, to save lives and cure disease, of course. What else would we be doing? The reason that we don't ask the question

---

and does not reflect the importance of the patient's own view of the problem in defining what the medical problem consists of; see the discussion of Siegler's (1982b) "moments" in the physician-patient encounter in chapter 4.

10. These teaching sessions and case consultations have all occurred within community teaching hospitals. It is worth noting that these students and residents constitute the audience for which Jonsen, Siegler, and Winslade 1986 is primarily intended. I should add, however, that experiences as a visiting professor and lecturer in other settings, both university and community, have convinced me that these findings may be replicated elsewhere.

out loud or discuss it among ourselves is that the answer is obvious." If my suspicions are correct, this is the point at which the rescue fantasy exerts its most deleterious effects. For to ask the question that Jonsen, Siegler, and Winslade propose—What can and should a medical intervention accomplish in a given case?—is tantamount to admitting that in many instances we lack the power to cure disease and save lives. I think it may well be comforting for the medical team, on its daily rounds among desperately ill and unfortunate patients, to avoid looking too directly at this unpleasant rejection of the rescue fantasy. If instead they talk of blood gases and peak-and-trough levels of aminoglycosides, the rescue fantasy is allowed to live on and cast at least a weak glow over their proceedings.

The problem is that a significant number of "ethical dilemmas" regarding life-prolonging treatment remain essentially insoluble so long as the question of medical goals remains unasked, and they virtually answer themselves as soon as that key question is raised. As this statement may seem simplistic and can be conclusively proven only by looking at a long series of case studies, I shall offer only one example. One of the cases presented to me as a teaching exercise by the third-year medicine clerks involved an elderly patient with a spreading malignancy who was in considerable pain. She had expressed some wishes previously about the aggressiveness of her anticancer treatment but was now in a depressed state of consciousness and could not enter actively into the decision-making process. Her family was distraught at her pain and wished to discontinue some of the treatment that the patient had previously requested. Not unnaturally, they claimed that they knew the patient better than the physicians did and that they felt confident she would not have consented to the treatment protocol had she known she would be in such pain. The attending physician and residents were approaching the problem as choosing between the two sets of conflicting wishes; and given both that they personally agreed with the plan for more aggressive care and felt that the patient's pain was unduly influencing the family's choice, they had thus far felt justified in overruling the family's request.

A few questions along the line proposed by Jonsen and his colleagues revealed two important conclusions that had not previously received any discussion within the medical team. First, the students could agree that the possibility for cure was nonexistent and the prognosis for life extension poor, either with or without the aggressive anticancer therapy. Second, they recognized that the problems of pain management had never received more than cursory attention within the array of therapeutic decisions. (Moreover, they had to admit that they had not, as part of their didactic training in internal medicine so far, received any instruction on the various modes of pain and symptom control that are now commonly employed in hospice units.) They quickly reached the conclusions that the team had been devoting too much attention to "treating" the cancer and not enough to alleviating the symptoms. They also began to realize that their dilemma might disappear if they did succeed in better addressing the patient's unmet needs for pain control. First, the patient herself might regain sufficient mental capacity to clarify her own wishes. Second, if the family saw that the medical team was attending to their primary concern—pain—they might become more amenable to a further trial of life-prolonging treatment. Of all the ways to get a handle on the case—that is, to intervene at one point in such a manner as to produce positive changes at several later points—better pain management emerged as the best candidate. Even so, the sheer inhumanity of the previous neglect of the patient's pain never entered the discussion.[11]

As the case was initially presented by the students, the rescue fantasy seemed to have seriously misled the medical team, made up of competent and humane people. The questions they chose to address were, "Should we try to prolong life or not?" and "Should we listen to the patient or to her family?" These questions fit the standard ethical guidelines as to how such decisions are supposed to be made. But they also served to obscure the unpleasant fact that the medical team lacked the power to affect this cancer much one way or the other. The patient herself may not have wanted to hear about this degree of medical impotence, and the rescue fantasy may initially have been as much a function of her needs as the physicians'.

The patient's pain came to serve two essential functions in the physicians' thinking about the case. First, it justified ignoring the wishes of the family, who were emotionally distressed because of the patient's pain and therefore unable to reason clearly about medical issues. Second, the pain may have served to keep the rescue fantasy alive even when the patient's poor prognosis and lack of response to treatment threatened to undermine it. The thinking behind the self-image of the team may have unwittingly and

11. This reinforces the point made regarding the "Debbie case" in chapter 5. By focusing attention on the termination of life-sustaining treatment as the major ethical issue, medicine has neatly avoided focusing on its own abysmal record in the area of humane symptom control. This point is made forcefully in Wanzer et al. 1989. It is symptomatic of the problem that the paper by Wanzer and colleagues devotes several pages to documenting the need for improved care of the dying and then appends brief discussions of assisted suicide and active euthanasia; the lay media (and most ethics commentators) picked up immediately on the two concluding sections and largely ignored the bulk of the article. See also Angell 1982.

imperceptibly developed into something like this: "The poor lady is experiencing tremendous pain. If we were weaker, we would give in to our natural inclinations and allow her to die more peacefully and quickly. But she turned to us in her need precisely because she expected us to be tough in carrying out her wishes. So we must steel ourselves to the unpleasantness and go on doing what we know is for the best, and what she herself wanted." That is, their ability to see her in pain, and to go on unflinchingly with the aggressive therapy, may have become a perverse test of their "power." That this so-called power was basically a cover-up for their impotence could emerge only when key questions about medical goals were raised.

It is not surprising that these surmises based on personal experience are not widely confirmed by published research, since to my knowledge no one has suggested that the rescue fantasy is a feature of ethical decision making worthy of explicit study. They suggest that a number of life-and-death cases hinge on problems with discovering and implementing the patient's own requests, and in those situations the authoritative guidelines and reports cited above will be of help. But in at least as many other cases, the problem is rather a failure to discern what medical interventions are possible and useful and to address the particular goals to which they are aimed.[12]

The terminology *rescue fantasy* suggests the error that occurs when physicians overestimate what medicine can do for a seriously ill or dying patient. Clearly, however, physicians might also underestimate what medical intervention can accomplish; this, at any rate, is now a standard complaint in geriatric medicine regarding the withholding of care from the elderly.[13] The physician abuse of power associated with underestimating what medicine can do is usually a form of relabeling, in which apparently authoritative reasons for inaction are given to cover up the physician's not wanting to deal with the patient.

A controversial but nevertheless illustrative example of the relabeling charge occurs in the British Medical Association's recent report on eu-

12. A similar point about geriatric medicine distinguishes between medical strategies that seek accurate diagnoses aimed toward possible cure and the (more fitting) strategies that seek to maximize patient functional ability; see Williams and Hadler 1983.

13. See chapter 12 for a discussion of withholding possibly beneficial treatment in the name of cost savings. In Brody 1987d (pp. 161–70) I address briefly a major dilemma of geriatric medicine: whether to accept that the elderly are near the ends of their lives and that many treatments will not work, and so lay itself open to charges of ageism; or to insist on aggressive treatment for all the elderly and thereby administer many treatments that will prove to be inappropriate or harmful.

thanasia, in which the BMA condemned the Dutch policy of quasi-legal voluntary active euthanasia. The BMA charges, not that active euthanasia is inherently immoral, but rather that it is clinically lazy. The claim is put forth that through a combination of symptom control and emotional and spiritual support, the physician can almost always provide relief of whatever is distressing a dying patient and might otherwise lead that patient to ask to be killed. But to do this the physician has to be willing to listen carefully to the patient's view of his predicament and indeed to share in the patient's anguish. In effect, the BMA charges (fairly or unfairly) that the Dutch physicians have opted for the easy way out by their willingness to end the patient's life quickly. If the BMA case could be fully supported—obviously the Dutch physicians take a different view of the matter—we would have an interesting example of the medical power to relabel as desirable and professionally responsible what actually amounts to a case of undertreatment and patient avoidance.[14]

The abuse of power inherent in the undertreatment of the seriously or terminally ill is different from the rescue fantasy in one important way: it is much less likely that patients will be willing collaborators, consciously or unconsciously, in the perpetuation of the practice. This in turn suggests that the guideline of shared power should be the most potent protection from the abuse of undertreatment. I have been arguing in this chapter that the basic problem with the rescue fantasy, on the other hand, is the problem of aimed power. Ultimately, however, proper care of the seriously ill or dying patient demands all three characteristics of the responsible use of power. The physician must discern the appropriate and reachable goals and choose medical interventions proportionate to them. The patient must be informed of the range of choices within responsible medical practice and encouraged to participate actively in the decisions. And, perhaps hardest of all, the physician must own the use or nonuse of power and try to avoid potentially destructive, unarticulated pacts with the patient to overstate the true extent of medical power. This point takes us back to the issue of truthful disclosure; but where the rescue fantasy exerts its power, there may be no explicit untruth or lack of disclosure. Rather, the physician and patient may effectively agree between them to talk about certain aspects of the treatment and avoid or skim over discussion of other aspects. It is not a "believing" or a "thinking" so much as an "acting as if." It is therefore

14. This report was published by the British Medical Association in April 1988; for further discussion, see chapter 5.

much harder to discern the line between those styles of communication that conceal essential truths and those that simply allow the patient to hang onto needed hope. In owning the true degree of powerlessness over the disease process the physician may feel as if she is letting the patient down too hard and too fast.[15]

Now to summarize the arguments of this chapter on the power implications of care for the seriously ill or dying patient:

1. *Aimed power* requires that physicians carefully specify the realistic goals toward which medical therapy is directed, and the appropriate means to achieve them. Physicians must be aware that the stresses of day-to-day practice and the fragmented nature of much of modern technological care will undermine this sort of thoughtful management and assessment unless they constantly remind themselves of the need for it. They must avoid thinking that the good intentions and noble goals of medicine suffice to define the goals and ends for specific patients. They must avoid both giving in to the rescue fantasy and inappropriately writing off elderly or less desirable patients.

2. *Shared power* becomes a special challenge in a group of patients whose serious illnesses render them powerless. The authoritative reports on care for these patients have listed numerous helpful strategies to allow the degree of patient empowerment that is optimal under these circumstances. Of special concern within a primary-care orientation is the value of anticipatory decision making, such devices as advance directives, and enhancement of discussions within family groups in support of realistic planning. An avoidable tragedy is that of the patient whose present crisis and deterioration could readily have been anticipated but for whom decisions must now be made in a vacuum because the physician failed to mention this contingency to the patient when the patient was fully capable of making some key choices. To the extent that the seriously ill patient is vulnerable or pow-

15. The general tone of these remarks would suggest that the physician who has little power to alter a disease state, based on a sound assessment of available medical technology, should be forthright in admitting this to the patient, and instead should focus their joint efforts toward relieving symptoms and improving the quality of life during the time remaining. It is only fair to mention the work of Siegel (1986, 1989), who would defend the need not to lie to patients but would nevertheless insist that a much more positive statement of possible outcomes is necessary to mobilize the patient's inner resources fully and to achieve the best results. Further research will be needed to determine whether this disagreement represents only a difference in physician style or whether more substantive issues in patient care are at stake; see, for example, Thomas 1987.

erless, effective sharing of power entails finding ways to involve the patient at earlier stages when capacity is preserved and empowering the family or others who can act on the patient's behalf.

3. *Owned power* requires a high degree of physician self-awareness and reflection, particularly with regard to transference and countertransference issues. Physicians must be willing to face squarely the ways in which they are using power and to acknowledge emotional distortions (like the rescue fantasy or the desire to avoid unpleasant patients) that might interfere with rational analysis of the medical goals and options. In appropriate circumstances, patients may need to be confronted with some of these issues, especially when the rescue fantasy becomes a matter of physician-patient collaboration.[16]

16. This confrontation demands that the physician own his role in perpetuating the rescue fantasy and not simply accuse the patient of being unrealistic; acknowledge the positive aspects (hope and optimism) as well as the negative aspects of the patient's request for continued aggressive treatment; and find alternative modes of treatment that preserve the positive aspects as much as possible, so that the decision is never to stop treatment but rather to switch to a more appropriate plan of treatment.

Bernice M. has had multiple sclerosis for ten years. Now sixty years old, she lacks the strength or stamina to do most of the activities that have made life enjoyable and meaningful for her. Two years ago she attempted suicide by taking an overdose of medication; she was, however, successfully treated and returned home. The psychiatric care that she received after that did not alter her fixed state of depression; and the psychiatrists declared that although depressed, she was able to make rational decisions. Last month she completed a "living will" declaring that she did not wish to be kept alive by artificial means, specifically by mechanical ventilation; at the same time she executed a durable power of attorney and appointed her husband as her surrogate to make medical-care decisions on her behalf.

Yesterday, her husband and daughter were away from home for several hours. When they returned they found Bernice unconscious on the kitchen floor, her breathing very slow and shallow. Her bottle of benzodiazepine capsules (a Valium-like substance used to control muscle spasms in multiple sclerosis and other neurological diseases) was empty.

In their first panic the husband and daughter called for the paramedics, who found Bernice breathing only three or four times a minute when they arrived; they began resuscitation and rushed her to the nearest emergency room. By the time they got to the hospital, Mr. M. and his daughter had had time to reconsider, and they now demanded that resuscitative efforts be stopped and that no mechanical ventilator be used. They were overruled and these treatments were instituted; Bernice, still unconscious, was taken to the intensive care unit.

Today the hospital ethics committee has been asked to help resolve the ongoing dispute between the primary-care physician and the M. family.

(Bernice is still unconscious and dependent on a respirator.) Mr. M.'s argument is that he has in hand the durable power of attorney entitling him to make a decision to disconnect the ventilator, as well as the living will showing that that choice indeed accords with Bernice's wishes. Moreover, the suicide attempt itself was a clear statement that Bernice wished to die and that she found her present state of existence unacceptable. The physicians have told Mr. M. that because of prolonged lack of oxygen to her brain, the chances are quite high that even if Bernice recovers consciousness, she will be even further disabled than she had been previously; and he considers this yet another reason to withdraw the respirator.

The primary physician agrees with the logic of these points so far as they go but feels obligated to demur. He states that only at such time as he is certain that the continued coma and dependence on a respirator is due to hypoxic brain damage rather than to the effect of the medication overdose will he agree to discontinue the ventilator. Because the benzodiazepine has a long serum half-life, it could still be accounting for all the patient's symptoms, and it will take another twenty-four to thirty-six hours to be sure that the drug is out of Bernice's system. He distinguishes between his duty to follow Bernice's wishes if he decides that she is terminally or irreversibly ill and a solicitation that he aid and abet her suicide attempt. He refuses to do the latter. He even questions, under the present circumstances, the moral validity of the advance directives that Bernice had recently executed. It is quite possible that she already had in mind her suicide attempt when she executed them, and he asks whether the documents themselves constitute evidence of preexisting suicidal ideation—hence evidence of incapacity to make a rational choice at that time.

Why might the ethics committee find Bernice M.'s case troubling or complex? Certainly at one level it should be easy to resolve. A patient, judged competent by her psychiatrists, executed clear advance directives; her duly appointed surrogate has refused treatment for her; and evidence from several sources shows that this refusal is entirely consistent with Bernice M.'s prior and consistent wishes. It therefore seems a gross violation of patient rights and autonomy to continue treatment for any period of time.

But this simple appeal to patient autonomy and advance directives seems at least incomplete. Many courts, as well as distinguished expert panels (Guidelines Committee 1987), have held that a death from the refusal of life-sustaining treatment should not be construed as suicide; but taking an overdose of medication at home is blatantly a suicide attempt, however good one's reasons for it might be. A number of distinguished physicians would argue that in some circumstances, the physician might morally assist a patient's suicide by providing the means to carry it out (Wanzer et al. 1989). But few would suggest that the physician who has not agreed in advance to aid in a suicide attempt ought to be dragged into it as an accessory after the fact.

Ultimately this question seems to come down to a power struggle. Does the patient's power to choose her own treatment (through a surrogate if she herself is later incompetent) extend to the power to force physicians to implement or enable a type of death to which they morally object? Is the physician's power to refuse to aid in a suicide attempt being used responsibly when it forces a patient to remain alive, to face a quality of existence she finds horrid, by the use of medical means she finds repugnant?

The thesis of this chapter is that power struggles like this frequently accompany decisions on life-sustaining therapy for incompetent patients, but that the language of substituted judgment and best interests often employed in these cases may obscure this fact. In particular, that language may be used to suggest an *objective* standard for decisions and hence conceal the fact that considerable personal discretion has been, and indeed must be, employed by the various decision makers, physician and surrogate alike.

The Evolution of the Issues

The historical evolution of this set of ethical issues runs through several stages. In part this evolution parallels the development of the "new" ethics as discussed in chapter 4; but to some extent it has been influenced by other social and political factors in the 1980s.

It is generally thought that these issues did not arise during most of the history of Western medicine, because physicians had so little power to alter the course of serious or terminal illness. This assertion has to be greeted with at least some skepticism. For example, the account of George Washington's death provided by his attending physicians indicated that the general was alert and coherent during most of his fatal illness and at one point expressed a clear wish to be allowed to die peacefully without further medical meddling; the record suggests that this wish was not honored (Blanton 1931, pp. 305–06). Nevertheless, as a rule, questions about withholding or withdrawing life-sustaining treatment received little discussion.

In the 1950s and 1960s, medicine entered what Jonsen (1986a) has called the age of rescue. New technology, including respirators, cardiopulmonary resuscitation, kidney dialysis, organ transplants, and various wonder drugs suddenly offered the hope of extending life where none had previously existed. During this period it would have seemed ungrateful to question the use of these technologies or wonder if patients would ever be better off forgoing them.

The partial disillusionment with technology corresponded to the arrival of the new ethics, with its emphasis on patient autonomy, in the late 1960s and the 1970s. Although philosophers are fond of insisting that medical ethics and medical law are distinct disciplines, and what is legal does not determine what is ethical and vice versa, it nevertheless remains true that a series of court decisions, starting with the 1976 *Quinlan* case in New Jersey, established the tone for this period of thinking on a patient's right to refuse life-sustaining treatment. These court decisions occupied a prominent place in most books on medical ethics published during that period, especially the influential President's Commission report (1983).

The series of court decisions that affirmed and extended *Quinlan*, ultimately to more than sixty separate rulings in at least twenty states, was notable for relative unanimity on certain key points, even though some subsidiary issues (for example, when physicians should be required to seek court approval before withdrawing treatment) were hotly debated. In retrospect, this apparent unanimity may have created a premature sense of national consensus; and yet public opinion polls reinforced this sense by showing that 80 percent or more of the population endorsed the so-called right to die in its various manifestations.

The points of near unanimity among the "Quinlan series" are strikingly consistent with the "new" ethics of patient autonomy:

1. Competent patients have the right to refuse any medical treatment, life-sustaining or not.

2. When a patient loses competence, this right to refuse treatment can be exercised on the patient's behalf by a family member or other appropriate surrogate.

3. The death of a patient as a result of withholding or withdrawing life-sustaining medical treatment can be clearly distinguished legally from either suicide or homicide.

4. The right to refuse treatment is not treatment-specific. In particular, artifically administered nutrition or hydration is no different from any other form of medical treatment, despite the fact that it could be considered "food and water" and hence "ordinary" or morally required care.

5. The surrogate's decision is most trustworthy when it can be shown to adhere closely to the specific wishes or preferences previously expressed by the patient when he was competent. The surrogate's decision becomes more subject to outside review or overruling when the patient's own wishes

are harder to discern. The most difficult cases are those in which the patient
has never previously been competent (newborn infants and mentally retarded adults).

6. Although the state (and presumably medicine) has a duty to protect
and prolong life, not all life requires equal efforts in this regard. In particular,
permanent unconsciousness, a terminal prognosis, an irreversible illness,
or unremitting pain and suffering all create a prima facie presumption that
a patient's or surrogate's request to forgo life-sustaining treatment is a
rational choice. (Many would deny that this means that life in those states
is of lesser value, but it seems undeniable that the duty to prolong life is
lessened in those circumstances. Ultimately, any question of the value or
the quality of one's life is left to the autonomous individual rather than to
either the courts or the medical profession.)

With the end of the 1980s, matters seem to have arrived at a new phase,
perhaps epitomized most clearly by the case of *Cruzan* v. *Harmon* in Missouri, the first "right to die" case appealed to the U.S. Supreme Court.[1]
The *Cruzan* ruling by the Missouri court is striking in breaking markedly,
and with little by way of supporting argumentation, with the entire *Quinlan*
series of decisions. Indeed, the divergence from the consensus can be seen
at almost every point. In *Cruzan* the Missouri court felt that the notion of
a right to refuse life-sustaining treatment (based in turn on a constitutional
privacy right) had been greatly overblown by previous courts and that the
state's duty to preserve life had been correspondingly undervalued. A persistent vegetative state was not evidence of the rationality of ending treatment; it was instead an indication of special vulnerability requiring more
diligent state protection of the life of the patient. Nutrition and hydration
are clearly different from other medical treatments, and much more stringent tests must be met before these could be withdrawn. Last, the refusal
of treatment by a surrogate must be viewed as an extension of the *parens
patriae* power of the state, and not in any meaningful way as an extension
of the autonomy of the formerly competent individual.[2]

1. This chapter was completed prior to the Supreme Court's decision in *Cruzan* (June
1990). The Court refused to set any national standard for treatment withdrawal decisions
and upheld Missouri's right to set a very strict standard if it chooses. It is therefore still
worthwhile to look at the factors that led the Missouri high court to trounce the Quinlan
doctrine. For an analysis of the legal impact of the final *Cruzan* ruling, see Weir and Gostin
1990.

2. Annas (1989) has commented perceptively that these positions of the Missouri Supreme
Court seem anomalous and counterintuitive (at least to those brought up on the *Quinlan*
series teachings) to the extent that one views the Missouri court as trying to say something

The *Cruzan* case is not an isolated phenomenon. Federal efforts in the "Baby Doe" arena—the Reagan administration actions, the 1984 federal law on medical abuse and neglect (Rhoden and Arras 1985), and the U.S. Civil Rights Commission report (1989)—all fit philosophically with a distrust of familial and surrogate decision making on behalf of newborns with serious birth defects. A few other court decisions, notably *O'Connor* in New York (Annas 1988a), had also deviated from the *Quinlan* principles, although not as strikingly as had *Cruzan*. With active euthanasia being openly practiced in the Netherlands, and with the Hemlock Society working to legalize active euthanasia through referendums in California and Washington, the court may have felt that the entire notion of a right to die had got out of hand and needed to be severely curtailed. And to those who pointed to the narrow 4–3 margin of votes in the *Cruzan* ruling, others were ready to reply that a substantial number of court rulings in the *Quinlan* series had been based on similarly narrow margins—again suggesting that the *Quinlan* series had hinted at a level of consensus that did not in fact exist.

The shift in perceptions and attitudes that resulted in *Cruzan* has, for our purposes, two distinct elements. First, one can discern within medical ethics a growing dissatisfaction with the patient-autonomy ethic, at least as applied to the practice of surrogate decision making. It began to occur to some commentators that either medicine as a profession or society at large ought to have some basic values that are relevant to life-and-death treatment decisions. The idea that *any* treatment refusal was morally compelling simply because it was the patient's autonomous choice (or an extension of it) was called into question (Siegler and Weisbard 1985; May et al. 1987; B. Brody 1988a; Gaylin et al. 1988). This element parallels the "newer" medical ethics, which seeks to move beyond an exclusive reliance on patient autonomy and toward a renewed sense of the values of the profession of medicine as well as a more communitarian ethic generally.

There is, however, a second element that seems a part of the political life of the United States in the 1980s rather than an intellectual feature of debates within medical ethics. This is the growing strength of the right-to-life movement under two presidential administrations dedicated to cultivating the support of that political-religious lobby. What had in the 1970s

about Nancy Cruzan, a young woman in a persistent vegetative state being kept alive by tube feedings. If on the other hand one views the decision as an effort to establish an analogy between right-to-die cases and abortion cases—previously decided in Missouri in the *Webster* decision, also reviewed by the U.S. Supreme Court—then the reasoning becomes more coherent, even if ultimately mistaken.

been the view of a vocal and committed but small segment of the population suddenly became stated national policy in the 1980s, with the president of the United States endorsing these views and taking care to appoint to the Supreme Court only justices who could be counted on to promote them. This in turn created a sociopolitical climate in which it seemed very middle-of-the-road to question the extent to which an individual's right of free choice could be allowed to take precedence over the preservation of life—whether one was talking about a fetus or an adult. This change in the sociopolitical climate (I would assert) was unaccompanied by any shift in the intellectual ground in the abortion debate: no distinctive philosophical or religious arguments were introduced, and no new empirical data emerged to show that the practice of abortion (or of forgoing life-sustaining treatment) had unanticipated deleterious consequences. The shift was purely one of political power.

It is most important here to focus on two points at issue between the "new" and the "newer" ethic: substituted judgment and the assessment of quality of life. Superficially, there has been agreement across the board that quality-of-life judgments are to be distrusted. Indeed, that *Quinlan* series courts ritualistically denounced the notion of quality of life while proceeding to make blatant quality-of-life judgments (such as that sapient life is more worthy of preservation than unconscious life) should be a strong clue that the *Quinlan* consensus was much shakier than it appeared. There has been much more disagreement about substituted judgment, with the *Quinlan* era relying strongly on the notion and the *Cruzan* era strongly questioning it.

Substituted Judgment and the Fallacy of Objectivity

The general acceptance of the notion of substituted judgment by the post-*Quinlan* courts fits perfectly with the ascendency of the "new" ethics. If I am now capable of autonomous choice and can foresee a later time when I will be incapable of it; and I direct now that I want to be treated at that time in a manner consistent with my enduring values and preferences, then it would appear that honoring my presently stated choice in that later set of circumstances is a way of respecting my autonomy. So long as we make minor allowances for problems of inaccurate interpretation of stated wishes, conflicts of interest of surrogates, unanticipated circumstances, and so forth, any ethic that claims to value autonomy would seem naturally to find advance directives of this sort controlling. And by logical extension, if I have not actually stated my wishes in that future situation but those close to me can infer my wishes by a reasoning process that others would find acceptable, respect for autonomy would seem to require that those inferred wishes be honored no less than my stated wishes would have been. Anyone offering arguments to the contrary would seem to be motivated by a vitalist or sanctity-of-life position, which would deny even to competent patients the right to refuse any life-prolonging treatment whatsoever.

To see both what is morally informative about the substituted-judgment standard as well as what may be confused about it, it is helpful to return to one of the earliest and most influential cases in the series of decisions that were influenced by Quinlan. In 1977, the Massachusetts Supreme Court ruled that Joseph Saikewicz, a sixty-seven-year-old mentally retarded man with acute myelogenous leukemia, need not undergo chemotherapy (which was thought to have a 30–50 percent chance of extending his life by two to thirteen months and which also had significant toxicity).[3] The court stated that it was employing a substituted-judgment standard in determining what Saikewicz's own preferences would be were he able to make a choice for himself (pp. 430–31).

Paul Ramsey, in criticizing the Saikewicz decision, elected to focus on one sentence in the ruling: "The decision in such cases should be that which would be made by the incompetent person, if that person were competent, but taking into account the present and future incompetency of the individual as one of the factors which would necessarily enter into the decision-making process" (p. 431). To Ramsey, this convoluted sentence proved conclusively that the court had no idea what it was talking about— or rather, that the substituted-judgment standard was merely a coverup for free-ranging subjectivity (Ramsey 1978). Ramsey here foreshadowed the reasons why the New York high court rejected the substituted-judgment standard in a later case involving a mentally retarded adult; to ask what an incompetent person would decide if competent is tantamount to asking, "If it snowed all summer, would it then be winter?" (quoted in Gutheil and Appelbaum 1983, p. 9).

And yet this criticism, though clever, fundamentally distorts the reasoning the Massachusetts court actually employed:

---

3. Superintendent of Belchertown State School v. Saikewicz, Mass. 370 N.E. 2nd 417. (Page numbers for quotations are supplied in the text.) At the time, medical commentators focused on one fairly minor portion of the Saikewicz decision, which would have required judicial review for all cases of that type. The medical press generally denounced this stipulation and referred back to Quinlan, which had suggested that physicians and families rather than courts should make decisions on behalf of incompetent patients. In later Massachusetts cases that court considerably softened its judicial-review requirement, and in retrospect Saikewicz seems to fit coherently within the Quinlan series.

One would have to ask whether a majority of people would choose chemotherapy if they were told merely that something outside of their previous experience was going to be done to them, that this something would cause them pain and discomfort, that they would be removed to strange surroundings and possibly restrained for extended periods of time, and that the advantages of this course of action were measured by concepts of time and mortality beyond their ability to comprehend. (p. 430)

This passage reads less like unbridled subjectivity and more like a disciplined effort to imagine what the experience of chemotherapy would be like for a man with a mental age of three who had lived all his life in an institution. Unless one had previously concluded (as Ramsey had) that the only means of serving the interests of an incompetent patient is to try to extend life no matter what the costs in suffering, one is likely to find this line of reasoning worthy of consideration.

Later critics of the substituted-judgment concept focused on a 1981 Massachusetts decision in a psychiatric case (Gutheil and Appelbaum 1983).[4] Presumably, a substituted-judgment standard (in which the court decides what X would have chosen for himself could he have done so) is quite different from a best-interests standard (in which the court decides what it thinks would be best for X). By contrast, Gutheil and Appelbaum argue that it is inevitable that substituted judgment will collapse into best-interest decisions. In particular, if X was previously competent and stated that he would wish for Y, the decision to provide Y for the now-incompetent X is based on the assumption that the circumstances now are substantially the same as those which X envisioned when he made his preferences known. But this cannot be true, since the question of substituted judgment would never come up unless circumstances were substantially different—at least in the sense that a competent individual has become incompetent, and probably in other ways as well.

What is most worth noting here about these criticisms of substituted judgment is the degree of subjectivity attributed to those applying the standard. Ramsey (1978) found this subjectivity unacceptable and preferred

4. In the Matter of Guardianship of Richard Roe III, Mass. 421 N.E. 2d 40. Gutheil and Appelbaum intend their commentary to demonstrate that substituted-judgment reasoning always collapses into best-interest reasoning. However, because the Roe decision dealt specifically with the sticky issue of psychiatric treatment for an incompetent patient, and because that court introduced several dubious elements of substituted judgment that had not been a part of the Saikewicz ruling, it seems impossible to apply Gutheil and Appelbaum's comments beyond Roe.

an objective standard: always extend the life of the incompetent patient. Gutheil and Appelbaum (1983) call for frank admission of subjectivity as inevitable in any such decision. What the critics seem to have in common, however, is a sense that what makes substituted judgment attractive to the courts is precisely its apparent objectivity. Show the courts that this appearance of objectivity is illusory, they seem to be saying, and the courts would soon lose interest in substituted judgment. And yet the Massachusetts court in *Saikewicz* forthrightly noted the inherently subjective quality of substituted judgment: "We should make it plain that the primary test is subjective in nature—that is, the goal is to determine with as much accuracy as possible the wants and needs of the individual involved" (p. 430).

Criticizing the substituted-judgment standard from a different direction, Rhoden (1988) tends to agree with the irreducible subjectivity of the judgments that must be made. It is mostly family members who speak on behalf of the incompetent patient; and in most of the *Quinlan* series of cases the courts have found good reasons to agree with the family's choice. Typically, a court looks for signs of antipathy, conflict of interest, or other factors that might make one family member an inappropriate decision maker on another's behalf. Finding none, it then proceeds to uphold the family's wishes—and also to justify them according to the substituted-judgment doctrine. In cases where there has been a straightforward declaration of preference by the previously competent patient, the substituted-judgment rationale is highly persuasive. In other cases, like those criticized by the authors noted above, the substituted-judgment model can be made to fit the facts of the case only with considerable strain. Rhoden's proposal is to consider dropping the substituted-judgment standard in favor of a family choice standard, whereby family members would be allowed to decide on behalf of an incompetent relative unless evidence could be brought forth showing a specific reason to disqualify them.

There are two problems with Rhoden's proposal. First, what about persons who have no family? What instructions should be given to the guardian or whoever is forced to make decisions on their behalf? To say, "Make the choice that she herself would have made had she been competent to do so," may be easy or difficult according to the circumstances; but at least it offers a bit more guidance than, "Choose as her family would have chosen for her had she had a family." Second, the family who are gathered around the seriously ill, incompetent patient may be in need of guidance just as any guardian would; and the substituted-judgment standard, whatever its legal status, may provide that guidance. Some preliminary data suggest that families make decisions that more closely match the decisions made by competent elderly persons when they are given substituted-judgment guidance instead of more generic instructions (Tomlinson et al. 1990).[5]

It therefore seems possible to conclude that the *Saikewicz* court was on to something morally important when it described its decision procedure. And yet the label *substituted judgment* continues to cause trouble. According to later formulations of surrogate decision procedures (Guidelines Committee 1987), the *Saikewicz* case offered just about the worst possible illustration of the concept of substituted judgment. Substituted judgment makes the most sense when applied to a previously competent adult who had communicated at least some consistent values and preferences, if not specific choices, regarding health care. It makes the least sense when applied to someone who was never competent and whose health-care wishes are largely unknown. In retrospect, one can say that the *Saikewicz* court made a best-interests determination, not a substituted-judgment determination.

In conclusion, if the *Saikewicz* court made the correct choice, it might be because they construed substituted judgment to mean something like, "Do not take patients for granted. Do not assume any patient fits into a standard mold. Strive to understand each patient's individuality, to empathize with the patient's suffering and distress, and then to act on that understanding" (Welch 1989, p. 1634).

Best Interests and Quality of Life

A search for objective criteria has also motivated some calls for the use of the best-interests standard.[6] This has been especially true in neonatology, where substituted judgment is implausible. The various federal initiatives around Baby Doe cases, whether categorized as prohibitions of discrimination against the handicapped or as prohibitions of medical neglect (Rhoden and Arras 1985), all share a common trust in a best-interests

5. Although there are conceptual problems with getting rid of the substituted-judgment standard in favor of a family privacy standard, one interesting study tends to offer empirical support for the latter. When a group of elderly people in rural Kentucky was intensively interviewed, the overwhelming majority both wished and expected that their families would make medical-treatment decisions for them if they became incompetent. They wished this not because the family could be trusted to make the same decision they would—indeed, they could not say now what they would want then—but because whatever choice their own family made would therefore be the correct choice (High and Turner 1987). It would be interesting to repeat this study in other geographic regions and with other populations to see how widespread this sense of family solidarity is.

6. A helpful observation is made by Welch (1989), who notes that the concept of best interests first emerged in those areas of property and estate law where the items in dispute could be measured in monetary terms. It is therefore easier to see how the concept of best interests could convey, to the legally informed observer, an aura of objectivity that it does not possess when transported into the medical arena.

standard that can be rendered medically objective.[7] It is assumed that there are a few exceptional situations where medical treatment will not serve the child's interests; in all other cases, medical treatment should be mandated and parental wishes thereby rendered irrelevant.

By contrast, quality-of-life judgments are held to be intolerably subjective and primarily a disguised way of ridding the world of classes of people deemed by the majority as not being of sufficient social worth. Ritualistic denunciations of quality-of-life thinking therefore appear frequently in the federal Baby Doe guidelines and in such court decisions as *Saikewicz*. These denunciations serve to hide the fact that quality-of-life judgments are unavoidable in trying to reach humane medical-treatment decisions on behalf of seriously ill patients. The Baby Doe law, for example, stipulates that withholding treatment is not medical neglect if the child is irreversibly comatose, if treatment would only prolong dying, or if treatment is virtually futile and inhumane. It is hard to analyze these exceptions as anything other than quality-of-life assessments (Rhoden and Arras 1985). Similarly, the reasoning of the *Saikewicz* court seems unavoidably (and appropriately) to revolve around the question of the quality of Joseph Saikewicz's life with and without a course of chemotherapy.

Some competent individuals, making a choice about medical treatment, might decide in such a way as to exclude all quality-of-life considerations. A religious person, for example, might feel a duty to live regardless of the dysfunction, suffering, or other consequences of prolonged ill health. Yet it seems that most people give some weight to the probable quality of their lives were they to pursue the various treatment options. This being the case, it is hard to see why quality-of-life considerations, properly understood, should be excluded from decision making for the incompetent, unless we wish to deprive the incompetent of the sorts of care that the competent routinely choose for themselves. The key, then, is *properly understood*. Would it not do simply to stipulate that quality of life, in this context, means the sorts of things competent people take into account in deciding

---

7. In this regard the latest report of the U.S. Commission on Civil Rights (1989) presents an interesting irony. The courts had overruled previous efforts to regulate Baby Doe decisions under the rubric of "discrimination against the handicapped" because there was no compelling evidence of systematic bias infecting the decisions that were being made. The 1989 report attempts to document just such bias among the pediatricians and hospital staff that inform parents about the life prospects of their deformed newborns. But if this bias is indeed present to the extent argued, then it is hard to discern any objective medical standards that would govern how such infants ought to be treated if they are not to be discriminated against.

how much continued life is worth *to themselves* and excludes all crude
utilitarian judgments of social worth or value of one's life to others?

This strategy may indeed define quality of life in a morally coherent
way, but it may not define the optimal decision strategy for cases involving
incompetent patients. One of the problems with the best-interests-of-the-
infant formulation is that it seems, on reflection, morally arbitrary to insist
that the infant is the only person whose interests ought to be considered
(Arras 1984; Brody 1988a). At the very least, it would seem that parents
and families might have some vital interests worthy of being assigned some
moral weight, even if the interests of the parents do not overrule those of
the infant except in very unusual cases (Strong 1983a).

An American and European panel of authorities on ethics took quite a
different approach in addressing issues concerning the never-competent
group of patients, which includes newborns. The panel argued that in
typical medical decisions at least five categories of interests may be present:
(1) the patient's; (2) the surrogate's or family's; (3) the physician's and
those of other caregivers; (4) the health-care institution's, where continuing
or withholding treatment may have religious, financial, and legal implications and may expose the institution to unfavorable publicity; (5) society's, including both the use of economic resources and the need for
research to help future patients (International Working Conference 1989,
p. 703). The panel went on to suggest:

> Normally, the patient's interest should be regarded as paramount. . . .
> It is important to remember, however, that in the cases most com-
> monly encountered, the various interests are not necessarily in conflict.
> Often the patient's own interest is integrally interwoven with the
> interest of the family and the community. Part of the physician's
> clinical wisdom consists of responsibly weighing interests and cre-
> atively resolving apparently irreconcilable conflicts (p. 703).

Such a statement would be quite unusual coming from an American
ethics panel; the reference to the physician's "clinical wisdom" seems too
close to medical paternalism for comfort, and the idea that the physician
should wisely and creatively balance all of these interests sounds too much
like a prescription for "playing God." Still, there is a lesson here: exclusive
focus on the patient's best interests, far from leading to moral purity, could
actually be a form of moral laziness. To be sure, if the only way to promote
the interests of the family, community, and society is to violate fundamental
interests of the patient, concern for the patient must come first. But what

if all of the vital patient interests have been protected and minor modifications in procedure or behavior could end up serving the interests of the family or the community? Would we say that the physician had made the ethically optimal decision if she merely watched out for the best interests of the patient and failed to take this opportunity to maximize the interests of other concerned parties?[8]

Power on Behalf of the Incompetent Patient

The responsible use of power on behalf of an incompetent patient occurs when the medical decision has the following characteristics:

1. The wishes and preferences of the patient (if previously competent) are acted on as far as possible, taking into account the inevitable changes in circumstances.

2. The patient is treated as a unique person, and the medical options are assessed in terms of their impact on that person.

3. The concerns and interests of other involved parties are addressed and promoted in so far as possible without compromising the vital interests of the patient.[9]

This formulation helps clarify some issues that the language of the "new" ethics has sometimes obscured. First, it should be obvious that decisions on behalf of the incompetent patient are inherently subjective. Even if there is a clear ("objective") statement of prior wishes, some interpretation is required to be sure that the present circumstances are the same as those envisioned by the principal at the time the choice was made. In the most common cases, the expression of wishes are rather vague, and considerable interpretation may be needed to reach a conclusion. The idea that *any* standard—substituted judgment, best interests, or quality of life—offers a medically objective answer to such questions misperceives the nature of the decision.

---

8. A case example here might be the declaration of brain death in a situation where the family is grief-stricken, angry, and in a state of denial. Looking only at the (now nonexistent) interests of the patient, the "right thing to do" is to stop all medical treatment immediately. Continuing to ventilate the body overnight, however, might allow the family to come to grips with reality and accept the death. Yet continuing treatment for three or four days, if the family seemed to need this much time to adjust emotionally, might intolerably strain the morale of the hospital staff and unacceptably waste community resources. It seems that the optimal course of action is to try to balance all these considerations and not simply to focus on the "best interests of the patient."

9. Among the interests of other involved parties is the interest of the medical profession in not having to provide interventions that are futile or that violate other professional norms or values. See chapter 11 and Tomlinson and Brody 1990.

Second, it is now clear that each of the proposed standards offers a morally plausible base. Substituted judgment calls attention to the patient's wishes and preferences and insists that we treat the patient as a unique person. The best-interests standard insists that a person not be used as a means to others' ends. The quality-of-life standard also focuses on the individual and on the consequences of medical treatment from that individual's perspective. But if the above statement is defensible, then each of these standards is ultimately an incomplete rendition of the duties of the physician and the surrogate.

Third, the statement provides justification (as well as limits) for the central role of the family in most surrogate decisions. The family is often the group to which the wishes and preferences have previously been expressed. It is usually in the best position to appreciate the patient's personal uniqueness. It is the group most intimately involved in the patient's care and whose major interests seem to deserve the most attention. Turning power over to the family without restriction, however, is irresponsible, because there can always be conflicts among the family's wishes, the patient's previously expressed choices, and the patient's vital interests.

Fourth, the statement indicates a need to balance several values and not to place exclusive weight on respect for patient autonomy. In this regard it is analogous to Fried's four "rights in personal care" (discussed in chapter 4). This helps answer the question of what to do when the physician knows exactly what the patient, if competent, would have chosen in the present set of circumstances and knows that that choice is quite foolish and entails grave consequences. The substituted-judgment doctrine would require choosing the foolish option on the patient's behalf. Gutheil and Appelbaum (1983) suggest that a judge faced with such a case would in fact not make the foolish choice; instead she would choose what seemed best for the patient in the long run and then offer a convoluted argument cramming best-interests reasoning into a substituted-judgment mold. I suggest that in such cases the tension may be between honoring autonomy in a narrow and legalistic sense and honoring the patient's uniqueness as a person with unique needs. Returning to Fried's language, it is a tension between the duties to respect autonomy and humanity.[10] Weighty reasons are required

___

10. It may be in this regard that I differ most from the notion of "beneficence-in-trust" proposed by Pellegrino and Thomasma (1988). Their discussion is quite congenial to most of what is said in this book, particularly their assertions of the limits of autonomy, the importance of discerning the values inherent in good medical practice, and the appeal to virtue as well as to rights and rules. I understand their beneficence-in-trust, however, as a way of incorporating the principle of autonomy within the principle of beneficence by stating

to justify overruling an autonomous advance directive; but in the sort of case envisioned, the weighty reasons would be forthcoming.

The power formulation of the duty to an incompetent patient suggests that the problem with the older doctrines may be lack of owned power. Both the surrogate who decides on behalf of the incompetent patient and the physician who advises or counsels that surrogate wield considerable power. Accepting that one has such power, and thereby assuming the obligation to account for how the power has been used, would seem to be a suitable way to minimize the chance of abuse of power to the incompetent's detriment. By contrast, if the doctrines of substituted judgment and best interests are seen as denying the need for subjective judgment and interpretation and as appealing only to objective evidence, then the use of power is papered over and accountability is thereby diminished. And if the standard is seen as requiring exclusive focus on the interests of the patient, one may in exercising one's power do considerable and wholly avoidable harm to others without being called to task for one's narrowness of vision.

that one must understand and appeal to a person's choices and preferences in order to know how to do good for that person. That is, the evil of paternalism lies not in overriding another's autonomy but rather in using the wrong yardstick—one's own values and preferences—to decide what is to another's benefit. I have argued in this book that I see no need to conflate or to reconcile the principles of autonomy and benefit. Depending on the sort of case under discussion, they may be competing considerations or they may coincide. Thwarting another's benefit and interfering with another's autonomy may be two distinct ways of abusing one's power; and I see no particular advantage in trying to reconcile the two principles in any across-the-board fashion. For more on this admittedly casuistic approach to moral thinking, see chapter 15.

Debates over withholding life-sustaining treatment have been going on for more than a decade, but discussions of the meaning and implications of the futility of medical interventions have emerged only more recently.[1] Since analytic philosophers are trained to define terms and clarify distinctions, it was not surprising that an important literature arose during the 1970s on the definitions of terms like *euthanasia* and on the validity of such distinctions as between active and passive euthanasia. But even in the early 1980s, the term *futile intervention* was most often treated as if its definition were self-evident.

One reason why explicit discussion of what counts as futility in medicine might be avoided is that acknowledging that any intervention is futile tends to run counter to the rescue fantasy. In this chapter, though, I will address a different dimension of the problem—that any adequate discussion of the various definitions of futility soon involves us in questions of which powers the society as a whole is willing to grant to the medical profession.

The Importance of Futility

Before turning to the complexities of defining futility, I wish to discuss the implication of defining it for medical ethics.[2] The point in determining that

---

1. I am indebted to Tom Tomlinson for the discussions that have shaped much of the material in this chapter, growing out of our collaboration in Tomlinson and Brody 1988, 1990. In some of that work, we used the phrase *futile therapy*; I am indebted to Loretta Kopelman for pointing out to me that that is an oxymoron—hence the term *futile intervention* in this chapter.

2. Discussion of futility issues has been spotty in the medical-ethics literature until recently. President's Commission 1983 discussed the lack of a duty to provide futile interventions for infants with severe illnesses but suggested that patients had a right to request futile

intervention X is futile in the situation of patient Y is the implication that the physician may then legitimately withhold X without Y's consent or cooperation. Indeed, if the physician nevertheless administers X to Y, he could be accused of a failure to adhere to basic standards of quality medical practice; and this failure would be adjudged even if Y were fully informed about all scientific details and voluntarily requested X. Thus, labeling X as futile effectively renders the decision about whether to administer X an exception to the general duty to respect patient autonomy in therapeutic choices.

This implication arises in turn from a conception of medical practice in which *practice* is employed as a technical term, after the form used by MacIntyre (1981).[3] I think that medicine is best conceptualized as a practical craft that applies scientific knowledge to individual cases toward the end of a right and good healing action. The patient's voluntary consent (among those patients capable of giving such a consent) is necessary but insufficient to ensure achieving that end (Pellegrino and Thomasma 1981). There is also the question of whether the best available scientific knowledge in a given case would proclaim the action under consideration to count as a net benefit. Patients themselves obviously ought to have some say about what counts as a benefit and what does not. But medicine as a practice also has some say in deciding what treatments generally count as benefits— for example, why treating cancer with laetrile is different from treating cancer with standard chemotherapy. Calling medicine a "profession" suggests that society has been willing to grant the professionals a great deal of autonomy in determining among themselves what counts as knowledge and truth within that field of endeavor (Freidson 1970).

In the most straightforward cases—a cancer patient demanding laetrile,

---

cardiopulmonary resuscitation. Guidelines Committee 1987 went a bit further in acknowledging the lack of obligation to provide futile intervention but favored a narrow, physiologic definition of futility (to be discussed below). More recently, discussions of futility in the medical literature have tended to focus on cardiopulmonary resuscitation; see, for instance, Blackhall 1987; Tomlinson and Brody 1988; Murphy 1988; Youngner 1988; Taffet et al. 1988; Schiedermayer 1988.

3. "By a 'practice' I am going to mean any coherent and complex form of socially established cooperative activity through which goods internal to that form of activity are realized in the course of trying to achieve those standards of excellence which are appropriate to, and partially definitive of, that form of activity, with the result that human powers to achieve excellence, and human conceptions of the ends and goods involved, are systematically extended" (MacIntyre 1981, p. 175). For a more detailed discussion of the implications of *practice* for medicine, see Brody 1987d, pp. 31–34, and Pellegrino and Thomasma 1981. For our present purposes it suffices to note that a practice has inherent within it certain standards of excellence independent of the uses to which that practice may be put by society.

or a patient with a demonstrably healthy gallbladder requesting surgery to remove it—there is no difficulty in saying that the physician is under no obligation to comply with the patient's request. The conception of patient-centered primary care developed earlier implies an important difference between decisions of problem assessment and decisions of therapy. The more traditional view held these two decisions to be equivalent. In both diagnosis and therapy, the physician, using gathered data and background scientific knowledge, would decide on the "right" diagnosis and therapy; the patient, having then been informed of the reasons, retained the autonomy to accept or reject what was offered (in diagnosis, by seeking another opinion or another physician; in therapy, by refusing the offered treatment). Patient-centered primary care altered this formula to allow a more direct play of patient autonomy in the process of problem assessment: that is, the physician cannot be said to assess accurately and adequately the nature of the presenting problem unless the patient is involved in the discussion and (upon negotiation) fully assents to the physician's appraisal.[4] But the same sharing of involvement did not, in that model of primary care, extend to therapy. True, if the patient indicates problems with the physician's first choice of scientific treatment, the sensitive primary-care physician will generally be comfortable with rather marked modifications of the "standard" protocol—for instance, seeking a possibly effective once-a-day drug if the patient's employment or activities renders the more ideal three-times-a-day regimen impractical. But in the final analysis, the physician must decide unilaterally whether a treatment possibility comes up to the mark as proper, scientific medical practice. The point of calling the physician a professional is that this judgment, while invariably including some idiosyncratic elements, ought to be based primarily on views that would be widely shared by properly trained physicians as a group.[5]

Is this feature of the primary-care model an internal inconsistency—specifically, a creation of a haven for physician paternalism within a model that claims to be antipaternalistic? I do not think so. On the one hand,

4. This makes the term *problem* much more general than the term *diagnosis*. The latter remains arguably the sole realm of the physician, even under the primary-care conception.

5. This is not to suggest that physicians never employ therapies which are not widely agreed upon as efficacious within the profession. Every physician probably has a collection of "empiric" treatments that are administered to selected patients without any scientific basis for the efficacy that seems to have been observed for them in the past. The use of such treatments falls within the professional limits I have been suggesting so long as (1) the empiric nature of these remedies is frankly acknowledged (that is, the physician does not reason from their success to a more general theory of healing which is at odds with accepted theories of biomedicine); and (2) the risk in the use of these treatments appears very low.

when a profession claims to be aimed at service to individuals (or more properly, to individuals' life plans), a great deal of personal autonomy must be included to assure that the problems as assessed by the professionals really are the problems as each patient sees them. This respect for autonomous involvement extends to the *effects* of therapy: if the professional's tests suggest that the patient has gotten better but the patient says that he is worse, this discrepancy must be investigated and negotiated; in primary care, at least, the physician cannot unilaterally impose his own criteria for resolving problems.

But this does not mean that equal patient involvement should extend to the selection of a therapy or of a set of therapies. The moral value at stake here is the internal integrity and coherence of a professional practice and the maintenance of its internal standards of excellence. This moral value is important to patients, in turn, as a matter of honesty, for they presumably go to physicians to seek the power to assist them in times of illness. If patients felt that the only powers involved were charismatic and social, it might be fine to insist on the fully shared power to pick and choose the best therapy. But so long as patients accept that a part of the physician's power is Aesculapian, then they must also accept that a practitioner within the Aesculapian craft is the only person qualified to say what is or is not an appropriate exercise of the craft. Someone who calls himself a physician, but who is constantly willing to compromise on valid modes of treatment in order to satisfy the wishes of each patient, is a fraud.[6]

When an intervention is futile, the physician may and indeed should withhold it regardless of the patient's request. This calls for a definition of futility that is independent of the physician's situational decision to withhold the intervention; else the definition is wholly circular.

Definitions of Futility

A necessary step in defining futility appears to be the specification of an appropriate goal of therapy. An intervention would seem to be futile or worthwhile only relative to some goal. To take some crass examples, no intervention seems futile if a legitimate goal is the personal enrichment of the physician in a fee-for-service financing system. By contrast, if the only legitimate goal of therapy is a total and immediate cure of the underlying disease process, then almost all interventions are futile. But this obvious point—that the futility of an intervention can be judged only relative to

6. An extreme example is the "Dr. Feelgood" who freely hands out tranquilizers and narcotics to all comers. This physician is practicing bad medicine even if each patient is fully informed about the risks and benefits of these pills and voluntarily accepts the treatment.

some specified goal—is not taken into account in some accepted definitions of futility.

Let us turn to three possible definitions of futility:

An intervention is futile if and only if it fails to produce any *physiologic change* in the patient.

An intervention is futile if and only if it fails to produce any *benefit* for the patient.

An intervention is futile if and only if it fails to promote any *reasonable purpose of treatment* in the patient. This may be the case under several circumstances: (1) the probability of benefit is unacceptably low; (2) the magnitude of benefit is unacceptably small; (3) the harm is much too great relative to any benefit.[7]

How are we to assess these alternatives? At first glance, the therapeutic-reasonableness approach seems unacceptable. Labeling an intervention as futile will ultimately mean that the physician can decide unilaterally to withhold it. But the usual views of patient autonomy would argue that only the patient can decide when a magnitude of benefit is too small, or when the probability of benefit is too low, or when the harm is too great to make the treatment worthwhile *for her*. But before rejecting the thera-peutic-reasonableness definition on those grounds, let us see what can be said for the other two proposals.

The physiologic definition has been the more widely accepted. Its key attraction seems to be its objective, value-free status. What counts as an acceptable benefit is obviously a value-laden judgment. By contrast, whether intervention X produces physiologic change Y in patient Z would seem to be a matter for scientific, empirical inquiry independent of any personal values.

This attractiveness, however, is based on a fallacy. That no sense of futility can ever be value-free in the required sense is driven home by the goal-relativity stipulation. One can always ask, "Futile relative to what goal?" and some values will have to be employed in the selection of the relevant goal from among the set of all possible or conceivable goals. Applied to the physiologic definition, it means that virtually no "futile" intervention

7. The physiologic definition is that employed in Guidelines Committee 1987. The benefit definition may be inferred from Brett and McCullough 1986: they argue that the physician may decide unilaterally when the treatment offers no benefit, but if there is to be a weighing of benefit against harm, the patient must be involved in decision. The therapeutic-reasonableness definition seems to be implicit in some studies of cardiopulmonary resuscitation, such as Bedell et al. 1983, even if it is not fully developed there.

produces no physiologic change at all; but it does fail to produce the physiologic change that is desired.

Consider the administration of intravenous insulin to a patient suffering from cardiopulmonary arrest. It is wrong to say that the insulin will have no physiologic effect, for its effect on certain body cells could be measured. But the insulin is futile for cardiopulmonary arrest because insulin does nothing to restore spontaneous heartbeat or respiration. In other words, the physiologic effect that the insulin produces offers no benefit to the patient: it does not right what is wrong. These judgments may be uncontroversial, but they are value judgments nonetheless. A defender of the physiologic definition will object at this point that I have created a straw man. Of course, all such judgments are value-laden; but the point is that the value judgments implicit in the physiologic definition are much less controversial than those required by the other two definitions. It is on those grounds that physicians should be allowed to make such judgments unilaterally.

But this objection would seem to be giving up too much. First, at least some judgments of patient benefit and therapeutic reasonableness may be every bit as uncontroversial as the judgments based on physiologic futility. Second, if the relevant distinction is between judgments the physician should be allowed to make unilaterally and judgments for which the physician ought to seek the involvement of the autonomous patient, there is no clear or persuasive reason to think that these judgments will divide neatly along the lines of less controversial versus more controversial. There would appear to be some extremely controversial judgments that still fall within the physician's technical purview, whereas other uncontroversial judgments might be of the sort that ought to be shared between physician and patient.

Consider now the benefit definition. The point of this definition is that physicians may appropriately withhold an intervention that offers the patient no benefit whatsoever; but as soon as there are benefits to be weighed against harms, the patient is entitled to have a say. This seems plausible, because the sort of effective deliberation that physicians ideally expect of patients as part of informed consent usually takes the form of weighing risks against benefits for the various alternative treatment plans. Moreover, this definition seems more compatible with the goal-relativity stipulation. For intervention X and patient Y, there could be a set of practicable goals of X, $(x, y, z, \ldots n)$. The claim, according to this definition, is that none of the members of the set $(x, y, z, \ldots n)$ count as a benefit for patient Y.

This definition begins to look less satisfactory, however, when we recall a fundamental value that stimulates the search for a conception of futility: the coherence and integrity of medicine as a practice. For this definition appropriately to demarcate those decisions which physicians ought to make unilaterally, benefit must be the only relevant factor in considering what treatment to offer a patient (and what treatments deserve a legitimate place within the medical armamentarium). But this is certainly not the traditional view of the profession itself, which has always held avoiding harm to be at least as important a value of practice as offering benefit. It thus appears suspicious to claim to be valuing the integrity of medical practice when one allows benefits to be considered but refuses to allow judgments of benefit-harm ratios.

A far-fetched example may help illustrate this point. Suppose that some sports medicine enthusiasts discover a super anabolic steroid that markedly increases athletic prowess for a period of ten years, after which it causes unavoidable deterioration followed by death. Suppose further that the various amateur and professional athletic associations are indifferent to the use of this drug or even promote it—sad to say, a supposition that does not strain credulity. Should physicians offer this drug to their athlete-patients?[8]

By the benefits definition, physicians apparently would have no business unilaterally deciding to withhold this "star now, die later" drug. For what is at issue is the balance between the immediate, substantial benefit and the long-term, substantial harm; and it would seem that only the autonomous patient could legitimately make such a judgment. But this conclusion seems to neglect the core professional values that ought to characterize medical practice. Why is it not more consistent with those values to announce, "We physicians will not dispense this sort of time bomb to human beings no matter how much they say they want it, and that is the end of the matter"?[9] If it accords with professional integrity not to require phy-

---

8. A common psychological trait among successful athletic competitors of the 15–25 age group is an extreme focus on the present and the short-term and an utter neglect of more distant future consequences, which would be considered highly irrational or pathological in almost any other person. It is thus not too farfetched to imagine such athletes requesting this Mephistophelian drug.

9. This is an argument used by some physicians to prohibit the practice of active euthanasia. To the extent that I disagree with this apodictic pronouncement on active euthanasia, it is not because I object to statements in this form (that is, that such-and-such a practice is too harmful for the medical profession to countenance its use). Instead it is because I do not believe that the distinctions between what is prohibited and what is allowed, either theoretically or practically, are clear enough to allow such a doctrinaire stance. See Brody 1987d, pp. 167–70. Incidentally, it might be objected that the examples of the "star now, die later" drug and active euthanasia are irrelevant to this chapter, since no one is calling those modalities futile.

sicians to honor a patient's request for an intervention that offers no benefit, even though that intervention may be harmless, it certainly accords equally (if not more so) not to require physicians to administer something that is disproportionately harmful, as weighed against short-term benefit.[10]

To summarize, the first two of the three proposed definitions are seriously flawed. The physiologic definition appears to offer a value-free judgment, but this turns out to be a false appearance; indeed, when the value dimension is tacked on, this definition effectively collapses into the second. The benefits definition misrepresents the core professional values which the concept of futility is partially designed to protect. Perhaps, then, the therapeutic-reasonableness definition merits a second look to determine whether it is as paternalistic and as neglectful of the rights of autonomous patients as it appeared at first glance.

Several points might be made in defense of the therapeutic-reasonableness definition. First, it coheres well with the sort of activity that medicine is—the craft of applying scientific knowledge to individual cases to produce a right and good healing action. Admittedly, to determine what counts as a good healing action will often require consulting the patient's own life plan and values. When one weighs risks and benefits of treatments, what counts as a net benefit for one patient might not for another patient with a different life plan.[11] But there might be cases in which there is sufficient evidence to say, even before consulting the life plan or desires of the individual, that the healing action could not be right and good. And that would be precisely when the probability of success almost vanishes, or the magnitude of benefit is miniscule, or the risks are massively disproportionate to the benefits. Where these characteristics apply across virtually the entire range of relevant life plans, physicians would seem to have good grounds for declaring that that treatment (for the targeted condition) has no place in the craft of medicine.[12]

But the point is to establish that physicians ought to have the unilateral authority to decide not to employ those modalities.

10. It might be objected that I have tipped the scales by using young athletes as the case example for they must be irrational to agree to take the "star now, die later" drug. But this begs the question: it may well be that the fact that no rational patient would ever request treatment X is a *sufficient* condition for regarding X as futile. It is not a *necessary* condition because a treatment may be rational for certain patients although the medical profession might still have a strong reason for not making a practice of offering or endorsing such treatment. Active euthanasia would fall into this category if its critics are right.

11. Mark Siegler has used the example of a ballerina with asthma, whose disease is well controlled by corticosteroids but only at the cost of producing muscle weakness as a side effect. Only the ballerina can determine whether the benefits of having easier breathing when she dances outweighs any incapacity produced by the muscle weakness.

12. An obvious example might be a treatment that prolongs survival although the patient

Second, this concept of the basic nature of medicine helps show why a relatively vague term like *reasonableness* is unavoidable. If medicine were primarily a science of human biology or physiology, then we could legitimately demand a more precise specification of what counts as a failure to produce a favorable outcome. But medicine is not that sort of activity. It is instead a craft that relies on scientific knowledge but also seeks to apply that knowledge to individual cases. And since most scientific knowledge takes the form of general or statistical statements, there is always some uncertainty when it is applied to individual circumstances. In this setting, it is hopeless to expect a protocol or algorithm; nevertheless, experienced and skilled practitioners of the craft could generally agree on what is reasonable and what is not.

Third, in practice, physicians ultimately would have to fall back on a reasonableness standard when their decisions were challenged. Consider those physicians who oppose any unilateral withholding of resuscitation from a terminal patient and argue that patient consent is mandatory even when resuscitation would be futile. These same physicians would have to admit that they make decisions unilaterally to stop resuscitative efforts after they have seen no response after perhaps thirty or forty-five minutes. Why, then, is patient consent not required for that decision? Should not patients have the option to demand one or two hours of resuscitation even though the physician predicts it would be futile? At some point, the only answer is, "We admit that the statistical chances of patient benefit are not empirically known to be zero; but it isn't *reasonable* to go beyond what we have already done." And this seems to be an admission that at some point, physicians are unilaterally entitled to withhold therapy based on its predicted futility.[13]

Fourth, the supposed conflict between unilateral physician determinations of futility and respect for patient autonomy may well be spurious. Consider the standard procedure now recommended in the various con-

is certain to remain in a persistent vegetative state; arguably this treatment provides no benefit no matter what one's life plan happens to be. I would favor extending the definition of futile intervention to include any therapy offered to patients who have been accurately diagnosed as being in persistent vegetative state, and I agree that medicine does not feel its tools are being properly used in extending the life of such patients. On this point, see Wikler 1988; for opposing views, see B. Brody 1988; May et al. 1987.

13. Rhoden (1988, p. 427), an attorney, seems to agree when she states, in criticizing physicians' tendency to overtreat the dying, "Doctors should be able to terminate treatment when its failure or probable failure (in human, not merely biological, terms) becomes apparent." As she makes clear in the article, she opposes physician assumption of exclusive decision-making powers and is strongly opposed to physician paternalism. Attorneys in general are puzzled as to why physicians feel that they need patient consent to withhold predictably futile therapy (I owe this observation to Frank Marsh).

sensus reports for do-not-resuscitate orders in circumstances where the best available medical evidence shows the likelihood of success to be near zero. The physician is obligated to share these facts with the patient and then ask the patient whether she wishes a do-not-resuscitate order to be given. If the patient agrees, all is well. But if she disagrees, it is not at all clear that the result is triumph of patient autonomy. Instead, it seems probable that the patient is not making a truly rational or autonomous choice. Perhaps she did not understand the information presented. Perhaps she understands the information but fails to see how it applies to her case. Perhaps she thinks that if she agrees to the do-not-resuscitate order, other treatments will also be withheld. By definition, it would be almost impossible for the patient to give a coherent account of any life plans or goals that would rationalize her request for predictably futile therapy.

It is important to notice that in this situation the patient herself cannot be blamed for the apparent irrationality of her request. The physician, not the patient, began the process of irrational thought by giving the patient a clearly mixed message: the therapy in question cannot be of any benefit to you but I feel obligated as your physician to offer it.[14] If the patient responds to this irrationally, the physician must accept most of the blame. This in turn means that feeling obligated to offer a patient the choice of a futile intervention ought not to be seen as promoting patient autonomy in any useful fashion.

I can only conclude that there are some significant advantages to the therapeutic-reasonableness definition when contrasted with the other two. The difficulty that remains, then, is to determine where to draw the line for legitimate applications. So long as the data show that the probability of benefit or the magnitude of benefit is extremely low or the risk is vastly disproportionate to the benefit across the range of relevant life plans, we can defend a physician's unilateral decision to withhold that therapy. But wherever those things are true in relation to some life plans but not others, then the physician, as servant to the patient's life plan, would be obligated to consult the patient's own wishes and values before making the final determination. How can the two cases be distinguished?

14. This point is closely related to the commentary in chapter 6 about including remote risks in informed consent. The point then was that the mere disclosure of additional information does not necessarily promote patient autonomy. Here, the point is that including the patient in a decision does not necessarily promote meaningful autonomy either. Judgments about such abstract principles as patient autonomy must be fine-tuned by much closer attention to the nuances of medical contexts, and discussions of power in medicine provide one avenue to become more aware of the relevant nuances.

The Importance of Owned Power

Elsewhere in this book, in providing an account of how patient rights can be protected without stripping the physician of legitimate medical power, I have relied on the guideline of shared power (as in explaining the doctrine of informed consent). But it seems that shared power will not do the job here. For the issue is precisely when physicians are justified in *not* sharing power but rather in making unilateral nontreatment decisions.

Another candidate from the list of proposed guidelines for the responsible use of power is *owned power*. Even when power cannot be shared, the patient has some protection from its abuse when the rules stipulate that it must be employed openly. Admittedly, rogues might enjoy abusing power openly. But physicians are not rogues; their self-image requires that they be able to see themselves as benefiting patients.[15] Hence a practice that amounts to withholding important benefits from some patients is unlikely to endure when physicians are forced to go public with it and accept full responsibility for it.

The goal of owned power, when applied to judgments of futility, appears to require disclosure at two levels. First, the physician must inform the patient or family when an intervention is being withheld on the basis of futility. This is different from seeking consent; it is simply a courteous disclosure of relevant information. The physician accepts full responsibility for the decision and in no way seeks to involve the patient or family in the decision-making process, but nevertheless he makes clear that the decision is being made without any attempt at concealment or misrepresentation. This stipulation runs counter to some of the motives cited in defense of unilateral futility judgments, such as, "If resuscitation is predictably futile, why shouldn't the physician just write a do-not-resuscitate order and spare the patient or family the depressing news? Why rub it in that things are going so badly?" By my guidelines, the fact that some patients might be transiently depressed (an argument traditionally used to withhold even crucial "bad news" from patients) is much less important than the danger that "sparing" patients and families could allow futility judgments to be made that would not withstand public scrutiny.

The rejoinder might be that it is wrong to withhold bad news—such

---

15. The focus on primary care recommended in chapter 4 adds a further check on abuse of the physician's power in this regard. So long as the patient herself helps determine the nature of the medical problem, she will be involved in a negotiation that will ultimately help determine which interventions are thought to be futile and on what grounds. In theory, it might appear that the patient has power to influence the definition of the problem but not the choice of therapy; in primary-care practice, defining a problem and choosing a therapy may be much more closely intertwined. For examples, see Poole and Anstett 1983.

as a diagnosis of cancer—when that news is essential for the patient to make decisions concerning further medical care and other life activities. But a patient's autonomy is not served by informing her of the withholding of futile interventions; presumably, no decision is there to be made, as no acceptable therapeutic outcome could be produced. But it is not completely true that patient autonomy cannot be served by disclosure of futility judgments. A patient might disagree with the physician's assessment of futility and request a second opinion, for example. Or a patient's reply might show that the patient is still in a state of deep-rooted denial regarding the hopeless prognosis, and the physician (in the name of benefit, not autonomy) might decide to humor the patient for now and delay further discussion of the issue. (In such cases, owned power does lead to at least a modicum of shared power.) By contrast, a serious threat to patient autonomy would be the sort of misrepresentation that occurs when a decision that is out of the patient's or family's hands is presented in the language of consent, as if their involvement is being sought and they are to be expected to have some responsibility for the outcome.[16] But that is the point in carefully distinguishing the duty to disclose a futility judgment from the duty to seek consent.

The second level of disclosure required by owned power is for the medical profession to establish an open process for defending judgments of futility for certain classes of patients and interventions. A model might be Blackhall's (1987) published defense of the claim that cardiopulmonary resuscitation is futile in a number of situations, such as metastatic cancer, widespread infection, or gastrointestinal hemorrhage. Open dissemination and discussion of the criteria for determining futility and the application of those criteria to specific diseases should help assure that any unwarranted assumptions are challenged and that all relevant life plans are taken adequately into account.

Blackhall does a good job of citing the relevant statistical data, but her study also points out the problem that has so far plagued discussions of futility in the absence of an agreed-upon definition. It is not enough to say that a certain percentage of patients failed to have an acceptable result from resuscitation. An "acceptable result" has been variously interpreted in studies as having restoration of heartbeat at cessation of the resuscitation procedure, being alive twenty-four hours after resuscitation, or surviving long enough to go home from the hospital. The value assumptions as well as

---

16. An extreme case of this is when hospital staff approach the family for "permission" to remove "life"-support equipment from a patient in whom brain death has been diagnosed.

the empirical observations must be candidly reported if the goal of owned power and full public dialogue is to be met.

My conclusion, then, is that the legitimate exercise of medical power ought to include the power to make judgments of futility. Physicians may unilaterally elect to withhold an intervention when it can reasonably be predicted to produce no acceptable therapeutic outcome. Whenever possible, such decisions should be based on value judgments and empirical data that can be presented for public discussion and challenge. Individual patients (or their surrogates) should be sensitively informed when such futility judgments are made regarding their care.[17]

An important reason for empowering physicians to make futility judgments relates to the role physicians may have in containing medical costs by preventing the expenditure of scarce medical resources on treatments that can be predicted to be of no benefit. Obviously, this presumes that physicians ought morally to be placed in a position to be agents of cost containment by making individualized case judgments. This assumption matters little for this chapter, where I have primarily considered duties owed to individual patients; but in the next chapter I will discuss the ethics of the gatekeeper role and the physician's social duty for a just distribution of resources.

17. The same restriction mentioned under *transparency* in informed consent (chapter 7) should apply here as well, however. At every medical visit, the physician fails to offer the patient a virtually infinite number of futile interventions, and no one imagines that she is obligated to inform the patient of this. Transparency would require that if the physician considers offering a treatment and then decides not to do so on grounds of futility, she should follow the general rule of "thinking out loud" and mention it. An interesting corollary of this approach would be that today, a physician deciding to write a do-not-resuscitate order for a hospitalized patient for reasons of futility would feel obligated to mention that fact. But in the future, after such decisions become much more routine, then physicians would not even think of the possibility of resuscitating and hence would not feel obligated to mention it.

Physicians have long been seen as a relatively powerful group, but there is one sort of power physicians appear to possess now that they acquired only recently: the power to deplete the public coffers in the name of healing. This power stems from an explosion of expensive medical technology, so that the routine or standard of care for many common ailments is many times more expensive than it was even thirty or forty years previously, and from the growing conviction that the quality of care available to the wealthy ought to be available to the average citizen as well (Thurow 1984).[1] The power of physicians to break the bank while seeking to do a thorough job is a serious-enough problem in countries that have in place a national system of financing medical care and thus some built-in mechanisms to apply brakes to escalating medical costs. It is even more difficult in the United States, which has steadfastly avoided the creation of a centralized medical-financing system. Data published in 1988 revealed that during a three-year period when the percentage of the gross national product (GNP) devoted to medical care was held constant in most highly developed nations, the United States stood alone in displaying a significant increase—at a time when unprecedented efforts were being made to control costs in the United States by prepayment of hospital services, increased use of capitation, and other means (Schieber and Poullier 1988).

Much has been written and remains to be written, at the level of political

1. According to a Harris/Harvard Community Health Plan poll, Americans believe everyone should have the right to the best possible health care, the same that would be afforded to a millionaire (91 percent), and that health insurance should pay for any lifesaving treatment, even if it costs a million dollars to save a life (71 percent). *Business and Health* 7 (November 1989): p. 8.

and social policy, about what to do about containing medical costs in the United States, but those matters are beyond the scope of this book.[2] I will focus on the role of the physician in whatever scheme may eventually emerge, and on what this will do to the physician's power and the nature of the physician-patient relationship.

So many conflicting forces are now working upon health care in the United States that it is difficult to predict the shape of future change. A few scenarios, however, seem general enough to cover some of the major possibilities:

1. The United States will continue to avoid a national health plan and will rely on continuation of a fee-for-service approach or slight modifications thereof. Government will continue to provide coverage for those among the poor or elderly not covered by private insurance. Physicians will continue to call almost all the shots within this system. Presumably, through education and voluntary action, they will become better skilled at identifying and adhering to cost-effective modes of medical practice.[3]

2. The United States will develop a nationalized scheme somewhat like that of Great Britain or (more likely) Canada. Cost containment will arise through central budgeting. Local hospitals will get only so much funding and will have to ration services accordingly. Presumably, as in Britain or Canada, the result will be more funding for primary care and chronic-illness care but less funding for highly expensive technology needed in caring for the sickest patients who stand the least chance to benefit.[4]

3. The future of American medicine belongs not to either physicians or government but to the large corporations. The corporations took over most other production and services in the United States at the beginning of the twentieth century; it is a temporary aberration that medicine missed out on their control. That trend, however, is speedily being reversed as larger and larger chains buy out hospitals and health maintenance organizations (HMOs). Some combination of government regulation and market competition will control excessive costs, but that will matter little to physicians.

2. I will assume for the purposes of this chapter that the United States has not purchased more health with these increased expenditures, as a good deal of evidence goes to show; various health indices in the United States are no better (and for minority populations are often noticeably worse) than in many other developed countries which spend less on health care per capita than we do.

3. A recent statement of scenario 1 is the "health policy agenda for the American people" proposed by the American Medical Association (Boyle et al. 1987).

4. Arnold Relman, editor of the influential New England Journal of Medicine, seems to have become a convert to scenario 2; see, for example, Relman 1989.

They will basically become corporate employees, and almost all vestiges of what we now quaintly call "professionalism" will disappear when they have no choice but to define their own interests and the corporation's as identical.[5]

4. The government and perhaps corporations will control many aspects of health care, including increased centralization of financing, but the physician will retain a pivotal role in the system. In this scenario, physicians are relied upon to help control medical costs. Unlike in scenario 1, the physicians do not do so simply because they are enlightened or good-hearted; they do so because they work within systems like HMOs (and have been trained to work within such systems), which offer some specific financial incentives to control costs. The federal or corporate role is primarily to assure that all citizens are enrolled in one of these HMOs and that adequate funding is available; the decisions of the HMO physicians primarily determine the balance between benefit to patients and control of costs.[6]

What are the power implications of these scenarios for physician, patient, and society? Scenario 1 finds great favor with organized medicine precisely because it would probably further enhance physician power; cost control arises out of a sort of noblesse oblige and not out of any diminution of the options open to the medical profession as a group (though various forms of peer review may limit the options of the individual practitioner). For that reason, few outside of organized medicine seem to think there is any chance of this scenario coming to pass. Although economists may disagree about many features of medical cost containment, they appear unanimous on one point—that serious cost constraints and fee-for-service practice are fundamentally incompatible.[7] It is the retention of a fee-for-service structure in the face of the technology explosion and increased access to medicine for all citizens that has brought about the present predicament.

Scenario 2 has traditionally been seen by organized medicine in the

5. A principal exponent of this scenario is sociologist Paul Starr (1982). There is, however, more recent evidence of waning corporate influence, at least in the falling off of the trend toward for-profit health care; see, for example, Ginzberg 1986, 1988.

6. Scenario 4 may not be incompatible with scenario 2. A recent recommendation for a variant of scenario 4 is Enthoven and Kronick 1989. On the virtues of a closed system, see Cassel 1985; Daniels 1986. On incentives to control costs, see Pellegrino 1986; Brody 1987a; Like 1988; Ellsbury 1989; Stephens 1989b, and the section below on the primary-care case manager.

7. This statement seems true for the sort of fee-for-service system in place historically in the United States. Canada has managed to control costs reasonably well while retaining a fee-for-service method of paying physicians; but hospital care is not fee-for-service, and a complex regulatory system of fee controls and volume controls is necessary.

United States as representing an unacceptable loss of physician power. The thinking is that unless physicians have power over the financial aspects of their relationships with their patients, they will lose the power to use appropriate medical means to treat their patients optimally. This argument flies in the face of any dispassionate analysis of the power possessed by physicians within a socialized or welfare-state medical system or of the general quality of care those systems deliver. The British National Health Service may appear to be an example of this threat given the long wait for many procedures that are commonplace in the United States. At least, Britain is the most common hobgoblin raised by U.S. medical politicians who wish to preach the evils of "socialized medicine." But the British system is seriously underfunded: only about 6.6 percent of the British GNP goes to health care, compared to the 8–10 percent typical of Japan and much of Western Europe. Canada maintains a GNP of about 8.5 percent and few would claim that Canadian health care is worse than ours.

Scenario 3, on the other hand, does seem to envision a genuine loss of power for the physician and a corresponding increase in power for various corporate managers. At any rate, in that system the relationship between physician and patient would probably largely be dictated by the corporate structure and policies, and both the patient and the physician would lose power to shape their relationship toward their respective ends.

Scenario 4 sets out a strategy that seems to hold promise for genuine cost control—at least the experience with well-managed HMOs to date strongly suggests that they can control costs adequately while delivering care equal in quality to that of fee-for-service medicine.[8] In general, physician power is maximized within this scenario, but unequally. The gainers in power are the primary-care physicians who function in the role of gatekeeper. The losers in power are the subspecialist physicians who assume care only of those patients whom the gatekeepers refer; if the subspecialists waste money or fail to take care of patients as the primary-care physicians think they should, they will find themselves without referrals and without jobs. The question, then, is what this means for the power of the patient in the relationship—specifically, whether a shared-power model is compatible with the physician-gatekeeper man-dated by this scenario.

8. The emphasis is on *well-managed*. Many HMOs and similar organizations first formed in the early 1980s, when money was spent on health care with few restrictions, were poorly managed; these are only slowly being weeded out as the fat is being cut from the system through more stringent cost controls. I am indebted to William ("Terry") Kane for insights in this regard; see also Hudson and Brody 1989.

The Division of Labor Model

One reaction to scenario 4 is that it must be rejected because it would lead to unethical medical practice. The problem is that the gatekeeper role creates a potential conflict of interest between physician and patient. This line of argument goes roughly as follows:

1. Under older reimbursement systems, there was no conflict of interest; the physician was paid when he helped (or attempted to help) the patient.

2. Under new systems of prepayment and capitation, a conflict of interest has appeared. The physician might get extra reimbursement for denying services to patients (such as for discharging patients more quickly from the hospital or denying referral to a specialist).

3. The physician, however, is morally obligated to serve the patient first and foremost, not the interests of society or a health-care institution.

4. Because the gatekeeper role sets up precisely such a conflict, it constitutes unethical medical practice.

5. Since gatekeeping is unethical, physicians cannot act as agents for cost control; instead they must act so as to try to secure for their patients any beneficial therapy, regardless of cost.

6. It is undeniable, however, that costs of medical care must somehow be constrained in the United States.[9]

7. Therefore, somebody other than physicians must act so as to deny certain categories of costly care to certain categories of patients. This must be an administrative and bureaucratic function separate from personal medical care.

This argument proposes a division-of-labor model (the physician serves the patient; the administrator serves the whole society by constraining costs) which has several initially attractive features. It allows each party to do what it was trained to do best (after all, physicians are not trained as economists). It retains for the physician a comfortable purity of motive and incentive. It seems to ring true psychologically: all of us know how we function under the duress of strong financial pressures and how easy it is to rationalize behavior that would objectively appear unacceptable.

There are nevertheless some major problems with the division-of-labor model. To begin, let me compare it with the four scenarios proposed above.

9. Again, a major assumption underlying this chapter is that simply cutting out waste will not eliminate the cost problems in American medicine. The bulk of the economic, health-policy, and medical literature supports this view; for an opposing view, see Angell 1985. Schwartz (1987) argues that no cost containment system will work in the United States unless some way is found to slow drastically the progress of medical technological innovation.

Only scenario 2 combines retention of physician discretion with central economic planning so as to make something like the division-of-labor model a working reality. But many defenders of that model (at least within organized medicine) would find scenario 2 unacceptable in any form. Moreover, one strong argument in defense of a strict division of labor is the ease with which physicians might otherwise come to rationalize denial of service on economic grounds as if it were a purely medical judgment. An elderly candidate for renal dialysis, for example, might be told he has been refused treatment because his heart can't take the strain of dialysis, whereas in fact he could get some benefit from dialysis but society hasn't funded enough machines to go around. But this charge has been documented with examples from practice in countries that adhere to scenario 2, notably Great Britain (Schwartz and Aaron 1984), so translating this ethical purity of motive into a working political program might be harder than it would at first appear.

Another rebuttal to the division-of-labor model is that it confuses a potential conflict of interest with an actual one. Where gatekeeping represents an actual and significant conflict of interest, it may be an ethically corrupt role; but it is not clear that this is necessarily true in all gatekeeping arrangements. Let's turn again to the example of Great Britain and the general practitioner's (purported) unwillingness to refer elderly patients for dialysis. Where does the ethical problem arise—from the fact that the general practitioner acts as gatekeeper? Or the fact that Britain is willing to spend only about 6.5 percent of its GNP on health while other developed nations devote 8 or 9 percent? In the United States, a corresponding difficulty is presented by the bonus that some HMOs pay to physicians who succeed in holding down costs. Such a bonus scheme has been attacked as an almost certain sign of unethical practice. But what does that bonus amount to? If HMO A pays a physician who avoids ordering marginally beneficial computerized-tomography (CT) scans a bonus of one hundred dollars at the end of the year, and HMO B pays a physician one hundred dollars each time he refuses to order a CT scan that the patient or a consultant has requested, are those ethically equivalent situations? Before judging whether an actual conflict of interest exists which is strong enough to be ethically worrisome, one would have to know both the size of the financial incentive and the directness with which it is linked to denial of services to identifiable patients. But these observations would lead to the conclusion that gatekeeping is wrong *under some circumstances*, not that gatekeeping is wrong across the board.

A quite different line of argument opposes the consequences of the division-of-labor model to those of the gatekeeper model, using a utilitarian view of social justice. Other things being equal, a cost-containment system is most just when those who are denied some treatment are those who stand the least chance of benefiting or will derive the least benefit. According to this argument, this ideal distribution of benefits is very unlikely if the division of labor model were used and the administrators making the judgments had no personal medical knowledge of the cases. In such a system, given the political realities, we would most likely end up with the sorts of exclusion rules that (it was alleged) held sway in Great Britain, such as "No one over age 55 is a candidate for renal dialysis" (Halper 1985). But any such rule is an extremely ham-handed way of sorting out benefits. Inevitably it will allow treatment for some seriously ill or dying fifty-year-olds who can benefit very little and leave out some hale seventy-year-olds who might benefit a great deal. By contrast, a physician gatekeeper is in a much better position to make the finely honed judgments about who can or cannot benefit from a particular treatment and to what degree.[10] In short, it is contended that the gatekeeper model will maximize social utility much better than would the division of labor model.[11]

At this stage in the discussion it may be helpful to put aside the list of arguments for and against each model and ask how the power concept might aid our understanding of the issue. Clearly, the division-of-labor model arises from a fear of misuse of the physician's power. One aspect of "the dark side of the force" would certainly be the physician's power to enrich himself without benefiting the patient. This danger may involve all aspects of physician power: the Aesculapian power to know what treatment will work; the charismatic power to sway the gullible or fearful patient; the social power to demand compliance and payment and to stigmatize the patient who will not cooperate; and the cultural power to determine the "truth" about which diseases are present and which treatments should

10. There is a sparse but suggestive literature on the ability of physicians to make these sorts of judgments. One example is the ability of physicians to adapt to overcrowding in an intensive care unit by moving out those patients who least need that level of care, without measureable increases in mortality or morbidity (Singer et al. 1983; Selker et al. 1987). A second example, also in intensive care units, is the close correlation between informal staff judgments of prognosis and the prognoses arrived at by a sophisticated, quantitative scoring system, APACHE 2 (Kruse et al. 1988).

11. This point is lost on some who oppose the gatekeeper model on the grounds that it interferes unduly with patient autonomy. Veatch (1986), for example, writes about the allocation of scarce medical resources almost as if medical technologies came with labels specifying which were effective and which were not. He neglects the need for individual case judgments of how effective specific treatments are likely to be for specific patients.

be used. The physician-gatekeeper who is being paid to keep costs down, and who will make more profit if the patient receives less service, is clearly susceptible to this temptation.

Earlier I showed the inadequacies of several ethical concepts (such as a pure autonomy/beneficence model) to give proper guidance regarding potential misuses of physician power. These concepts failed to recognize the real power features of the physician-patient relationship or else served as comforting verbal formulas to deny power without really changing anything. I will now assert that the division-of-labor model displays precisely this sort of inadequacy.

The inadequacy is perhaps most obvious when we ask why this fear of misuse of power suddenly has arisen with the push toward cost containment. Is it really true (as the division-of-labor model implies) that physicians under the old fee-for-service system had no incentives to enrich themselves at the expense of patients? Studies of the rates of unnecessary surgery in a variety of settings, or of the increased frequency with which physicians order X rays and electrocardiograms when they own the machines in their offices and can charge directly for the tests, suggest that the physician's role before cost containment was hardly ethically pure. A frequent rejoinder to this point is, "Yes, but at least in those days the physician made extra money by doing more things for the patient; the gatekeeper is more problematic ethically because she is likely to do less, not more." This comment betrays a subspecialist perspective which is inimical to the primary-care model. First, any good primary-care physician knows precisely how much damage can be done by doing more rather than less. Second, although the primary-care physician may order fewer tests, hospitalize less, and refer more seldom to subspecialists, she is likely to compensate by spending more time with the patient and closely following the course of illness in return visits. To charge that this type of practice amounts to doing less suggests an unjustified bias that only by employing high technology is one "doing something" in medicine. As the inauguration of a gatekeeper system generally means that the primary-care physician gains power and the subspecialist loses power, it might seem that it is this factor, not any actual risk to the patient, which prompts this rejoinder.

Thus, a power analysis indicates one serious objection to the division-of-labor model, since it is not clear that this model will avoid the potential conflicts of interest that are said to make the gatekeeper model unethical. (At any rate, I feel safe in stating that no reimbursement system has yet been invented which rewards the physician when and only when he has done something that is of real benefit to the patient.) But a further analysis of the physician-patient relationship and the powers in it leads to a deeper objection—that the pure patient-advocacy role envisioned by the division-of-labor model is unattainable. The model assumes that the administrator will play the social utilitarian and keep costs down while the physician plays the patient advocate and tries to get every conceivable benefit for the patient (subject, of course, to the constraints on resources imposed by the administrator, which are outside the physician's control and therefore do not threaten his moral purity). We have a clear picture as to what it would mean for the administrator to play his role—though perhaps in the heavy-handed way noted in a previous objection. But do we really understand what it would mean for the physician to play her role, with the degree of moral purity and singleness of purpose that the model seems to call for?

To see what it would take for the physician to be purely a physician advocate "without regard to cost," it will help to recall that perhaps the scarcest (and hence most costly) resource at the physician's disposal is not money but time (Gillon 1988). The physician who takes the division-of-labor model seriously must take care never to have more than one patient at a time. She must never see patients according to a daily appointment schedule.

Most physicians do use an appointment system and allocate, say, ten minutes for each routine office visit. And most physicians will on occasion deviate from that system in times of special need. If a patient expresses deep emotional anguish or appears to be suicidal, the physician will spend extra time counseling and evaluating; and if the physician suspects that a patient's "gastritis" is a sign of a myocardial infarction, she will immediately arrange for hospitalization and will phone some orders straight to the hospital unit. These actions put the physician behind schedule and cause the other patients to wait longer. What, then, do we make of the physicians's behavior when, at the end of ten minutes, she goes on to see the next patient? It can hardly be the case that this patient will not benefit at all from extra time. Even a few minutes spent reviewing the instructions for taking the medication or reassuring the patient about the physician's concern about his symptoms might produce much better results. So if the physician does not take that extra time, it must be because she has made a judgment that the slight extra benefit this patient might derive is not worth the cost to her other patients—or indeed to the physician, if this delay causes her to get home an hour late. But trading off benefits among different patients is precisely what gatekeeping is supposed to do. It violates the patient-advocacy role alleged by the division-of-labor model in a fundamental way and illustrates real conflicts of interest: "If I spend as much time with each patient as he wishes, I'll have no time for my personal life; if I restrict my practice to only as many patients as I can see each day without time constraints, I'll suffer serious financial losses."

If the allocation of the physician's time seems too mundane to apply to the concept of pure patient advocacy, take instead the allocation of effort or of procedures or tests. Maybe repeating a battery of tests would reveal a new, unsuspected diagnosis. Maybe continuation of the course of anti-biotics for an extra week would reduce the chance of a later recurrence of infection. Maybe if I sent all my healthy patients for an annual total body CT scan I might one day spot curable cancer at an early stage in one of them. At any rate, a "pure" patient advocate would worry about such things. But the average physician does not worry about them, and when asked to justify this failure to provide possible extra benefit for the patient would do so on grounds of reasonableness. The physician has done as much for this patient as seems reasonable; it is time to devote her resources and efforts to somebody else's problem.[12] But this, again, is gatekeeping.

To summarize, the power to make trade-offs among patients (based, one hopes, on sound judgments of relative likelihood of benefit) is a power that is inherent in medicine as generally practiced. The idea that we should somehow eliminate that power because it can be misused to the patient's detriment is unrealistic. It is not illogical but it would impose such radical changes on medical practice as to be utterly impractical. Therefore the division-of-labor model, which suggests that that power can and ought to be eliminated, is either an unrealistic call for utopian reform of medicine or (more likely) a mere verbal formula to preserve the fantasy of moral purity while ignoring the inconvenient realities.

The Primary-Care Case Manager

The discussion thus far has shown that the division-of-labor model ulti-mately fails in its effort to brand all physician gatekeeping as unethical. The discussion has not, of course, shown that gatekeeping is always ethical; indeed, it has shown that significant abuses of power are possible. This brings us back to the central question of this book: given that the physician's power cannot be eliminated or easily counterbalanced, what would count as responsible use of power in a gatekeeping setting?

In approaching this question, it may help to describe the role of the case manager. This role is not restricted to physicians. Indeed, as some

12. On the circumstances under which physicians can be justified in making unilateral judgments about which treatments provide reasonable degrees of benefit for various classes of patients, see the discussion of the reasonableness standard of futility in chapter 11.

insurance carriers begin to move toward managed-care systems, the operating assumption is that nurses will make the best case managers, for three reasons: they can be hired much more cheaply than physicians; they do not think like physicians and thus are less likely to advocate big-ticket expenditures; and they may be more willing to identify their personal interests with the interests of the company that hires them. Partly because of the implications of the third reason, I will discuss the role of case manager as it would be adopted by a primary-care physician rather than by other health professionals. I make the assumption that the ethics of that role will be more defensible when the case manager is employed by, or contracts with, an organization dedicated to providing health care for a population of patients rather than one concerned solely with financing and reimbursement. Of course, within such an organization (like a staff-model HMO) there might well be nonphysician primary-care providers, such as nurse practitioners, who could serve as case managers; for them, the ethical implications of the role will be the same as for the physician.

The case manager takes responsibility for making ongoing care decisions on behalf of a patient or family. He makes these decisions from the vantage point of the one who provides the bulk of the care as the first-contact primary-care practitioner; this entails both personal knowledge of the patient and face-to-face accountability for most of the decisions that are made. (I think it important to emphasize that in this model of the case manager's role, most decisions to allow or deny[13] expensive tests and referrals are made in conversation with the patient; they are not made in an isolated office where the patient is represented only by pieces of paper.) The goals that motivate the good case manager are the long-term health of the patient and advocacy for the patient's interests. (Being a direct-care provider, the case manager is motivated by the same emotional factors discussed earlier, including a need to feel that patients are grateful for the care they have received.) The attitudes that guide the decisions about the appropriate use of health-care resources on behalf of the patient include an awareness of

---

13. In order to assess the real power of the gatekeeper, it is important to recall what "denial" of care by an HMO actually means. In a system that allows at least some private, fee-for-service medical practice, no one can prevent any patient, whether enrolled in an HMO or not, from obtaining any care he wishes to pay for himself. Hence the patient denied a service by an HMO gatekeeper has been denied insurance coverage for the care, not the care itself. Of course, the middle-class enrollee can better afford to purchase the care privately than can the poor patient. Ironically, it is usually the educated, middle-class patient who complains loudest about an HMO "denial," because that patient is most aware of the other options.

the potential harms as well as the potential benefits of technological interventions; focus on prevention as well as treatment; belief in the value
of comprehensive and continuing rather than fragmented care; and emphasis on maximizing function instead of on diagnosis and cure when
dealing with the chronically ill and the elderly.

The term *gatekeeper* seems to raise an ethical red flag in a way that the
term *case manager* does not. What is the difference? In an organizational
chart of a health-care delivery system, the gatekeeper and the case manager
are often, if not usually, the same person. The main point of the relabeling
is to signal a different set of personal motives and attitudes. It seems
generally taken for granted, in published discussions of the gatekeeper role,
that the services being denied to the patient are invariably beneficial and
that the only true reason the gatekeeper might close the gate is financial
(whether for private gain or for the gain of the organization or the national
system). The term *case manager*, by contrast, serves as a reminder that
technological interventions have a potential for significant harm and that
individualized judgment is required to assess the balance of benefits and
harms in particular cases. Hence many recommendations against additional
interventions will be motivated primarily by beneficence toward the patient.
The motive of saving money for the organization may well be present but
is hardly the dominant theme.

The differing connotations of the two terms suggest that the physician-
gatekeeper will think like the stereotypical subspecialist—that more care
is better care and that good medicine requires rigorously excluding every
possibility of disease no matter how remote. For such a person to act with
a bias toward controlling costs, he must go against his training and experience and employ a variety of rationalizations to make himself more
comfortable with this dissonance; and presumably only an obvious fiscal
carrot or stick could compel him to behave in this unnatural fashion. By
contrast, the physician–case manager is generally a primary-care physician
who favors a "high-touch" instead of a high-tech approach and is convinced
that spending time talking with patients will often clarify issues of treatment
and prevention much better than a battery of tests and procedures can.
For this physician, in most situations, there is no conflict between quality
medicine (as she was trained to practice it) and cost-effective or cost-
conscious medicine. Serving the interests of the patient and trying efficiently
to promote the patient's health while sparing him iatrogenic disasters is an
ideal that the case manager can embrace openly and enthusiastically. The
case manager is indeed happy that embracing this ideal generally means

that money can be saved (compared to care for the same medical conditions administered by the stereotypical subspecialist); but the money saving need not be the primary reason for pursuing the ideal.[14]

The importance of this line of thinking becomes more clear if we recall the earlier discussion of the physician-patient relationship (chapter 4). I argued there that a proper conception of primary medical care, which ties the physician's task to the need to understand what meaning the patient attaches to his own experience of the illness, may be essential in developing a shared-power model of that relationship. I have reached a similar conclusion in this chapter: one way to reduce the ethical tension inherent in gatekeeping, and thereby to use the power of the physician both to promote the patient's individual good and to promote the social good of cost containment, is to move toward the case manager conception with its primary-care orientation. I then add as a further refinement the transparency model of informed consent, which by requiring that the physician think out loud encourages the physician to make it explicit to the patient whenever cost factors substantially affect management decisions.

The physician—case manager that emerges from this discussion is one who has no reason to conceal his true motives from himself and thus is less likely to conceal what is going on from the patient. As the regular caregiver, he will display in a variety of ways his willingness to pay extra attention or provide additional services when the patient is experiencing an acute need. That means that on another occasion, when he recommends that the patient forgo a test or procedure he considers unnecessary or deleterious, the patient is more likely to credit this bit of gatekeeping as an acceptable and understandable facet of the total care.[15] If, by contrast,

14. An illuminating exchange of comments that reinforces this point is Scovern 1988; Hudson and Brody 1989; Scovern 1989. Scovern, a physician formerly employed by an HMO in the Eastern United States, described the unsatisfactory conditions under which he was required to work and the negative implications this had for the quality of care that patients received. The conclusion suggested was, first, that HMOs are generally bad and, second, that this physician did something morally praiseworthy by resigning. Physicians more familiar with HMO management then replied that the bad outcomes were partly attributable to the fact that Scovern was trained mainly as a subspecialist and naturally felt out of place in a setting that required the services of a primary-care physician. Scovern objected to this assessment, claiming that he had worked many hours in an emergency room and hence was fully qualified. A review of the primary-care model discussed in chapter 4 will show that emergency-room medicine is a far cry from ideal primary care. Ironically, Scovern's self-defense only served to point up that he had no idea how primary-care medicine is supposed to function. (Of course, he should not be blamed for the managerial incompetence of an HMO that hired a physician with his qualifications to serve in a role for which he was not suited.)

15. I am indebted for this point especially to Dr. A. C. Markus, a British general practitioner who spoke at a conference on U.S. and British approaches to medical ethics in New York in

the patient is being denied a substantial benefit as a result of this gate-keeping, the physician, by adhering to the transparency standard of in-formed consent and disclosure, is likely to allow the patient to see that the matter requires more discussion. And because education and negotiation are basic interpersonal skills that this physician stresses as a result of his training, there is a greater likelihood that the discussion will lead to a satisfactory and amicable resolution consistent with the patient's right to quality health care.[16]

So far my analysis of the ethical role of the physician in cost containment has followed the power approach, focusing on the concepts of shared power and owned power as they are elaborated in the concept of the primary-care case manager. Ethical analyses based on more widely accepted ethical principles end up in much the same place, although with a different em-phasis. Most analyses of the gatekeeper role, for example, conclude that fully informed consent is an adequate defense against the charge of potential conflict of interest and therefore the ethical physician will disclose to the patient any features of the insurance plan or the physician's employment that conflict with the patient's individual interests (Marsh 1985; Levinson 1987). This conclusion, as far as it goes, seems hard to challenge. And yet it leaves a good deal unsaid that emerges from the power approach—notably, the centrality of the primary-care conception in defining a role that takes patient advocacy seriously while still accepting cost efficiency as a mark of good medical practice. Why the primary-care physician who has been trained as described above would be a different sort of gatekeeper is a matter on which the more traditional bioethical analysis is silent.

This observation leads in turn to two obvious challenges to the approach taken in this chapter. The first is that the focus on the primary-care phy-sician appears to neglect the other essential actors in the drama. Do I mean to suggest that specialist physicians engage in unethical behavior when they try to control medical costs? Or that only primary-care physicians can be expected to be cost-conscious?

I do not intend to slight the contributions of specialist and subspecialist

June 1987, cosponsored by the Hastings Center, the Royal Society of Medicine, and the New York Academy of Medicine.

16. For this reason, perhaps the most serious moral charge that could be leveled against a managed-care system is that it works actively to discourage this sort of disclosure by its physicians. The case of a class-action suit against a Pennsylvania HMO in which this violation was alleged caused me to suggest (Brody 1989b) that it should be seen as prima facie unethical for any primary-care physician to accept employment with a managed-care system that restricts disclosure of information on how gatekeeping decisions are made.

physicians. Clearly their efforts are essential for quality patient care; no primary-care physician could function as a true patient advocate without ready access to highly skilled specialists.[17] There are numerous ways in which specialists can work to control costs; doing procedures on an out-patient basis when it is safe to do so and thereby saving inpatient costs is but one example. Still, the primary-care physician deserves special mention for at least two reasons. First, in an HMO or similar organization with both primary-care case managers and cost-conscious specialists on staff, the system will probably work to the patients' benefit only when there is teamwork and open communication among all physicians. (The quality-assurance committee within such an organization is an example of a useful mechanism to review cost-containment decisions for possible adverse impact on quality of care.) It is fair to assume that the primary-care physicians will take much of the responsibility for making the staff work as a team. Second, as the physician of first contact, the primary-care case manager will generally be the one with the heavier burden of disclosure and education, charged with assuring that the patient understands how decisions are made within the system and what role issues of cost play.

A second challenge to this analysis argues that the case manager role, described in glowingly positive terms, is an even greater threat to the rights of patients than is the dreaded gatekeeper. The latter, presumably a stuffy bureaucrat in a three-piece suit, is bound to arouse patient suspicion and distrust, and that will tend to keep the gatekeepers honest: patients will be quick to appeal any adverse decision through various administrative or legal channels. But the avuncular case manager is precisely the sort of person calculated to disarm the patient. Harking back to the kindly family doctor of a small-town America now passed, this physician would seem to have the power to make all kinds of decisions that are detrimental to the patient yet to which the patient would be afraid or embarrassed to object. Most patients, given the choice, would prefer to avoid any unpleasant confrontation with their personal physician; and if pressed, they would admit to a fear that the antipathy this might arouse in the physician might lead to them getting worse care in the event of a future emergency. This

---

17. It is possible, however, to overestimate the *quantitative* need to rely on specialist consultation and referral. Numerous studies of family practice settings have shown that as few as 5 percent of patients may present problems that the skilled family physician is unable to manage on her own. Nevertheless, the needs of that 5 percent are extremely important, and no conscientious primary-care physician would be willing to practice in a setting where appropriate specialty backup was unavailable (with the obvious qualification that rural medical practice places limits on what support can realistically be expected).

cautiousness of patients renders the kindly case manager a greater threat to patient rights and autonomy than the more acerbic gatekeeper.

This challenge is important because it goes to the heart of some of the assumptions underlying this book. It is granted that physicians generally have the power to interfere paternalistically with patients' choices and to serve their own selfish needs while outwardly conforming to the standards of appropriate patient care. The question is how to respond to this power disparity between physician and patient—by empowering the patient or by defanging the physician. This challenge seems to favor the latter course. The gatekeeper, by this line of argument, is rendered relatively powerless because his machinations and his motives are forced out into the open; the case manager is left too powerful because he can conceal his actions behind a kindly veneer. But if the challenge is allowed to stand, the conclusion is that patients' rights and autonomy must be protected at all costs, even if it means that what could have been a humane and compassionate relationship is replaced by an adversarial and bureaucratic one. The goal of medical ethics is seen as defanging the powerful physician, even if he then is not the sort of person from whom we wish to seek help when we are ill. But in that case we are allowing a view of medical ethics to undermine the fundamental ends of medicine itself.[18]

Recall that the primary-care model of the physician-patient relationship was selected because it brought some important *ethical* features to the relationship—notably, enhancement of patient involvement in the therapeutic and decision-making process. The role of case manager presumes the retention of these ethical qualities within the context of a compassionate and supportive interpersonal relationship. But the case manager is also supposed to control costs, when this can be done by withholding non-costworthy, marginal treatments. And to allow the case manager to carry out this new responsibility, additional power is granted him—the power to limit reimbursed access to specialists and special procedures. (This additional power has been necessitated by the relative powerlessness of the primary-care physician within the overall architecture of the U.S. health-care system, as reflected in the relatively low incomes of such physicians; see chapter 13.) But these arguments are designed to show that adding this new responsibility to the primary physician's role is not fundamentally at odds with the patient-advocacy attitudes of the primary-care physician.

18. It is worth recalling here the argument that a proper ethic for medicine must grow out of a proper appreciation and analysis of the type of activity that medicine is, not out of a contrived application to medicine of concepts developed in other spheres of human activity (Pellegrino and Thomasma 1981).

In sum, the argument has been designed to show (1) that some sort of gatekeeping is inevitable in modern medical practice, (2) that under some circumstances, gatekeeping is ethically problematic, and (3) that if the task of gatekeeping were to be assigned to the primary-care case manager, its ethically problematic features would be minimized and its patient-advocacy features enhanced. This second challenge—that the case manager is un-trustworthy precisely because of his benign nature—suggests two possible errors in thinking. Either the line of argument summarized above has been rejected and the critic views the transition from gatekeeper to case manager as a cosmetic change; or the critic has elevated respect for patient rights and autonomy so far within the hierarchy of ethical principles that he does not care whether the physician-patient relationship is stripped of such other features as beneficence and compassion.[19]

The Scenarios Reconsidered

Ideally, a full discussion of how society ought to provide and fund medical care for its citizens would include many elements, of which the relationship between individual physicians and patients would be only one. Many phi-losophers would say that such a discussion requires a well-elaborated theory of social justice. Issues of justice will inevitably play a role and ought to render certain aspects of the health-care system nondiscretionary. For ex-ample, all but the more extreme libertarians would presumably acknowl-edge that the poor ought not be denied basic health care because of inability to pay. Other elements of the system will be discretionary and will depend on political decisions made by voters and their representatives. For example, the decision in Oregon in 1988 not to provide Medicaid funding for organ transplants may have been wise or unwise but seems to have fallen within the discretionary category; that is, no one in Oregon can reasonably claim that their basic human rights were violated by this action of the state legislature (Welch and Larson 1988). But in turn, a full discussion of both the discretionary and the nondiscretionary elements of the system will

---

19. Yet another objection can be added, that this line of argument amounts to an undue glorification of the primary-care physician, whereas available evidence (at least in the United States) does not support the notion that the average practitioner will do a good job in all the ways required by the case manager model. It is important to return here to a point raised in the chapters on informed consent, that any serious ethical analysis of the concepts involved is likely to turn into a platform for the reform of medical education and medical practice. I think that the data are clear that *some* primary-care physicians are capable of making thoughtful case judgments and of communicating openly with patients in the ways required by the case manager model. If *all* of them are not, it may be more important to review current education and practice patterns than to dismiss the concept out of hand.

require a thorough analysis of the power relations among the various segments of society and the involved institutions and professional groups. A brief review of the four scenarios from the beginning of this chapter may provide some helpful comments.

The scenarios—a reformed fee-for-service system; nationalized medicine; corporatized medicine; mixed corporate and federal funding, with capitation, stressing the case manager role—differ in the degree of power retained by the medical profession. The second and third signal a major net loss of power, and the first and fourth are contingent on the continuation of power. As already noted, the loss of power attached to a national health service does not automatically mean that physicians cannot provide good care for patients or be effective patient advocates. No one knows how physician power will fare under a totally corporatized structure; but preliminary investigation suggests that corporate control would prove a bigger threat to both physician and patient power than government control. But in either scenario, when it comes to balancing benefits to the patient against extra costs of care, a variety of decisions will be made at levels of the system to which patients have no direct access.

This does not mean that patients have no power to influence those decisions. In the National Health Service of the United Kingdom, for example, the health budget for a particular region or community may be fixed by a centralized authority; but how that budget is divided within the region (such as for acute hospital care versus nursing-home care) is a matter over which a local governing board has considerable discretion, and citizens have several means of access to those boards. Therefore, in either a nationalized or a corporatized system, a patient denied beneficial services in the name of cost control has a route of appeal and retains the power to pursue it. My main point, however, is that when the patient exercises that right of appeal, she does so in the role of citizen, from a position of equality among all citizens. With the total health budget fairly fixed, any extra care provided to citizen X means less care for some citizen Y; and the members of the appeals board (governmental or corporate) have no duty to pay more attention to X's plea than to Y's, or vice versa. Any decision to support X's claim over Y's ought then to be made according to some impersonal criteria such that if the lots of X and Y were reversed, Y would get the nod over X. The members of this appeals board cannot function as personal advocates for one patient without introducing substantial unfairness into the process.

In the first and fourth scenarios, such decisions are still made outside the physician-patient encounter. For instance, a state government may still decide that organ transplants will not be covered by Medicaid, and physicians in that state would have to abide by that law (though, of course, they could lobby along with their patients to change it). But because those scenarios delegate more cost-control functions to the individual physician and thereby allow that physician more discretion than do the more centralized scenarios, more decisional power is retained within the physician-patient relationship. Ideally, this would mean that a patient caught in the benefit-versus-cost bind could appeal directly to a physician who is committed to serving as a patient advocate. This duty of patient advocacy is tempered by an institutionally imposed duty (backed up by an appeal to distributive justice) to constrain costs. But at least the patient has an identifiable agent to whom to turn, and that agent cannot (consistent with professional responsibilities) regard the patient as just another citizen making a claim that must be adjudged solely on impersonal grounds.

Admittedly, there will be much that is impersonal in the judgment this physician will make. If the data show that diabetics with a certain grade of peripheral vascular disease do poorly on renal dialysis, this particular diabetic patient may be denied a referral for dialysis on those grounds alone. The moral obligations of the personal physician, however, ought to carry him beyond this general appeal to scientific data so long as he views his commitment (in Charles Fried's terms) as that of "servant to the life plan of the patient."[20] The personal physician cannot discharge his task simply by assessing a symptom or disease in scientific and impersonal terms; he must ask about its particular significance for this patient and her life plans and goals. This moral commitment suggests that in the personal physician the patient has a special advocate. This advocate is committed to try to secure extra benefits for the patient whenever it is unclear whether those benefits are worth the costs (unless, of course, the patient freely forgoes them). And, in those cases where the benefits are clearly noncost-worthy, the advocate is committed to a course of open explanation and negotiation, which often can lead to a creative compromise.

So far I have tried to show that the two scenarios that preserve physician power (the first and fourth) contain some necessary ingredients for the exercise of physician power on behalf of the patient, where the patient may be relatively powerless owing to the emotional ravages of illness or to lack of information. But do these scenarios assure both a reasonable level of cost efficiency while maintaining both the patient-advocacy role and quality care? Here I would argue, for the reasons I have indicated, that the fourth

20. For a review of this concept, and of Fried's four "rights in personal care," see chapter 4.

scenario is clearly superior to the first. The first scenario, which would be advocated by representatives of organized medicine, contains two serious power imbalances that threaten the ethical goals. First, cost containment comes primarily as physicians voluntarily and unilaterally promise to clean up their act and eschew spendthrift medicine. But so far this approach has seldom worked, and costs have continued to rise out of proportion to any consequent patient benefit. Second, the status quo in fee-for-service medicine distributes power within the medical profession unevenly, at least to the extent that reimbursement is a rough guide to relative power. The most generously reimbursed physicians are those who perform the types of highly technical, invasive procedures that have often been overutilized and count as the big-ticket items in the health budget (not solely because of physicians' fees but also because they utilize high-cost facilities and equipment and require a large ancillary staff). The bottom rungs of the medical ladder are occupied by the primary-care physicians whose main tools are thought and time. This means that the more powerful physicians are more likely to be those who have two qualities that tend to make them unsuited for the role of patient advocate–cost container described above. First, they have a financial incentive to overutilize expensive interventions; and second, they are likely to adopt a view of the medical craft which focuses on the technological cure of disease rather than long-term relationships with patients according to the primary-care model advocated in chapter 4. The latter means that their skills in advocacy and negotiation are likely to be less well developed and more peripheral to their own views of their medical roles.

I would argue for all these reasons that the fourth scenario is best suited to balance the goals of patient advocacy, cost containment, and quality care. It fits the shared-power ideal at two especially important levels. At the physician-patient level, it promotes shared power by encouraging a primary-care conception of the physician's work. At the institutional level, it allows nonphysicians much more power than would the first scenario, while still retaining a wide scope of physician discretion. Assuming that the organizations that would be funded under this scenario resemble the better-run HMOs and preferred-provider organizations (PPOs) now in existence, the incentives under which physicians will work (and which encourage cost constraint) will be heavily influenced by representatives of government, industry, or whoever ultimately pays the bills. These representatives in turn have a type of public accountability that the physicians lack. To run such an organization effectively, power must be shared between the physicians and the nonphysician managers. Allowing either side to accumulate too much power will assure that the plan will eventually become noncompetitive: too much physician power will probably lead to out-of-control costs; too much managerial power will lead to inability to retain high-quality physicians and to deliver satisfactory services to the patients.

Although I advocate the fourth scenario, it is my view that some elements from the second scenario have to be included for the fourth one to work properly. I do not believe that the United States can achieve the goals of its health system so long as it retains the multiplicity of third-party payers that now afflicts it—fifteen hundred by one estimate, each with its own rules and its own red tape. Americans are slowly coming to realize that they are paying almost double what the dreaded "socialized-medicine" systems pay for administrative costs: U.S. hospitals must bill each payer separately and must keep track of each capsule, bandage, and box of tissues to be sure it is billed to the correct patient's account (Himmelstein and Woolhandler 1986; Evans et al. 1989). In addition to these excess administrative costs, the multiplicity of payers encourages all actors in the system to increase their profits not by providing better or more efficient services but by shifting costs and trying to go to the deepest pocket for reimbursement of each item. (Along with this cost shifting inevitably comes skimming, trying to secure for one's own clientele those patients who are under the umbrella of the most generous payer and to avoid caring for those patients whose reimbursement is lowest—usually the most disadvantaged patients.) As the payers see what cost-shifting games are being played against them, they change their rules to forestall profiteering—often on a year-to-year basis, sometimes on a month-to-month basis. But that in turn means that the rules of the fiscal game are changing so fast that the better HMOs and PPOs cannot possibly make rational decisions as they try to devote themselves to providing quality care. Rational decisions in medical care seem to require some predictability and stability of the financing structure, which under the present competitive marketplace system is rapidly being lost.

I can only conclude that the present patchwork system in the United States must eventually fall apart of its own weight, and that so-called reforms that simply patch the patches (such as the catastrophic-illness coverage under Medicare added toward the end of the 1980s) cannot rescue the system (Dickman et al. 1987). Although a single, national health insurance pool may never come to pass in the United States, some form of centralized and streamlined administration appears inescapable (Himmelstein et al.

1989). These views, however, are rather more controversial (and less well informed by specific expertise) than my previous arguments on behalf of the fourth scenario, and I would not insist on them as a well-formulated solution.[21]

21. It has been widely argued that the problem in determining a just way of financing health care in the United States is that we lack a theory of social justice in health care worked out in sufficient detail to do the job required. I have tried to show in this chapter that it is at least possible that a careful analysis of the social and political context in which ethical judgments must be made might be at least as suggestive for future research as an elegant but abstract theory. I have here sided with those who avow that as much ethical knowledge can come from well-considered and well-grounded case judgments as from ethical theories (Murray 1987). For more discussion of this matter, see chapter 15.

Doctors have unusual control over their incomes. A significant number of them use that power to make much greater incomes than even the average physician. . . . Neither the peculiar value of their services nor the need of patients to go to respected, prestigious members of their communities requires they be given additional economic power. The argument should not so much focus on the particular question of whether two, three, or five times the average worker's earnings is the proper income level for doctors; instead it should account for these disparities of power. It is utterly hypocritical for doctors, health-care administrators, academic analysts, and policy makers to close their eyes to the level of doctors' incomes amidst an otherwise vigorous concern for making health care worth the increasing money we pay for it. (Menzel 1983, pp. 228–29)

This passage, taken from a chapter on physicians' incomes in a book on moral questions in medical cost containment, is a refreshing departure. It is one of the few passages in books or articles on medical ethics to identify the physician's power as a crucial ethical issue. And the book it is taken from is the only one (to my knowledge) that devotes an entire chapter to the ethical problem of the appropriate income for the physician.

In American society, the linkage between power and income is often taken for granted. Therefore, whereas works employing the more traditional medical-ethical vocabulary might well avoid the subject of physician income altogether, it is hard for a work that employs an explicit power vocabulary to escape the topic.[1] But it remains to be seen how an analysis of physician

1. Any explicit discussion of physician income as an ethical issue would tend to make physicians feel that their moral good faith was being challenged and to suspect that those

income as an ethical issue can be carried out in terms of the responsible use of physician power. Even Menzel devotes almost his entire chapter on the subject to an analysis in terms of *justice* and does not take the discussion of *power* much beyond the passage just quoted.

At least a few physicians have been less reticent than most ethicists and have addressed the moral dimensions of physician income. Occasionally one may find passages like the following in medical journals:

> Physicians who limit their office practice to insured and paying patients declare themselves openly to be merchants rather than professionals [and foster] the myth that physicians as a group are greedy and self-serving rather than dedicated and altruistic.... Physicians who value their professionalism should treat office patients on the basis of need, not remuneration. Physicians who do not do so deserve the contempt and censure of their colleagues. (Elias 1986, p. 391)

> [Physicians] will be safer and more satisfied... if, from an income basis, we are again part of the middle class of society, with opportunities to act out our compassion by providing care to the unfortunate who cannot afford our care. (Reitemeier 1985)

> The degree to which the public felt that physicians' fees were reasonable fell from 42 percent in 1982 to 27 percent in 1984.... A public opinion poll concerning physicians' incomes showed that 70 percent of the respondents felt that physicians were overpaid. (Stewart 1985, p. 335)

In this chapter, I will address the question of the appropriate income for physicians, and what counts as a responsible use of the physician's economic power. These questions can be asked in turn about two matters: the total income of physicians and disparities in income among medical specialties. Much attention has recently been focused on disparities as a result of the publication of the resource-based relative value study (Hsiao et al. 1988) and the adoption of the resource-based relative value scale

---

raising the challenge were simply envious of the money physicians earned. Therefore, "ethicists" working alongside physicians in health-care and academic settings who depend on physicians for their point of entry into the health-care arena have a strong interest in not raising this issue. A secondary reason (perhaps a rationalization) for avoiding the issue is that although physicians control up to 80 percent of health-care expenditures, they may put into their own pockets only about 10 percent. Therefore, those who wish to contain costs ought to focus on how physicians control hospital utilization and other expenditures and ignore the relatively small potatoes of physicians' personal income (Fuchs 1974). Menzel (1983) suggests that this reasoning is shortsighted.

(RBRVS) by the federal government to pay physicians under Medicare.[2] Therefore, it is important to note that such a device as the RBRVS raises two slightly different ethical questions. One is the straightforward question, which will be addressed in this chapter, of how much the various kinds of physicians get paid. The other is the question of which kinds of financial incentives may appropriately be paid to physicians in order to encourage cost containment or other socially desirable outcomes (which might not be desirable from the standpoint of the individual patient). That problem has already been discussed in the previous chapter and will not be further investigated here.

The Physician's Income and Aimed Power

Is it ethically appropriate for physicians as a group to make much more money than the average worker? This problem may be viewed as one of aimed power or of shared power.

The aimed power problem has to do with the "target income phenomenon" discussed at some length by Menzel (1983). Americans do not take kindly to the idea of a loss of personal income. They tend to view any decline in income from one year to the next as a sign of loss of personal worth or productivity. They will devote a good deal of energy to making sure that they make at least as much next year as this year, regardless of whether their accustomed income level is in any sense justified.

As Menzel has noted, physicians possess almost unique economic power to carry out this intention. To a remarkable degree, society defers to physicians both to decide how much they should be paid for which services and to determine when those services are truly needed. Under the present U.S. system, physicians can control their income levels either by increasing their fees for individual services or by performing more of those services

2. The RBRVS was developed under contract from the Federal Health Care Financing Administration by a team at the Harvard School of Public Health. Physicians of numerous specialties were interviewed about the relative amount and intensity of work as well as the level of training necessary to perform a wide variety of medical tasks. From these data, weightings were calculated to correct current physician charges. In general, the study found that such "cognitive" work as the standard office visit by a primary-care physician was underreimbursed while "procedural" work like most surgical procedures and endoscopies were overreimbursed. If the original version of the RBRVS had been put into effect for Medicare, it was calculated that payments to family physicians would have risen by about 60 percent while payments to thoracic surgeons and ophthalmologists would have dropped by more than 40 percent (Hsiao et al. 1988). The actual figures have already been modified as a result of physician lobbying, and it is uncertain at this writing precisely which figures will be implemented in the federal reimbursement system for Medicare scheduled to be introduced between 1992 and 1996. The American Medical Association has supported RBRVS in concept while questioning some of the calculations.

or both. Even in more tightly regulated systems, efforts to control physician income by restricting fees for services may cause an immediate increase in the number of services performed (Lomas et al. 1989).[3] And given the large role that physician discretion now plays in determining which medical services are appropriate for a given patient, it may be difficult to show in any scientifically compelling way that those additional services are unnecessary.

The phenomenon of target income might not be a problem if it could be verified independently that the fees charged by physicians in the past were fair, reasonable, and responsible.[4] And it might be of little concern if we were proposing to start afresh and redesign the physician reimbursement system for the future. But so long as we are dealing with the current U.S. realities, we are stuck with the historical record of physician income, which (absent other strong forces) will predictably generate an effort by physicians to maintain that level of income in the future. Hence physicians are going to be under suspicion of aiming their power in ways that are not properly respectful of the needs of patients. If physicians set out primarily to provide service to more patients, or a higher quality of service, others might not begrudge them higher earnings as a consequence. But if physicians set out primarily to make more money (although this motivation will, in all likelihood, remain unconscious), others might well be suspicious of their later claims that they provided more or higher quality services.

It is also important to see this question against the backdrop of a growing social consensus on the need to restrain the cost of medical care. If a physician were to behave in ways that tended to lower medical costs, one might well identify a problem of aimed power: should the physician use her power to promote social goals like cost containment, or should she try harder to meet the particular needs of the individual patient? The physician

3. Congress, in the Medicare budget for 1990 which provides for moving to the RBRVS system of physician payment, also established a "Medicare volume performance standard" to measure the growth of physician services. Presumably there will be an effort to sort out increased volume prompted by new technology or the aging of the population from increased volume that reflects physician effort to maximize income under an RBRVS.

4. Deciding when physician charges are fair would seem to involve several factors. Menzel (1983) argues that charges are fair which reimburse physicians for time, specialized skill and training, and the sacrifices undergone by deferring income during extended training; they are unfair if they are based on the idea that physicians deserve more simply because they treat such a valuable commodity (human life and health) or that physicians should have high incomes because patients wish to be treated only by a powerful, elite group. The designers of the resource-based relative value scale (Hsiao et al. 1988) agreed with Menzel but added another factor: the intensity of the service performed, or the stress that the physician undergoes while performing it, might also justify a higher fee.

in this case might be blamed for going too far in either direction, saving money or advocating extra patient services. Here the physician is being pulled between two competing moral goods and is viewed sympathetically. The situation is quite different when a physician is suspected of being motivated (consciously or unconsciously) by the target income phenomenon. One cannot have much moral sympathy for the physician whose conflict consists of, "Should I try harder to provide patients with the services that they truly need while keeping social costs at acceptable levels? Or should I try to make more money?" When this physician goes before the public in the role of patient advocate, requesting that additional services be provided for certain categories of patients, the public is much less likely to listen: it will see the point as not whether those services are needed by the patients but how much those services will enrich the physician.[5]

Advocates of the RBRVS might reply that this problem of mixed motives would be resolved if their proposal were implemented. A major factor in the target income phenomenon has been the ability of the physician to identify low-work-intensity services that are nevertheless highly remunerative. Most physicians work hard and long now and are unlikely to accept a major increase in work load simply to maintain a high income (when a relative drop in income would still leave them financially well off). Until now, almost every specialty had its procedures that took relatively little work but for which the fees, for historical or other reasons, were high. Under a RBRVS, all such "special" procedures would (in theory) disappear, and any physician who increased her income would have done proportionately more work.

This forecast, however, is less than reassuring. First, as the RBRVS is a new device, there is no empirical evidence that it will work as intended. If it succeeds as well as the last highly touted revolution in U.S. health-care financing—diagnosis-related groups—we might have cause for pessimism. Second, and more basic in terms of ethics, is the fact that a *resource*-based relative value scale is not an *outcome*-based relative value scale. The reason physicians should work harder is not because such efforts will earn them a special place in heaven; they should work harder if it will be of benefit to patients. But this is precisely what the relative value scale by itself cannot determine. The scale may tell us that we (as patients and insurers) have paid too much in the past for coronary artery bypass surgery and recommend that

5. There is ample evidence that this has been occurring for some years in U.S. politics and has steadily been eroding the effectiveness of physicians' lobbying on behalf of the public health. See, for example, the public opinion polls cited in Stewart 1985; see also Brody 1990a, 1990b.

we pay the surgeon only half that fee. But the surgeon will still be paid the same for an unnecessary operation as for a necessary one.

The argument so far has tended to show that the relatively high level of physician income poses an ethical problem. Physicians, being only human, will work to maintain that level of income; and as long as they are doing so the public will have a hard time determining whether the physicians' power is being aimed properly for the benefit of patients. But this argument does not automatically yield the conclusion that regulations are desirable to limit income or to disallow unnecessary services. Such regulations will be put in place whether we wish them or not, for reasons of cost containment, both by governmental agencies and by private industry. But before giving full ethical support to such regulations, one would need to determine that their intrusiveness relative to physician decision making and the physician-patient relationship does not impose more burden than the money saved is worth. And that requires difficult-to-obtain empirical data beyond the scope of this book, although some assumptions were offered in the previous chapter. Moreover, the right to use one's economic power to make more money seems comfortably enshrined in the American bastion of political values and relatively immune from alteration.

The income issue may also be seen as a problem of shared power. Here the connection is less direct. The problem has been addressed most eloquently by Hilfiker (1985). In describing why he found it necessary to give up an apparently successful practice in rural Minnesota to become a much less well paid physician in an inner-city poverty clinic in Washington, D.C., Hilfiker describes the various stresses of rural general practice and how the strategies he used to cope with them ultimately made things worse. One coping strategy was money. For a while, material wealth and the ability to take first-class vacations seemed to make up for the sleepless nights and the sense of professional isolation. But ultimately Hilfiker came to feel that the income differential had become a wall between him and his patients. The financial implications of practice made it difficult for them to approach him as they would have wished; and he was increasingly unable to approach them, as his life-style served to isolate him from their life experiences.[6]

---

6. Hilfiker's book can be as frustrating as it is illuminating. The author seems too prone to wallow in guilt, too willing to ruminate obsessively over small matters, and indeed too ill-equipped by his training to undertake a demanding rural practice. It may thus seem arrogant for Hilfiker to suggest that his personal tribulations represent a general warning to American medicine. At a talk that I attended, Hilfiker compared himself to the miner's canary. By this simile he admitted that he was more sensitive than the average American physician but therefore could serve as an ethical early-warning system. That is, the force that might drive

The power that his income gave him was not one that could effectively be shared with his patients, and the power therefore became a chasm over which they peered at each other as strangers.[7] Ironically, Hilfiker himself felt much more empowered to practice decent and compassionate medicine when he in effect accepted a vow of poverty to work in the inner city.

What may sound like an extreme point can be put more moderately, as suggested by Reitemeier (1985) in the quotation earlier in this chapter. It is not the case that the rich physician will be coldhearted and the poor physician compassionate. But as income creates a gulf in life experiences between physician and patient, the sensitive and caring physician will have to devote extra effort to bridge that gulf. And what about the physician who is unwilling to make that effort?

To summarize, there are at least two ethical problems (independent of straightforward issues of fairness and justice) with the relatively high income that physicians enjoy. This privileged economic status raises difficult questions about the ability of the physician to attend to the patient's interest and to serve as an effective advocate for the patient when additional services may be helpful. And it creates a power disparity between physician and patient that may be hard to bridge.[8]

An ethics of rights and rules may be ill suited to suggest appropriate action in the face of these observations. It is not clear how, in a society like ours, we could enforce lowered income for physicians as behavior required by minimal moral decency. Rather, these observations seem pertinent for the discussion of virtue and character in chapter 16. The observations have more to do with questions of excellence in medical practice and of what sort of person the good physician ought to be.

Disparities in Physician Income

Until recently, the widening disparity in income between primary-care physicians and procedure-oriented subspecialist physicians was little

Hilfiker to give up his practice might cause another physician merely to have a few sleepless nights; but the force is there nonetheless and has to be recognized.

7. Similar claims are made by Benjamin (1989), recalling his father's rural practice between 1920 and 1960: "From his farmhouse calls he knew the straitened circumstances of his patients. . . . Asceticism and the Puritan ethic necessitated that he drive a Ford. Intuitively, he knew that a more affluent lifestyle would drive a wedge between the healer and the sick and destroy his effectiveness" (p. 1191). Benjamin, a university professor, advocates the RBRVS as a means to erase intolerable inequities within medicine.

8. This argument is in large part a prudential one: if physicians wish to retain sufficient political clout to be able to act as effective patient advocates, then they ought to consider ways to limit excess income. It follows, then, that since political and social influence is at stake, the *perception* of excess income is every bit as important as any actual excess income.

known by the general public and even within medicine was the subject of anecdotal comments unsupported by hard data. Again, it is the recent debate over the relative value scale that has brought this issue to public attention.

The record shows that the difference in income among U.S. physicians began to increase dramatically around 1965, when Medicare and Medicaid were inaugurated and physicians began to expect to be paid for services that had previously been considered charity care. Since then the median annual income (after business expenses, including malpractice insurance, and before taxes) of hospital-based physicians and procedure-oriented subspecialists has risen at a much steeper rate than that of primary-care physicians (family physicians and pediatricians in particular). In 1988, the median annual income of anesthesiologists was $150,000 and of surgeons was $153,000, while that of general practitioners and family physicians was $80,000 and of pediatricians was $77,000. Since 1978, the median annual income of general and family physicians rose by 60 percent, while that of surgeons increased by 115 percent; surgeons earned 42 percent more than general and family physicians in 1978 but 91 percent more in 1988 (Gonzalez and Emmons 1988).[9]

The reasons for this disparity are primarily two. First, as has been widely publicized since the RBRVS was proposed, American medicine has tended to pay markedly higher fees for invasive procedures than for what are now coming to be known as "cognitive services." Physicians who cut and sew or who use complex machines are paid more for their time and effort than physicians who primarily think and talk. Second, procedurally oriented physicians have the option of using hospital facilities and equipment in much of their work; the hospital charges for use of the equipment and room while the physician submits a separate fee. The physician accordingly must cover little in the way of business expenses out of gross income. The

9. Many published figures in the United States do not reflect this wide disparity, because of the method of reporting. The "internal medicine" category used by the American Medical Association includes both general internists (whose income is presumably somewhat higher than that of family physicians and pediatricians but is still at the lower end of the scale) and subspecialists like cardiologists, who perform many invasive procedures and accordingly have incomes near those of some surgical specialists. Therefore, if internists are lumped together with other primary-care physicians, primary-care income is artificially inflated and appears to be closer to the average income of other specialists. (Median income for internists in 1988 was $100,000.) If the trends of income for family physicians and pediatricians and for anesthesiologists and surgeons between the early 1970s and 1988 are compared to the rate of inflation and to the increase in the cost of living, it becomes evident that the former groups actually lost real income during those years while the latter gained. I am indebted to my colleague, James Hudson, for those calculations.

primary-care physician, on the other hand, must pay a much larger proportion of gross income for space, utilities, nurses, receptionists, and other
costs of practice.

Since the striking disparity in income among specialties has not been
widely known, at least prior to the proposal of the RBRVS, it is not surprising
that it has been addressed in the medical-ethics literature even less than
the issue of physician income generally. Writers on ethics may have assumed that all physicians are probably overpaid and that it made little
sense to quibble over the relative degrees. They may have felt (in keeping
with a fundamental assumption of the relative value scale study) that the
pay differential for specialties was an internal matter for physicians to settle
among themselves so long as the total cost of medical care did not go up
as a result. And they may have believed that the ethicist should not appear
to play favorites among medical specialties. Since all physicians, from neu-
rosurgeons to pediatricians, should strive to respect patient autonomy,
promote patient interests, and treat patients justly, the ethicist should
address all specialties in equal terms. To argue that the income of primary-
care physicians should go up and that of ophthalmologists go down might
be seen as suggesting that primary-care physicians are more ethical than
ophthalmologists—obviously an ill-considered stand for a medical ethicist.

In chapters 4 and 7, I deviated from this conventional wisdom by arguing
that there was something ethically special about primary medical care
(properly conceived), particularly in terms of promoting a shared-power
relationship between physician and patient. I tried to avoid misunderstanding by pointing out, first, that many good subspecialists borrow techniques
from primary care and have a shared-power relationship with patients;
second, that many primary-care physicians, unfortunately, do not practice
that style of medicine; and third, that specialists who are unable to have
such a relationship because of fragmented or episodic contact with patients
can still be highly ethical by taking care to respect patients' rights and
interests. Nevertheless, I argued that what we have been calling primary
care in this book (regardless of who does it) plays a special role within
medical practice and that if this type of medicine were lost, or if patients
had less access to that sort of physician, the physician-patient relationship
would suffer. I therefore wish to extend this argument by contending that
reimbursement for primary-care services has important ethical implications.

The pre-RBRVS reimbursement system tended to discourage new physicians from seeking a career in primary care. This is particularly true to
the extent that the average medical school graduate has to pay back a debt
of about forty thousand dollars and hence is less likely to choose altruist-

ically when it comes to selecting a specialty. It has been estimated that schools are already training far fewer primary-care physicians than would be needed for a future medical system that swings toward a managed-care model (Mulhausen and McGee 1989). Continued underpayment of primary care relative to other specialties is almost certain to result in fewer patients having access to a well-trained primary-care practitioner.

The disparity in physician income also has a subtle effect within managed-care systems like HMOs. It is customary for the financial reserves in an HMO to be divided into three funds (after costs of administrative overhead are deducted): a primary-care fund, a specialty-care fund, and a hospital fund. The primary-care fund covers not only the salaries or fees of the primary-care physicians but also other services provided in the office or clinic: nurses, office laboratory procedures like urinalyses; and additional services such as nutritional counseling. The cost of the care paid for by the specialty-care and hospital funds tends to be driven, in part, by the fees earned by specialists. If a patient is sent off for lab tests or X rays, the fees charged by the clinical pathologist and the radiologist need to be paid. If the patient is referred directly to a specialist, that physician's fees must be paid. And if a patient is hospitalized, the chances become much greater that she will require additional laboratory and X-ray investigations, surgical procedures, or specialist consultation.

Other things being equal, this means that as the income curve for specialists rises more steeply than the curve for average medical costs overall, a greater proportion of the managed-care monies will have to be shifted to the specialty-care and hospital funds, leaving primary care relatively underfunded. This shift might mean less access to preventive services like nutrition counseling, less time to talk with the physician as schedules become more crowded and the HMO is unable to hire more primary-care practitioners, and reduced access to an advice nurse and other nonphysician services. In any event, the result is that those medical services most useful for empowering patients will be neglected.

I have already noted that subspecialists can deliver ethically superior care by adopting into their own practices many of the techniques described here as primary care. But this recommendation assumes that primary-care skills are well taught in medical school and residency training. Unfortunately, one tends to observe in academic circles the same power and economic disparity as in medical practice.[10] It is therefore an unusual medical

---

10. This becomes even more the case as state and federal funds for medical education are reduced and schools and residency programs must increasingly make up their operating

school which stresses the skills needed for good primary care to the same degree as it stresses basic science. And it is an unusual subspecialty residency program in which residents are taught things like patient interviewing and psychological counseling and support. So long as the American medical world proclaims by its income scale that it does not value primary care, it is unlikely that the teaching institutions will make much room for imparting primary-care knowledge and skills.

I have tried to make the case that the maintenance of the wide gap in income between primary-care and subspecialist physicians will have ethically deleterious consequences, for patients as a group will be disempowered in important ways. Is the answer, then, the RBRVS, which is designed to remove this disparity? The problem now is to reconcile the observations about total physician income from the previous section with the desire to narrow the income gap within medicine. I submit that the relative value scale, as originally proposed, cannot resolve the problem because it is designed to keep *total* physician income unchanged. But the arguments noted in the previous section led toward the conclusion that it would be a good thing for medicine if total income were lessened.

If physicians were told that they ought to take a pay cut in the name of enhanced virtue and character, then it would seem grossly unjust to assess primary-care physicians in the same way as subspecialists. The data show that primary-care physicians have already been taking a pay cut over the past fifteen years (while getting no public recognition for this). It is not simply a matter of justice; there are also good utilitarian reasons not to reduce primary-care income and thereby further reduce primary-care recruitment. But neither can it be said that primary-care physicians are underpaid relative to the rest of society; as a group they seem to be able to afford decent housing, clothes, cars, and other material benefits. At the same time, the relative value scale research project suggests strongly that the "excess" income earned by procedurally oriented subspecialists cannot be justified in terms of extra work, extra training, or extra stress; it is a

budgets from practice income. The highly paid specialist can make a comfortable income without putting in a full work week, thereby leaving plenty of time for teaching and clinical research. The primary-care physicians must devote the greater proportion of their time to practice in order to generate a comparable level of income; hence they have little time left over for teaching and research. Within the academic institution, then, it is almost inevitable that the influence of the specialty departments will grow and that of the primary-care departments will shrink (assuming that the primary-care physicians had any influence to begin with, which has hardly been the case within most traditional teaching hospitals).

historical oddity. There seems to be no justification for maintaining this level of income.

These considerations together lead me to advocate the following position:

1. The portion of the relative value scale that would reduce the income of subspecialists should be implemented as soon as possible across the entire field of medical-care financing.

2. Of the money saved by not paying these "excess" fees, a small increment should be paid to the primary-care physicians, based on a calculation of income needed to pay off the average debt incurred during medical education.

3. The remaining money saved should be used in the medical-care system to improve the services offered, especially to those now lacking access to health care.

This proposal would have several advantages. The overall income of physicians would drop relative to the general population without harming those physicians now at the low end of the pay scale. By removing artificial inducements to go into specialty practice, recruitment to primary-care fields would be enhanced. The chances that the RBRVS would lead to internecine warfare in medicine would be reduced; the specialists would see that those who call for a reduction in their income are not personally going to profit as a result. If it became publicly known that physicians as a group had taken a cut in pay and that the money thus freed up was invested in improved access to health care for the poor, the public image of physicians might improve and physicians would become more effective advocates for the interests of their patients.[11]

There are also some potential disadvantages. The small increment of increased income might not attract enough new medical-school graduates into primary care. In focusing on income levels of the various *specialties*, the RBRVS might miss the issue of what was paid for particular *services*. For instance, from the ethical stance advocated in this book, it would be highly desirable for a surgeon who spends more time talking with patients to be paid as much as or more than a surgeon who does additional procedures. But an increase in the fees for such visits would also lead to a net increase

11. I have argued this case in more detail in Brody 1990a. I here depart from the established position of my own specialty society, the American Academy of Family Physicians, which has advocated adoption of the original version of the RBRVS in toto. In Brody 1990b I argue that the AAFP stand is politically shortsighted.

in the income of primary-care physicians, who spend most of their time in conversation with patients. Perhaps a creative economist can redesign the RBRVS so that it still rewards cognitive efforts while lowering specialist income.

CHAPTER 14

THE

SOCIAL

POWER

OF EXPERT

HEALERS

So far I have addressed the power that physicians possess by virtue of being physicians. In this chapter I wish to argue that the physician's social power (and, to a lesser extent, cultural power) derives not only from physicianhood per se but also from membership in a particular social class, that of the affluent, professionally trained expert. I will suggest further that some ethical analyses in medicine will be flawed or incomplete unless this source of power (and of the abuse of power) is taken into account.

The Case of Opal

Opal, now two and a half, suffers from microcephaly, extreme developmental delay, grand mal seizure disorder, regurgitation with aspiration (partially corrected by surgery), feeding by jejunostomy tube, and recurrent respiratory infections requiring eight to ten hospitalizations a year. She was delivered by emergency cesarean section at four weeks past her due date. Her teenage mother was a heavy user of drugs throughout the pregnancy; her father (unmarried) also used drugs and was in prison by the time Opal was born. Opal's mother had had only sporadic prenatal care and showed up at the hospital in labor, initially unsure of her due date. The fetal monitor showed loss of fetal heart tones requiring emergency cesarean section.

Opal was in the nursery for six weeks and required respirator support. She also developed her seizure and reflux problems at that time. (Microcephaly did not become evident until Opal was eight months of age.) Her teenage mother initially took her home and cared for her with the help of the maternal grandmother. After a short time, the mother dropped Opal off at grandmother's house with a request to "take care of her for a while

while I get a break." She stayed away three weeks. Finally, the grandmother suggested that she assume legal custody of Opal; the mother and the father (contacted in prison) both agreed. Grandmother now takes care of Opal full-time; Opal's mother comes by to visit once a week or so.

The grandmother lives in a farmhouse in a rather isolated area. The house belongs to her male companion, who is a truck driver; he occasionally helps out by taking care of Opal for short periods. Opal also has an uncle in his early twenties who is seldom seen; once he came home for a while with a broken leg (suffered in a fight over drugs) and demanded that his mother take care of him while he was disabled. Income for Opal and the grandmother consists primarily of Social Security, state Crippled Children's funds, and Aid to Dependent Children. These cover most medical care but still leave grandmother with many unpaid bills. For example, as the previous summer was unusually hot, Opal had great difficulty with perspiration and secretions, and the grandmother and her male companion installed air conditioning in the house; they were unable to get the welfare grant for the added utility expenses and currently are in arrears to the power company for seven hundred dollars.

Grandmother spends almost her entire day taking care of Opal, who needs fairly constant attention for clearing secretions in her throat, feeding her, and administering range-of-motion exercises prescribed by the physical therapist. There are some school programs for handicapped children Opal's age, but the grandmother has not utilized them; she claims that Opal's frequent infections have made this impossible but also admits that she thinks she can take care of Opal better than anyone else can.

The primary physician and other members of the crippled children's team who make occasional home visits as well as see Opal in the hospital have noted that they consider the grandmother to be pathologically attached to Opal. The grandmother has virtually no interests or human contacts outside of Opal's care. She is totally unwilling to engage in any discussion of Opal's poor long-term prognosis, saying, "She won't die until I die." Although she generally uses denial to avoid the subject, she has said specifically on several occasions that if Opal did die she would not want to go on living herself. Dealing with these issues is also complicated by distrust toward the hospital and toward at least some caregivers. The grandmother has contacted a lawyer to discuss whether "mistakes" made by the physician who did the cesarean section caused any of Opal's problems (highly unlikely). During one hospitalization, Opal suffered a burn on the hand from the efforts of an inexperienced phlebotomist to warm the extremity before blood drawing, and this incident has also led grandmother to threaten the hospital with legal action. She does, however, seem to trust the primary-care pediatrician and the crippled children's team.

That group is now meeting in their weekly family assessment conference. They wish to try to intervene to do something about grandmother's clinging relationship with Opal, thinking in part that Opal could benefit from some school programs and that the grandmother could also benefit from giving up some of Opal's care and finding other interests. They hypothesize that this clinging relationship is meeting some deeply felt needs of the grandmother. She seems to feel guilty for having been unable to control her daughter better during the pregnancy, to keep her off drugs and get her to accept regular prenatal care. (Hence, presumably, the displaced anger in trying to blame the obstetrician.) Moreover, Opal, despite her inability to do any of the things that a normal two-year-old would, is in many ways, the perfect child. She will remain forever in a totally dependent status and will never challenge the grandmother's authority or control. ("Opal is the only kid in the family the grandmother knows will never do drugs," is how one of the team members put it.)

The discussion among the medical staff turns to mechanisms to accomplish the desired changes. One person suggests that legal pressure could be applied if there is a school program that could benefit Opal and the grandmother refuses to cooperate. "Is it illegal not to send a two-year-old to school?" another wonders. And a third says, "Look, we have a kid that is being well cared for and a grandmother who is happy. Who are we to mess with this?"

Power, Interests, and Experts

There are a variety of ways to approach this case ethically. Surely it could be asked what the plans ought to be if Opal suffers a crisis, is hospitalized, and questions of aggressive life-prolonging treatment come up. More to the point now, should the staff intervene regarding school placement and the overly clinging relationship between the child and the grandmother?

Both these issues will no doubt be addressed first by asking what would be in Opal's "best interests." Does grandmother reflect Opal's best interests in her decisions? Or is she so preoccupied with her own interests that she is a poor surrogate decision-maker for Opal? Is it in Opal's interests to be deprived of the training and stimulation that the school could provide? What about the additional infections she would be exposed to at school? Or the risk of upsetting the major caregiving relationship in Opal's life—perhaps the only thing that stands between Opal and the back ward of a state hospital?

How should the team resolve disputes about what is truly in Opal's interest? I have argued that the term *best interests*, if not actually meaningless, is at least extremely difficult to specify with any operational precision (Brody 1988a). As Humpty Dumpty would have it, the question is not what the term means, but who is to be master.[1] I suggest that almost any effort to state what would be in Opal's best interests is really a disguised way to promote some specific *adult* agenda, which entails a variety of value judgments about how "good" people ought to lead their lives.[2]

One such agenda is that of the particular social class and subculture to which Opal's family belongs. This is a way of life shaped by chronic financial inadequacy, uncertain employment, and constant battles with social bureaucracies designed by the middle class to treat the lower class as adversaries.[3] This way of life is further shaped by the relative inability to control one's environment or plan for the future and by the pervasive temptation of alcohol and other drugs as escapes from this grim realization. In this setting, certain kinds of human relationships make sense which would be dysfunctional in a middle-class world. And an infant like Opal may indeed have a value that would be unthinkable in social world that prizes good looks, mental proficiency, and accomplishments. According to this agenda, the decisions involving Opal ought to be made by those who are of her world and who have the closest family and emotional ties.

A quite different agenda is that of the upper-middle-class, professionally trained healers, or "experts." This is the group to which the physicians and the crippled children's team belong. They are committed to a worldview

1. For more on problems with the term *best interests*, see the extended discussion of decisions on behalf of incompetent patients in chapter 10.

2. This assertion must of course be qualified. It could be determined to be contrary to Opal's best interests right now to cause her such sensations as pain and hunger. But these basic and obvious interests of all sentient beings say little about the important decisions that must be made about Opal's care.

3. I am indebted to Leonard Fleck for pointing out the peculiar injustice of the bureaucracy Americans have created as a result of a patchwork of health-care entitlement programs. Many of those who lack health insurance in the United States are among the working poor and therefore pay taxes. These taxes go to support systems like Medicaid, which hire staff to make sure that only those truly eligible get benefits. Therefore, the working poor effectively pay taxes to make sure that they are excluded from the health-care system. Likewise, private insurance companies hire extra staff to make sure that only those eligible receive benefits; and that practice adds to the cost of private insurance, helping to price insurance out of the market for the smaller companies that employ most of the working poor. As noted in chapter 12, some have calculated that Americans could pay for health care for all citizens now excluded from coverage if they saved the money they now spend on administering this crazy quilt of systems (Himmelstein and Woolhandler 1986).

that prizes specialized, scientifically based knowledge and the dividing up of all human experience into problems for which one must consult the correct expert if one is to have any chance of being happy.[4]

Moreover, if these experts have psychological training, then of course they know the motives and intentions of the average citizen better than he does; and if he is so impertinent as to reject their advice, they can state precisely which mental pathology is responsible for his aberrant behavior. According to this agenda, what is best for Opal is what this group of experts says is best, and indirectly it is whatever creates the greatest chance of future employment for all members of the expert class, including special-education teachers, physical therapists, social workers, family counselors, and of course physicians.[5]

A quite different agenda would be that of the conservative group which has become increasingly vocal in U.S. politics during the 1980s. Their reaction to Opal's case would be one of disgust for all family members, whom they would censure as unemployed junkies ripping off the welfare system and having sex outside of marriage. Presumably this group would favor using any medical technology to keep Opal alive regardless of her prognosis; fight against using tax dollars to create any supportive services to aid her when she is well; call for locking up both her parents for as many years as possible; and blame the grandmother for her failure to discipline her daughter properly and teach her the proper values.[6]

4. A caricature of this view is that the ideal citizen is one who on getting up in the morning immediately checks whether any of the American Cancer Society's seven early warning signs of cancer has appeared overnight, runs the precise number of miles at precisely the target pulse rate that his sports medicine specialist has recommended after his graded exercise electrocardiogram, and then phones his nutritionist to see how much fiber he should eat for breakfast.

5. My analysis here draws heavily on Lasch 1979 and to a lesser extent on Freidson 1970; see also Illich 1976. On the irony of a society that is increasingly preoccupied with its health and as a result feels a decreased sense of well-being, see Barsky 1988. No doubt this paragraph in the text presents a vicious caricature of "experts"; but since many of my readers, like me, are among them, it is wise occasionally to remind ourselves how foolish we can look to those who do not share our comfortable presuppositions.

6. William B. Weil, in commenting to me on this case, has suggested that there is a fourth agenda, one of rights of the disabled. I would argue that that agenda is actually a hybrid, adopting sanctity-of-life elements from the third agenda and elements of liberal do-gooderism from the second. A common observation in the wake of the Baby Doe controversies in the early 1980s is that the movement for the rights of the disabled, previously a creature of the political left (because it advocated reallocating tax revenues to aid a self-proclaimed minority group), had suddenly made an uneasy alliance with the conservative right in espousing a sanctity-of-life ethic for the treatment of seriously deformed newborns.

Each of these three agendas has a different status within American society. The third has managed to rise several notches during the 1980s, with the success of a federal administration committed to it. But for our purposes the most important agenda is the second one. If anyone in the United States runs afoul of administrative or legal rules—particularly within the school or court systems—it is this agenda which is most likely to be forcibly imposed by the state apparatus. It is this class of experts which is likely to decide who should go to jail, who should be committed to a mental hospital, who should be enrolled in this or that school program, and for how long, and what counts as having achieved benefit from being there; and judges, teachers, and school boards are likely to acquiesce in whatever course of action the experts suggest.

Of course, all this has been heard before. It has become the stock criticism against medicine more generally and psychiatry particularly (Szasz 1974). The argument goes that these disciplines have almost no scientific credence but function simply as a means of social control imposed by the ruling class for its own benefit. To these critics, the Chief of Medicine (see chapter 1) is correct in assessing the real Aesculapian power of the physician as very limited. They contend that social power is the primary element of physician power and that the myth of Aesculapian power is used as a smoke screen lest the lower classes catch on.

This line of criticism may seem trite and simplistic, but it is also occasionally on target. Numerous examples could be given; for now it may be sufficient to consider the question of psychiatric testimony regarding the future potential of criminals for violence. It seems difficult to dispute that there is hardly any scientific basis for making confident prediction of future violent behavior. Rather, there seems to have arisen an unholy alliance between the courts and certain psychiatrists. The courts benefit by passing off difficult decisions about length of sentence and the sort of facility to which prisoners should be sent; they get to pretend that these decisions derive from objective criteria instead of from irreducibly subjective judgments for which the judges themselves would be held accountable. A few psychiatrists, who have made a career out of giving such testimony, would find their income and prestige in jeopardy were the lack of scientific validity for their conclusions ever discussed. A larger group of psychiatrists, who may have genuine sympathy for individual prisoners or patients and want to view themselves as aiding them, offer testimony of low potential for violence altruistically; and so they too, though for better motives, acquire an interest in obscuring the scientific basis of their predictions. The rest of us, who can be relied upon most of the time not to want to know what really goes on in courtrooms or in prisons are inclined to leave this unholy alliance to its own devices and not to question it.[7]

Yet focusing on these examples of the use of pseudo-Aesculapian power for social control will obscure the more subtle message of the Chief of Medicine story about the fine line between the use and the abuse of physician power. It is one thing for people to view themselves as victims of the abuse of power by physicians and other powerful groups in society; it is another for them to view themselves as active collaborators in that abuse of power. But ultimately the public must acknowledge their role, as the more thoughtful critics of physician power make clear.

As Lasch (1979) has eloquently stated, we Americans seem to have become, as a society, profoundly uncomfortable with and estranged from a set of functions and behaviors that our forebears viewed as natural and manageable. We have adopted an ideology of personal happiness which holds that life consists of a series of snares to be avoided and problems to be solved, and that only by getting the advice and aid of specialist experts can we solve those problems in such a way as to assure happiness. I view this as an ideology rather than a rational belief because the more experts we consult, the more unhappy we get. But of course we tell ourselves, in that case, that we went to the wrong experts or did not properly follow their advice: ideology always wins out over facts.

The power of this ideology can be seen in that efforts to reject it end up re-creating it in a different form. Many in American society view physicians as too powerful and call for a return of power over one's health to the individual. Among some groups involved in holistic cancer self-help for instance, it is an article of faith that cancer is easily preventable and curable and that physicians have a selfish interest in avoiding and suppressing these preventive and curative measures in order to make more money off cancer sufferers. But the movements dedicated to overturning the power of the expert healers—notably the so-called holistic or alternative medicine movement—tend to re-create the structure of the system they reject. People appear to become every bit as dependent on the counsel of these "alternative" experts as they were on that of the more traditional healers.

It is doubtful that we can replace this ideology with another, less dysfunctional and less neurotic one. It is therefore especially important to see

---

7. For representative views on psychiatrists' predictions of violent behavior, see Peszke 1975; Ewing 1983; Monahan 1984; Chiswick 1985.

how it feeds the temptation to abuse the power of the class of experts either for social control or for the personal gain of the expert class. *Personal gain* must here be construed as including the expansion of employment opportunities for like-minded experts by systematically expanding the number of experts that must be consulted before a "problem" can be declared "solved."

The difficulty of doing away with this ideology, however, can itself be used as a rationalization to avoid change, even where individual experts can make small modifications for the better. This difficulty requires a hard look at how physicians might abuse power in this fashion and what can be done to avoid that abuse.

Abuses of Expert Power

The abuses of power attached to membership in the expert class cut across all guidelines for judging the responsible use of power. Owned power becomes a problem when the role of the expert and the need to consult experts over every detail of day-to-day living are taken for granted. It is easy for the physician to deny under these circumstances that she has any such power since the self-image of the expert healer is to be helpful, not manipulative for selfish ends.[8] But power that is unrecognized is hard to channel into responsible uses.

Similarly, aimed power is resisted so long as the self-image of benevolent helper remains untarnished. If the power tends both to respond to the needs and desires of individuals and to cement the social authority of the expert class, the first aim of the power may be confused with the total aim. Justifications for the use of power will be offered which miss the problematic features of the case but sound superficially compelling. Worse, alternative strategies may be denounced in the name of the individual autonomy they are supposed to promote. Since the public willingly complies with the expert ideology, refusal by the expert to accept the assigned role could be seen as a violation of the autonomy of the client or patient and as an attempt to impose a new ideology on them out of paternalistic arrogance: "we know better than they do what they really need."[9]

8. "The elite cannot truly be thought of as men who are merely 'doing their duty.' In considerable part they are the ones who determine their duty, as well as the duties of other men. They do not merely follow orders; they give orders. They are not merely bureaucrats; they command bureaucracies. They may try to disguise these facts from others and from themselves by appealing to traditions of which they imagine themselves to be the instruments, but there are many traditions, and they must choose which ones they will serve. And now they face decisions for which there simply are no traditions" (Ladd 1981, citing Mills 1959).

9. An oft-cited example of this phenomenon is the clash between the modern physician,

Shared power is difficult to achieve so long as the physician occupies this expert role.[10] To empower the patient might, in some ways at least, threaten the social hegemony of the expert class and put experts out of their jobs. Despite this pull, most experts genuinely want to be helpful and see an overdependence as unhelpful to their clients. But the more subtle problem is that even given the urge to empower, the ideology may be so strong that the empowerment itself becomes a reinforcement of helpless dependence. It may, in the end, seem as if one can get power only by going to the right expert and following his advice precisely; one cannot get power simply by choosing to exercise it. In an age when people pay lots of money to attend seminars that purport to teach assertiveness and self-esteem, this danger seems real.

In chapter 3, I argued that some abuses of power might be called playing God. The expert may be tempted to use the power attached to his role not simply to carry out his role functions and assist those who seek his aid but to try to redesign the world—often by rewarding the "good" and punishing the "bad." Of course, if the power were appropriately aimed and owned, the expert would have to take explicit responsibility for doing this—and by implication would have to defend publicly his judgments as to who the good and the bad are and what gives him the right to decide their fate. The net result is that some patients get approved for disability or other benefits while others get turned down; some needy persons have opportunities and assistance opened up to them while others face a brick wall of bureaucratic inertia. No expert has to own responsibility for making any value-laden judgments because each of these acts can be justified in terms of the professional judgments within a particular field of expertise.

The challenge for physicians (and other experts) is to find ways to make their patients feel genuinely more powerful to control their own lives and health; to be more aware of the actual ends of their social and cultural power, not only the ends that bear the most benign interpretation; and to be willing to accept responsibility for the use of power with a realistic understanding of all its facets.

who has been trained to believe in patient autonomy, and the old-fashioned patient, who expects and indeed values paternalistic treatment from the doctor. To the extent that one can autonomously choose to be treated paternalistically, the physician's efforts to promote the patient's autonomy can themselves be denounced as unwarranted paternalism.

10. Ladd (1981) indicates that the sharing of power is a useful antidote to the possible abuses of social and political power by physicians. He fails to address, however, the problem of sharing when the power has been rendered culturally invisible. In this regard, shared power requires owned power as a prior condition.

The Rabkin Explosion

It is of little use to analyze the power of the healing experts in our society if the only conclusion is that the experts are bad people (or else that the society is bad). A further case study may help at this point to illustrate how complex the issues around power and expertise can be.

This case comes from an unusual source. People are by now used to the idea that books and articles on medical ethics might present controversial cases, which become the subject of heated debate. But it is a bit out of the ordinary for controversial cases to arise in literature and medicine journals.[11] Nevertheless, the growing field of literature and medicine now has one "hot" case study to its credit, and it may prove instructive here.

David Barnard, a professor of medical humanities trained in religion and psychology, contributed a case study which he titled, "A Case of Amyotrophic Lateral Sclerosis" (Barnard 1986). As a participant-observer, he followed "Dr. Valerie Walsh" in a series of visits with "Mr. and Mrs. Baker." Mr. Baker was seventy-seven when he developed progressive weakness and was diagnosed as having ALS. Mrs. Baker, seventy-three, became his caretaker in spite of her own medical problems of angina, diabetes, and arthritis. Dr. Walsh came to bond closely with the Bakers, who were in turn deeply and openly grateful for the care that she provided. But she also struggled with two ongoing problems. The first was her desire to clarify Mr. Baker's wishes regarding intensity of medical treatment, particularly the eventual question of intubation and mechanical ventilation. The signals given by both Bakers strongly suggested their desire to hold onto hope and not to face the grim prognosis. The second was the Bakers' insistence on remaining in their own home, at some distance from needed social and nursing services, and their resistance to efforts to place aides or other workers in the home following an unfortunate incident with an uncaring person. These limitations conflicted with Dr. Walsh's desire to provide the best care possible for Mr. Baker and to spare the strain on Mrs. Baker's health.

Eventually, after months of home visits that left Dr. Walsh feeling both isolated and frustrated, she was able to get Mr. Baker to articulate his desire not to receive mechanical ventilation; she also was able to arrange for a health aide to visit the home to help with the most burdensome physical

---

11. "Literature and medicine" refers to an emerging field within the medical humanities. Professors of literature have turned to the study of medical themes, teaching various works of fiction that portray medical themes and examining how language is used within the practice of medicine itself. The journal *Literature and Medicine* is the primary compendium of work in this field.

chores. Within a month, however, Mrs. Baker was dead of a sudden heart attack. Mr. Baker then had to be placed in a nursing home, where he died six weeks later.

When the case study was solicited for the journal *Literature and Medicine*, the issue editor, Joanne Trautmann Banks, had some questions about the case history format. To what extent was the study an "objective" account of events, and to what extent was it fiction? With this in mind, she requested a commentary from an authority on narrative theory, Eric Rabkin. Rabkin's commentary (1986) is perhaps most notable for violating one of the norms of commentaries in scholarly journals: it is markedly uncivil, even angry.[12] He concluded that Barnard had elected to ignore the needs of the Bakers in order to write a manuscript that glorified the caring physician; that Dr. Walsh had been driven more by a need to see herself as a hero-martyr than by a realistic appraisal of the Bakers' needs; and that between them Barnard and Walsh had lied to Mr. Baker about his disease and its prognosis and probably hastened Mrs. Baker's death.

Not unnaturally, given his background, Rabkin chose to analyze Barnard's text as a piece of fiction, and indeed Rabkin offered much internal evidence to justify that way of looking at the material. His analysis led him to conclude that Barnard was too self-effacing as narrator; if he was actually present in the home during some of the highly emotional exchanges he described, then his being there was a part of the narrative, and it was not honest to act as if he were merely the reader's window onto events. Rabkin also identified a number of passages that hinted at Dr. Walsh's personal needs—to do battle against a dread disease; to protect Mr. Baker from demoralizing news by being the sole judge of what he was ready to hear and when; to keep other potential team helpers out of the case while complaining that she was left to deal with the Bakers all by herself; and especially to accept the frequent and forceful expressions of gratitude and praise bestowed on her by the Bakers.

Rabkin suggested that two things should have been done. First, Mr. Baker should have been confronted earlier with his poor prognosis so that open planning could have taken place; and second, Dr. Walsh should have insisted on getting the Bakers to move closer to the center of the city, where more services were close at hand. Banks thus felt obligated to call

12. An example of the tone that runs throughout the article is an early sentence, "I must stress that I personally believe Barnard and Walsh in no *conscious* way acted to harm the Bakers" (Rabkin 1986, p. 43; emphasis in original). In context, this sentence can best be interpreted as saying: not only did they do evil things, but they were also too stupid to know what they were doing.

for another commentary on the ethics of these recommendations, and that was supplied by David H. Smith (1986). Smith faulted Rabkin for ethical inconsistency. Presumably the need to tell Mr. Baker the truth was rooted in respect for his autonomy. How, then, could Rabkin recommend violating Mr. Baker's autonomy by forcing him to leave the home that meant so much to him and his wife?[13]

These are the basic facts of the case and the central issues in the controversy that erupted around its publication. What light can the case shed on the question of experts' power?

An interesting role reversal developed in this controversy. Walsh is the physician, and Barnard seems to have accepted the role of the physician's apologist. It would therefore seem natural for them to impose their own views on the Bakers, paying scant attention to what the Bakers themselves say they want. And Rabkin, as defender of the patient against the power of the experts, might have been expected to call the expects to task. But the reality of the case is quite different. Dr. Walsh is the one who seems to be listening to the Bakers, telling them what they want to hear, backing off when they indicate they do not wish to deal with certain issues, and supporting their oft-stated wish to remain in their own home. It is Rabkin, by contrast, who urges Dr. Walsh to push her expert opinion of the matter onto the Bakers and force them to move to a more convenient location for sending a crowd of like-minded experts into the Baker home to take care of them. This observation by itself does not establish who is right and who is wrong (if anyone is either). But it does suggest that things may be muddier than they first appear. Taking sides with or against the experts is not enough to assure moral purity.

What should have been done in this case? Rabkin's telling observations suggest that Dr. Walsh's course was not driven by the most appropriate needs. But neither is it clear that Rabkin's suggestions are wise: people cannot be forced to move, accept home services, or face a harsh prognosis squarely.

13. Smith's commentary on patient autonomy seems correct as far as it goes; but it also appears to be a cheap shot in the context of the case. It seems reasonable that a more active confrontation with the Bakers, focused on the eventual need for additional home services and the threats to Mrs. Baker's own health, would have caused them to revise their initial views on accepting help or even on moving (after all, they did eventually accept an aide, after saying consistently that they would refuse). And in turn, insisting on being more forthright about Mr. Baker's actual prognosis would seem to be a vital element in this process of confrontation. Although Rabkin openly admitted his lack of clinical experience and skills, his recommendations nevertheless seem to have a clinical cohesion which Smith fails to recognize.

It is always much easier to be wise or creative in retrospect in such cases. What would have happened, though, if Dr. Walsh had paid more attention to her own conflicts about the Bakers earlier in the course of treatment? She was defending their rights and their privacy, she was having their praise and gratitude heaped on her, yet she still felt frustrated and fearful that things would not go well. This led to her increasing isolation from her medical team. What if she had seen this isolation and had decided to get the team more involved and to consult other physicians as to what her own feelings meant?[14]

Through this consultation, Dr. Walsh may have learned more about her own psychological needs and how they were influencing her treatment decisions. In addition, she might have evolved a positive plan for confronting the Bakers with the difficult care issues. Ideally, the confrontation would lead each faction—the Bakers and the healing experts—to own the part of the problem that only they could solve.

Dr. Walsh might have arranged for some colleagues on her medical team to accompany her on a home visit to make a less biased assessment of the home situation and of Mr. Baker's present and future needs. If after that visit no new plans could be formulated, the next step might be to return to the Bakers' home and tell them something like the following:

"Our team is frustrated. We are getting mixed messages about you and your situation and don't know how to interpret them.

"On the one hand, we know that you love each other, that you value your home life and your privacy, that Mrs. Baker is dedicated and unselfish in providing care, and that Mr. Baker has shown great emotional strength in coming to grips with a serious disease. These are all very important, and it ought to be our job as a health-care team to support and reinforce them.

"On the other hand, we know that a good deal of help is available for families in situations like yours, and we are puzzled as to why we have not been able to get you linked up with such help. We have heard Mrs. Baker express her own frustration with how things are going, and we know

---

14. A family physician found herself taking care of a close friend during a terminal illness. This physician feared that the personal ties could lead her to mistakes in judgment, but she did not use that as an excuse to withdraw. Instead she made special efforts to consult regularly with her colleagues to be sure that her management of the case was reviewed regularly by more impartial observers. I am grateful to Elizabeth Alexander, M.D., for this illustration. See the discussion in chapter 16 on compassion and the widespread fear that too much compassion will cause the physician to lose objectivity.

that she fears that her own health will be affected by the strain. And we are not sure that we have yet had a frank discussion about what Mr. Baker's future needs are going to be.

"We are frustrated because we have these two sets of messages—one saying that things are going well and the other that things are going badly. Until we get our own problem solved, we are afraid we will not provide for you the high-quality care you deserve. Can you help us work toward a resolution?"

If this approach seems like a reasonable alternative to the trap Dr. Walsh sensed herself falling into, it may be because the message is a complicated mix of owned power and owned powerlessness. The powerlessness is admitted: the health team cannot remake the Baker family into their image of the ideal client and cannot force the Bakers to place a higher value on receiving certain sorts of technical assistance than on remaining together in their own home without outside interference. The team cannot even get a clear idea of the problem is without their participation. The power is stated more subtly: there is a clear threat that if the Bakers do not discuss these matters and in the process talk about things that they have heretofore been unwilling to talk about, assistance will be withdrawn at some level. But this threatened use of power does not seem inappropriate, for professionals should be able to avoid giving care under circumstances in which they feel strongly that they cannot do a good job.[15]

If this team conference approach to the Baker's situation represents an ethically superior alternative to what actually occurred, then why was it not done or even considered? One hypothesis is that the three parties— Mr. Baker, Mrs. Baker, and Dr. Walsh—were locked in a serious but unrealized power struggle. Indeed, one might conclude that all three were guilty of the unowned, unaimed, and unshared use of the power that they possessed, thereby producing a tangle of cross-purposes.[16]

---

15. Of course, if professionals claimed that they could do a good job only in those circumstances where they were given enough control unilaterally to define both the problem and the solution in their own terms, then professional help would be too much of a threat to individual autonomy for American society to tolerate. My assumption, by contrast, is that professionals define respect for individual autonomy as part of what it means to do a good job (compare the patient-centered primary-care model discussed in chapter 4); and that the conclusion, "I can't do a good job in this case," is reached only after extensive dialogue with the would-be client.

16. I here omit the fourth party, Barnard, from consideration. For one thing, Rabkin has already given him sufficient grief to render him an unappealing target for further criticism. For another, Barnard's lapse was primarily in the area of owned power, in that he tried to efface himself as the narrator rather than acknowledge and reveal the role he played in the unfolding of the case. He portrayed himself at the start of his article (Barnard 1986) as a

Dr. Walsh never examined the types of power she did and did not possess in relation to the Bakers. For example, she agonized over her power to destroy Mr. Baker's hope by being too candid in discussing the prognosis of ALS, but she paid scant attention to the power she was assuming by taking it upon herself to decide how much he wanted to hear and when. She worried about an eventual bad outcome and several times referred to the Bakers as a "time bomb," but continued to make her routine home visits without asking whether they might be reinforcing the impression that no additional help was needed. She paid no attention to the potential for a power struggle between her and Mrs. Baker that was inherent in a female physician's making house calls.

Without having examined the power issues, Dr. Walsh could never be sure what she was trying to do with her power. How much was aimed at doing battle with ALS, which had killed a previous patient of hers just before she met the Bakers? How much was aimed at keeping up her own hopes, in the guise of keeping up Mr. Baker's hopes? (When she finally did bring up the subject of mechanical ventilation, Mr. Baker responded promptly and thoughtfully, with appropriate sadness; there was no clue from that exchange that the subject could not have been safely broached six months earlier.) How much was aimed at maintaining herself in the role of sole caregiver, the only one who could meet the needs of the Bakers?

Power is almost impossible to share when one does not know that one has it and does not know what one is doing with it. Therefore Dr. Walsh lost opportunities to empower the Bakers through her visits and her care. This failure assured that any power the Bakers exercised themselves had as much chance of being in conflict as in collusion with Dr. Walsh's power. The Bakers were in a bind: they were quite socially isolated and needed the comfort that Dr. Walsh's visits provided. They could not bring the power struggle out in the open without threatening that relationship. And so on the surface, all of Dr. Walsh's efforts were met with expressions of

---

"participant-observer" but then went on to write as all observer and no participant. It is perhaps revealing that Barnard's purported misstatement of the issues found an echo in the editorial comments of the issue editor of the journal. Rabkin took Barnard to task for calling his article, "A Case of Amyotrophic Lateral Sclerosis," as if this locution would guarantee the scientific objectivity of what followed—and as if what really mattered was Mr. Baker's disease, not Mr. Baker. In her brief editorial note that introduced the series of three articles, Joanne Trautmann Banks used the title, "A Controversy about Clinical Form." This again runs the risk of leaving out the human dimension of the account in favor of a comfortable scholarly analysis. If we are to take Rabkin seriously (even to disagree with him), the controversy is not over clinical form; it is over whether some professionals abused the people they were supposed to be helping.

praise and gratitude, but no one looked critically at those statements to see what issues might lie concealed below them.

The Bakers, on their side, had similar problems with power. Mr. Baker seems to have become quite absorbed in his illness. His calm resignation in the face of weakness and loss of independence was commendable. But there is almost no hint, in the passages recorded by Barnard, of any real concern for the toll the illness must be taking on Mrs. Baker. At one point Mrs. Baker complains bitterly that her husband is not trying to help himself. His reaction is to defend his efforts: it's not that he isn't trying, but his muscles simply will not respond. Any reaction from him like, "I know how hard it is on her, and I worry about her health," is absent from the record. Neither wish to admit that Mr. Baker is going to die soon. This means they cannot address the subject of what life will be like for Mrs. Baker after he is gone—whether she will be able to function well or whether his illness will have taken such toll on her that she will have to go into a nursing home. There is thus a sense in which Mr. Baker's power to cope with his illness is being directed against his wife, not just against the effects of the ALS.

Mrs. Baker's efforts to use her power mirror Dr. Walsh's. Mrs. Baker also has a strong need to be seen as the sole caregiver, even at the cost of being the hero-martyr. At one point she proclaims, pointing at her husband, "I'm going to get ten more years out of this if it kills me!" (Barnard 1986, p. 29). This statement is a tragic foreshadowing of the actual outcome of the case. Mrs. Baker also has a strong need to buoy her own hopes by not facing the serious prognosis of ALS. A statement by Mr. Baker that suggests resignation and acceptance is likely to be followed by an aggressively optimistic interruption from his wife. In retrospect, when Dr. Walsh withheld frank discussions about prognosis because she felt that her patient was not ready to hear them, we may wonder whether it was actually Mrs. Baker she was protecting. It is thus possible that Mrs. Baker used her power to maintain control and sustain her own sense of her role instead of trying to achieve the best outcomes for Mr. Baker and meet his real needs. This also made it inevitable that Mrs. Baker would become locked in a power struggle with Dr. Walsh.[17]

17. A revealing statement by Dr. Walsh, toward the end of the case, is, "I feel like I have no control over what's happening right now. I'm completely dependent on [Mrs. Baker], and she's doing an *excellent* job" (Barnard 1986, p. 40). An undercurrent in this passage is that Dr. Walsh thinks that she herself should have control and feels badly for not having it. (The obvious rejoinder is: the caregiver who is actually in the home should be the central figure, and the doctor should not feel threatened in her role by the strength and power of the

The way all parties used their power at cross-purposes makes it understandable why a better resolution was not reached—and why the outcome of the case might have been the best that could *practically* have been achieved. Still, when it comes to the appropriate use of power, the professional must assume a deeper responsibility than the client. It is perfectly excusable for the Bakers to be unclear on what their power consisted of and how it was being employed; it is less excusable for Dr. Walsh. My analysis suggests that all three guidelines on the responsible use of power would need to be consulted to avoid this sort of outcome in future cases.

The analysis suggests a further clue. If Dr. Walsh went wrong, it may be due in part to an inappropriate and unrealized *self-preoccupation*. She may have been too wrapped up in her needs to vanquish the disease, decide what should be told to the patient, and see herself as a certain kind of compassionate physician. Thus an important character trait for physicians to cultivate would be a way of avoiding, or at least identifying, self-preoccupation. I will discuss this under the heading of the physician's virtues and character in chapter 16.

Before embarking on a discussion of character and virtue in medical ethics, however, it will be helpful to consider some theoretical and methodological issues, since ethics can be conceived of in ways that render virtue and character (as well as power) largely irrelevant. This will be the focus of the next chapter.

---

caregiver.) Although Dr. Walsh implies that she resents Mrs. Baker's power, she lauds her work, thereby mirroring the praise and gratitude that the Bakers feel obliged to heap on Dr. Walsh at every opportunity.

CHAPTER 15

POWER

AND

THEORIES

OF MEDICAL

ETHICS

I n chapter 3, I suggested some reasons why medical ethics proceeded for some time largely without discussing power. Why has that concept now suddenly reappeared? Is it just coincidence that few philosophers pursued the ideas that John Ladd originally presented in 1980 (assuming that they even read them)? Or that while I was in the middle of work on the subject, a number of books and articles appeared which also called attention to the importance of power issues?[1] I will not guess at the causes of the reemergence of power talk, but I will now offer some reflections on recent developments in the theory and methodology of medical ethics. These developments do not require that one use power language, but they do provide an environment in which a proposal to reintroduce the concept of power will be more likely to find support and sympathy.

I have already underlined that I do not propose to dispense with the language of autonomy, beneficence, and justice while embracing power talk; but my acceptance of these standard terms may hide a methodological assumption about their significance within ethical activity generally. I contend that the activity of ethics is best described as a particular sort of ongoing conversation, and that the importance of both ethical principles and case studies or stories can be properly understood only within the framework of that conversation. Specifically, I propose for contrast two models, what Caplan (1983) has called the engineering model of medical ethics and what I call the conversation model.

1. Representative samples would include Zaner 1988; Drane 1988; Pellegrino and Thomasma 1988; McCullough 1988, 1989; Callahan 1989; Doerflinger 1989.

Engineering and Conversation Models

The engineering model is, admittedly, an extreme caricature useful mainly as a point of departure for further discussion of ethical method. Nonetheless, it is my contention that the model has more unconscious force than many philosophers may be aware of, and that it has guided thinking in medical ethics in the past fifteen to twenty years. According to this model, ethical reasoning about cases proceeds in largely deductive fashion. Abstract ethical theories like Kantian duty-based ethics or utilitarianism give rise to a small number of general ethical principles: respect the autonomy of those capable of rational choice; provide benefit and avoid inflicting harm; distribute limited resources according to some principle of fair distribution; and so on. These, when applied to specific case examples, yield reasonable deductions about appropriate action. Here is an example:

1. One should always respect the autonomy of those capable of rational thought.
2. In the case at hand, X is capable of rational thought.
3. In the case at hand, X has chosen to refuse treatment.
4. Therefore, one ought to honor X's refusal of treatment.

This model has a number of important implications for medical ethics. First, everything of philosophical importance occurs in the derivation of the ethical principles from the more abstract ethical theories. The application to those principles to specific cases is, by contrast, a mechanical exercise of little philosophical interest (except in the cases where equally valid principles come into conflict in especially interesting ways). It follows that philosophers interested in medical ethics learn very little from detailed case studies. Case studies serve as entertaining parables for getting the uninitiated (medical students and practicing physicians) to see the application and the importance of the ethical principles. Moreover, since the principles are relatively few and are specifiable in advance, it follows that which features of a case will be morally relevant or morally controlling can also be known in advance. One can know, for instance, that whether Jones is capable of rational decision making is going to be a matter of great moral relevance, and whether Jones is male or female is going to be of almost no moral relevance; and one can know this while knowing nothing at all about Jones or about Jones's case.[2]

2. For a rather extreme statement of how the nature and application of a moral distinction is independent of context, see Rachels 1986.

Further implications arising from the engineering model help reinforce its use among physicians who are sympathetic to the introduction of better ethical thinking into medicine. If one adheres to a hypothetico-deductive model of the scientific method, then the engineering model of applying medical ethics will seem, in outline, amazingly similar to the way in which general scientific laws yield specific judgments about particular instances. For example:

1. All metals expand when heated.
2. This sample is a metal.
3. Therefore, this sample will expand when heated.

Now, any philosopher of science would immediately provide dozens of reasons to reject this model as saying anything true or interesting about scientific methodology. But most physicians have not studied the philosophy of science, and almost all were taught in junior high school that this is indeed the way science comes to reject false hypotheses and accept true ones as theories. If that is so, then it may appear that medical ethics shares much of the rigor and the potential certainty of scientific reasoning. This makes it easier for these "scientific" physicians to accept ethicists as hardheaded thinkers worthy of respectful attention (in contrast to social and behavioral scientists, whose soft-headed theories—in the physicians' view—obviously have nothing in common with real science and whose predictions are always in the form of rough approximations, never certain truths). Moreover, the form of ethical reasoning, just like the form of hypothetico-deductive scientific reasoning, assures that any conclusions reached are not only true in the present instance but are true throughout history and across cultures, because they are logically deduced from culture-free general theories. This certainly must mean that the reasoning of ethicists is far superior to that of the social scientists.

My main point here is similar to one reason I suggested for ethicists' trying to get along without speaking of power. If an ethicist wants the scientific, hardheaded physicians to welcome her into their fold, and if she wants to prove to them that she is different from those social scientists who had previously made themselves unwelcome, then the engineering model of medical ethics is a useful approach. This thinking, in part, makes me suspicious of the ethicists' protestations that Caplan has set up a straw man with this model and that no real philosopher would ever stoop to such a simplistic mode of reasoning. Simplistic it may be, but it definitely has its uses, and the temptation to give in to it is strong even if one, philosophically, knows better or ought to.

The engineering model has implications also for the sort of decision forum that could be predicted to provide the best ethical advice in health-care settings. It leads, for instance, to a resounding rejection of the idea of a multidisciplinary hospital ethics committee. The argument against such a committee goes as follows:

1. Either there exist principles which yield good ethical conclusions when applied to cases, or there do not.

2. If these principles exist, then one does not need a committee. Anybody with a sound knowledge of the principles and of the facts of the case can as readily come up with the correct answer as could anyone else.

3. If these principles do not exist, then an ethics committee could never begin or end its deliberations, as it could not possibly know what features of the case to look at or how to reason from them.

4. Therefore, ethics committees are either unnecessary or ineffectual.

What is important to note about this argument is that it implicitly takes the engineering model for granted and denies the existence of any competing model worthy of study.

I can now contrast the engineering model with the conversation model (Brody 1989a). According to the latter, ethics is an attempt to answer the question, "What, all things considered, ought to be done in a given situation?" (Benjamin and Curtis 1986, p. 9). The only way to answer that question is to engage in an extended and rigorous conversation about the situation at hand. Western culture, over centuries of such conversations, has evolved a sense of what considerations are relevant in deciding what ought to be done. As products of that culture, we will look out for those features of a given case and attempt to reason from them, probably by analogy with other cases we are familiar with. Some of us will be better than others at this sort of reasoning, even though the mode of reasoning and the morally relevant features of the case are products of the whole culture and are not a matter of special technical expertise.

Jonsen and Toulmin's (1988) proposal that medical ethics is less akin to philosophical ethics than to the ancient practice of casuistry seems consistent with the conversation model. The term *casuistry* acquired a negative connotation in the late Renaissance which it still possesses to-day. But during earlier times casuistry was a logically rigorous and fully respectable method of approaching ethics by means of case studies. Instead of looking for a few ethical principles, casuists identified a multiplicity of moral maxims or rules of thumb. They then selected for each maxim a paradigm case that seemed to illustrate it in its most perfect form and with the fewest special circumstances that detracted from the understanding of its application. For many Americans, for instance, the apocryphal story of George Washington and the cherry tree has fulfilled this function of paradigm case with regard to the maxim, "Tell the truth." The casuist then proceeded to consider a variety of cases and to lay them out in orderly fashion around this paradigm case. A case that differed from it only in minor details would be shown as still illustrating the maxim clearly, whereas a case that had a number of novel circumstances would be described as farther from the center of the maxim. Eventually the casuist would come to borderline cases where the application of the maxim was very questionable or where there was serious doubt as to which of two contradictory maxims applied. For instance, the casuist might describe Kant's famous dilemma, "Do you tell the truth to a homicidal maniac who comes to the door brandishing a weapon and asks which way your friend has fled?" as between two maxims, "Tell the truth" and "Preserve others from harm."

Today, medical ethics is assumed to derive from philosophy. Jonsen therefore takes pains to note that although the classical casuists made free use of philosophical concepts when this suited their purposes and helped illuminate cases, they did not see their activity as fundamentally grounded in philosophy. (They made equally facile use of legal and theological concepts or arguments when that seemed to suit better.) Instead they appealed to the discipline of rhetoric, which (within the Aristotelian framework) dealt with sound and persuasive reasoning in those realms of human activity where only probability, not certainty, could be obtained. But even this much of a claim for "disciplinary grounding" may give a misleading impression of casuist activity; actually, the casuists "may not have thought much about method, as we understand the idea" (Jonsen 1986b, p. 68). There were indeed rigor and skill in their work, but it was the "skill of *interpreting the case*" (p. 68).

For modern use, one may provide an alternative to the casuist's reliance on medieval concepts of natural law. To the casuist, the maxims were given and could not be altered by the case study method. But by adding the idea that one might eventually come to revise the maxims or devise new maxims, as a result of testing the fit between the maxims and a wide variety of cases—so that the reasoning would be bidirectional—the casuist approach could be modified so as to make it more applicable to a secular pluralist culture like our own. This model of ethics allows the ethicist to utilize case studies without embarrassment as a central research tool instead of having to pretend that these are simply teaching devices necessary to get the attention of physicians who are unschooled in ethical theory.[3]

The casuistic or conversation model allows an important role for ethical principles and theories, but their role within the conversation model is quite different from what the engineering model envisions. Theories and principles are handy when one sits down to discuss a case. Principles like respect for autonomy and theories like rights-based theory or utilitarianism emerged because they were pithy and insightful summaries of morally relevant features that tended to arise over and over again in many classes of morally problematic cases. To date, in Western culture, no single ethical theory or principle has succeeded in establishing itself as the basic or primary ethical theory, to the extent that those appealing to a rival theory can be shown to be irrational or unreasonable. This seems to be because the class of features of cases or situations that may, under the right circumstances, be morally weighty or morally compelling is larger than the class of central ideas or principles that can be coherently and compactly included in any single ethical theory. It may be true, for example, that in many situations what one ought to do coincides with what would produce the most benefit. But it is also true that in some situations one ought not do what would produce the most benefit; and in other situations one ought to do something that will produce the most benefit, but the fact that it produces the most benefit is not the most compelling reason why that thing ought to be done. This means that utilitarianism is a plausible and appealing moral theory, and also that there will be important counter-examples to a utilitarian theory. The same could be said for Kantian respect for autonomy, rights-based theories, or virtually any other theory that has been proposed. The conclusion seems to be that the more of those theories one has studied, the larger one's stock of possibly morally relevant features to search for in a given case. But that is almost the same as saying that the person who is best able to think through a tough moral problem is the person who has attended most closely to the prior conversation about general moral problems that has gone on throughout the history of Western culture.

These observations suggest as one possible approach a broader appreciation of the potentials of an ethics committee. If the goal is the efficient application of a single, superior theory, then a single "expert" can outperform any committee. But if the goal instead is to have out on the table for

3. What would be required for this move would be to integrate with casuistry John Rawls's notion of wide reflective equilibrium. See Rawls 1971; Daniels 1979, 1980.

consideration as broad as possible a list of considerations or features of the case that may be ethically relevant, then a committee of many minds and varied backgrounds will probably provide a more comprehensive list than any one person alone.

Another way of making this point is to note that it is almost pathognomonic of the engineering model for someone to say, "First, of course, you have to get clear on the facts of the case. Then you proceed to . . ." Usually what follows is the application of some general theory to the facts. The assumption is that the "getting clear on the facts" is both pre-theoretical and ethically neutral. But the conversation or casuist model would claim that getting clear on the facts is often the most difficult feature of a case, and one can drastically change the moral weights of the alternatives either by introducing a new "fact" or by reexamining an old one in a new light. And often, in practice, adding or reexamining "facts" substantially means looking at the situation from the viewpoint of an actor who previously had not been given much consideration. A multidisciplinary committee is more likely to have people who can readily empathize with many actors in the drama, whereas any single person is more likely to fall into the trap of looking at a situation from the vantage point of only one or a few parties.

This is not a call for ethics committees as a moral panacea. There are many ways in which an ethics committee might fail to live up to the potential I have attributed to it. The members might be too quick to reach a consensus and unwilling to listen to the lone minority voice. The committee may be dominated by one person or ideology. It may be too prone to defend the interests of the institution. Insufficient data exist to say how many committees fall into these traps, and how often. My point is that a committee approach is congenial to someone who employs the conversation model, whereas the same approach seems like nonsense to anyone using the engineering model. If on further trial it turns out that the institutional ethics committee, as now constituted, has fatal flaws, the "conversationist" is more likely to tinker with that approach or try to invent something rather close to it to replace it than simply to trash the concept.

The conversation model and the more modern version of casuistry (that is, a form shorn of natural-law assumptions) admit that ultimately there will be a major role for intuition in deciding what features of a case are morally compelling and what reasons are worthy of acceptance. At any rate, the model denies any preexisting algorithm or formula that can decide these questions in advance of a specific case situation. What one thinks of this model will depend on what alternatives one sees open. If one thinks that other approaches do indeed offer eternal and culturally independent truths about morality, then this model will seem shoddily relativistic. If one thinks that the promise of certainty in both the engineering model and its first cousin, the positivist model of science, is a will-o'-the-wisp, then this model, which locates the relativism squarely within the cultural and historical context that gives shape to our conversation, may seem refreshing by contrast.[4] To paraphrase Richard Rorty, when physicians sit down to discuss a difficult case, they are in effect continuing a long conversation about morality that has characterized Western culture since its Judeo-Christian and Greco-Roman beginnings. When they ask, "What should we do in this situation, all things considered?" they take for granted that prior conversation and turn to it for clues to interpreting the present problem. Their conclusion will likewise be embedded in the history of their culture and will form a small part of that ongoing conversation. The skeptic will object that they cannot have any confidence that their conclusion is correct for any other culture or historical period. In the end, the reply to the skeptic must be, "What other conversation would it make more sense for *us* to be having *now*? If we are not to join in the conversation that characterizes our culture and our historical epoch, which *other* conversation *should* we join?" (Rorty 1982).

By the engineering model, ethical reflection is an intellectual, totally asocial activity. By the conversation model, applied ethics has an irreducibly social element.[5] It is not simply that ethical behavior, as Rawls (1971) defined the term, is what one rationally wants ones' associates to engage in. It is also that one comes to discover what counts as good reasons for the weight of competing considerations in particular cases only by a process of social dialogue, or by a process that closely mimics social dialogue.

The irreducibly social features of ethical decision making show up clearly when one considers what it is like to make an important, personal moral decision. We do not, generally, wish *only* to do the right thing or follow the rules. We wish also to be a certain sort of person. We want our lives to hang together as the connected stories of whole people, not as a disconnected series of snapshots of individual actions. When we try to decide

4. Murray (1987), in defending casuistry in the sense of interpretation of cases, points out that proponents of the engineering model cannot escape the fact that they too must use interpretation to decide how their general principles apply to specific cases; and the more general the theory, the greater the role that interpretation must play. Admittedly, interpretation can be done badly: "people can and do engage in logic-chopping and precious distinctions in order to evade moral responsibility for themselves or those whose interests they serve.... But to condemn *all* interpretation because it is on occasion misused is foolish" (p. 640).

5. At this point, what I am calling the conversation model may deviate from the methods of casuistry as the term is used in Jonsen and Toulmin 1988.

what to do, we inevitably ask questions like, "How will those whose respect and affirmation I most value respond to me if I do such-and-such? And how will I, in turn, react to their responses?" Often we actually go over such questions with someone else, rehearsing various options and seeing how those to whom we speak react.

In making important decisions we try to maximize self-respect. Rawls (1971) suggests that self-respect has two important elements. First, our actions conform to a reasonable and discernible plan for how we are going to live our lives (even if that plan consists only of a vague outline). Second, that plan must win the affirmation of those close associates whose opinions we value. If I am inclined to act in a certain way in a difficult dilemma and I discover in conversation that all my close associates would disapprove of me if I acted that way, I have a problem. I may still rationally decide to act in the chosen manner, reasoning that ultimately my associates will be persuaded that I was right all along or, in the most extreme case, that I need to find a new set of associates. But what I cannot do rationally is ignore the question of how valued associates will react to my behavior. This suggests that moral decisions presuppose both a sort of conversation and a set of social relationships that go toward defining one's identity as a person.[6]

If the trend in the theoretical side of medical ethics is away from the engineering model and toward a conversation or casuist model, then the time seems ripe for reintroducing or reexamining the concept of power in medicine. As we have seen so far, talk of power does several things. It highlights features of situations that otherwise might go unseen. It causes us to look at known features in a new light—in particular, to reexamine actions and intentions which initially appeared benign when seen from the vantage point of the more powerful individual in the relationship. It prompts us to see issues as reciprocal and mutually reinforced which may initially have appeared one-dimensional. And it imports into ethical discourse some useful ideas which previously had been largely restricted to the social and behavioral sciences. According to a model that tends to elevate the detailed study of the circumstances of concrete cases and downplay the importance of abstract theory or principle, these developments will seem helpful.

The conversation model might take a dim view of power talk if it were thought to be a proposal for a new abstract theory intended to replace the

6. For a further discussion both of Rawls's concept of self-respect and its implications for the social dimension of ethics, see Brody 1987d, chap. 3.

theories or principles of respect for autonomy, beneficence, and justice and the other mainstays of recent medical ethics.[7] If, however, power talk is simply a way to make sure that more relevant considerations are put out onto the table for discussion and that previously implicit aspects of cases are made explicit and opened to additional inquiry, then discussions of power issues can supplement talk of autonomy, beneficence, and justice in ethical discourse.

Power and Moral Reasoning

Like characters out of Molière, many medical ethicists have been pleased to discover that they have been talking casuistry all their professional lives without knowing it. But there still remains the task of distinguishing among different subtypes of casuistry (or conversation) and the modes of moral reasoning that each uses.

At first glance a discussion of types of moral reasoning may seem an inappropriate reversion to the engineering model. Many advocates of casuistry are comfortable in discussing intuition (or interpretation) as an inevitable ingredient of their approach, for which one need not be ashamed. They might want to say that reasoning will take us so far, and then intuition will have to take over. For instance, reasoning will allow us to clarify all the morally relevant features of the case at hand, but only intuition will allow us to determine the relative weights of the competing considerations. Thus, the question ought to be not which types of moral reasoning are employed but what is the proper mix between reason and intuition.

Though this point merits further discussion, I find the ready appeal to intuition too lazy a strategy. In everyday moral discourse when hard cases are under discussion, the term *intuition* may indicate not a move for which no reasons can be given but instead one for which the reasons are fairly obvious and uncontroversial and therefore remain unspecified or undiscussed. Therefore, instead of talking of the mix between reason and intuition in a particular ethical theory such as casuistry, I prefer to discuss the relative balance between two types of moral reasoning, which I call the *formal* and the *narrative*.[8]

By formal reasoning I refer to reasoning that proceeds like geometry, from axioms to conclusions, in a logical and stepwise fashion. The truth

---

7. Zaner's (1988) phenomenological approach to case studies in medical ethics does indeed seem to dispense with all such principles; see the discussion of Zaner below.

8. Here it may seem that narrational reasoning is simply a restatement of the conversation model alluded to above. As I will discuss later, however, I wish to claim that both forms of reasoning (formal and narrational) may be found within the conversation model.

and the meaningfulness of a statement depend on its deducibility from earlier statements, which have been found to be true or meaningful in their own right. The term *formal* suggests the existence of a reasoning framework independent of specific content. Before one knows any of the facts of a case, one can predict what general reasoning strategies one is going to use and how those facts, when they are given, will fit the reasoning strategy.

By narrative reasoning I refer to reasoning that makes sense of events and yields further conclusions, primarily by placing those events in a broader life context and then viewing the relationship among all the events that seem relevant. This reasoning is more holistic than linear; a statement becomes true or meaningful by virtue of its relationship with a set of other statements and not simply by logical deduction. In general, this mode of reasoning proceeds retrospectively after most of the facts are known. When one has assembled all the relevant facts—when one has told the most coherent story about the events in question—then a reexamination of the facts and their interrelationships will yield meaningful and interesting con-clusions. But before those facts (or that story) are known, there is not enough material available to construct a reasoning framework, because narrative reasoning occurs in context and is informed primarily by context, not abstracted from context.[9]

To illustrate further what these types of reasoning refer to, consider the role of the family in the treatment decision made by a patient. Formal reasoning might begin by stating the respective rights and responsibilities of patient and family members. It would be noted, for example, that the patient who is capable of choosing autonomously ought to have a right to make his own decision, and the family has no corresponding right to impose

9. There is a significant resemblance between these two proposed modes of reasoning and what Gilligan (1982) refers to as the masculine and feminine modes of reasoning in ethics. Her point is that our male-dominated culture has always devalued an approach to ethics that focuses care, nurturance, and relationships instead of on rights and rules and remains embedded in the human context in which events occur. It is wrong, however, to reduce the difference between formal and narrational ethics—or, put differently, an ethic of rules and an ethic of care—to a simple difference between men and women. For one thing, it is not clear whether the ethic of care is a women's ethic or is the ethic of whichever group within society happens to be relegated to inferior status. For another, the psychological investigations of Gilligan and her colleagues need to be supplemented with a full-blown theory of a "contextual" ethic of care and nurturance (presumably, a non-Kantian theory); once this is carried out, the care ethic might well prove to have persuasive arguments on its behalf that are independent of gender (Tronto 1987). I take the discussion in the first part of this chapter to be a sketchy outline of such a non-Kantian theory; and general critiques of Kantian meta-ethics are becoming more frequent within moral philosophy (see Rorty 1979; Hampshire 1983).

their wishes or values on the patient. If the patient ends up making a decision to forgo a possibly beneficial treatment because it would be a great financial burden to the family, we would initially suspect that the family had been guilty of undue influence. We would demand some evidence that the patient had previously and voluntarily assimilated those family values and preferences and made them his own before reaching this decision. But to assess that this is what had occurred, we would have to assume that we could know two things—the patient's voluntary preference and the family's preference—as independent "facts" at the outset of the case.

Narrative reasoning would proceed differently. When we have a momentous decision to make, we often ask ourselves how that decision would fit within our unfolding life story. Would it cohere in a meaningful and authentic way as the sort of action that the principal character of this narrative would be likely to perform? Or does it stick out as an incoherent and unexplainable aberration? Given that most of us want to view ourselves as people who care about our close associates and the opinion they have of us, it seems unlikely that we would finally make such a decision without checking their reactions. We normally do this by extended conversations, over time, in which we can verbally try on various alternative decisions to gauge the reactions of those we care about. It is not until we can assemble those reactions—and until we can practice *owning* the various decision options by hearing the words come out of our mouths—that we can decide what our true preferences are. Our preferences and values emerge from the narrative process; they are not "facts" that can be known prior to the process and independently of it (Brody 1987c).

Even though the patient may not know what his own true preferences and values are until he has allowed himself to be "influenced" by his family and other close associates, it is still possible in some cases that a selfish family can unduly manipulate a patient and impose wishes that the patient, under more propitious circumstances, would disown. Formal reasoning would approach the question of whether such manipulation occurred in the case at hand by analyzing the extent to which the patient voluntarily and intentionally adopted the family's wishes. Narrative reasoning would start by noting that issues of voluntariness and intentionality are difficult to discern within the close emotional networks that make up family relations. Indeed, the very terms suggest an ability to isolate the individual from the family that may be unrealistic. Instead, the best way to judge this case is to ask for a detailed story about this decision, the patient, the family, and previous decisions that they may have made. Narrative reasoning assumes that the story of a selfish family imposing its will on a vulnerable member and the story of a concerned and thoughtful patient rejecting personal benefit for the greater family good are quite different. The two stories may be confused with each other when the events are loosely sketched, but as the events are told in the full richness of the real-life context and history, it will be hard not to know which story is which.

It may seem that I am just restating old conclusions, since formal reasoning is equivalent to the engineering approach or standard analytic model whereas narrative reasoning embodies the casuistic approach. But this seems to me not to be the case. A review of three recent books on medical ethics that can all be said to reflect a casuistic approach will reveal strikingly different mixes of formal and narrative reasoning.

Consider first Richard Zaner's *Ethics and the Clinical Encounter* (1988). Zaner, drawing largely from phenomenology and a deep analysis of aspects of the history of medicine, calls for an approach that appears to reject the standard tools of formal reasoning in ethics, such as principles of beneficence and autonomy. His focus instead is describing a case with sufficient richness of detail and sufficient understanding of the views and motives of all involved parties so that an appropriate resolution will emerge from the telling. (It is indicative of Zaner's critique of the formal methods in the standard ethics texts that those texts commonly have four of five cases illustrating the theme of one chapter, and each case description might occupy one or two paragraphs. Zaner, by contrast, devotes an entire chapter to stating one case in the detail that seems to him necessary before any valid conclusions can be drawn.)

I have already alluded to the volume by Albert Jonsen and Stephen Toulmin, *The Abuse of Casuistry* (1988), from which much of the previous discussion of casuistry was drawn. In their description, casuistry seems to rely heavily on narrative reasoning, but some elements of formal reasoning are also important. The maxims that are embodied in the paradigm cases are formal statements that cut across a variety of real-life contexts. But once a cluster of settled cases has been assembled around the paradigm case that best illustrates the application of the maxim, discussion of new and problematic cases seems to involve formal reasoning as well as narrative reasoning. Ultimately, the careful listing of the precise analogies and dysanalogies between this case and other cases, with a careful weighing of their significances, is all that can determine whether this maxim applies to the new case and with what qualifications or reservations. Casuistry, however, is quite eclectic in method and will happily import reasoning from law, philosophy, or theology if those more formal methods seem to shed light on the problem at hand.

A final example is Baruch Brody's *Life and Death Decision Making* (1988b). Brody develops a model within the framework of pluralistic casuitry to approach decisions regarding life-prolonging medical treatment and tests out his model by carefully analyzing forty cases. He begins by listing all appeals that may be morally relevant in cases of this type, which he characterizes as appeals to consequences of actions; appeals to rights; the appeal to respect for persons; appeals to virtues; and appeals to cost-effectiveness and justice. Under each, he offers several subtypes. Under "appeals to rights," for example, Brody includes the right not to be killed; the right not to have pain or injury inflicted; the right to be aided against threats to life and health; the right to make one's own decisions; and the right to participate in decisions that affect a family member. He further notes that as these appeals will often conflict in difficult cases, it is also necessary to specify the extent to which each has a hold on us in various cases; and for each appeal he offers some general guidelines for assessing its degree of applicability. Under the right of a family member to participate in a medical decision, he lists two such factors: the relative incapacity of the patient to make his own choice and the degree of closeness of the family member. Therefore, by the time Brody gets down to cases, he has developed an extensive framework for moral analysis; the application of all these appeals and the weighing of each in the case examples often seem fairly mechanical. Again, a typical case description for him occupies one paragraph—something that Zaner would not consider a case at all.

In sum, in looking at three books that purport to rely on case study as the primary method of medical ethics, we find widely disparate degrees of employing formal and narrative reasoning, ranging from Zaner's almost total disregard of formal reasoning to Brody's heavy reliance on it. Murray (1987) offers a distinction between two aspects of casuistry that is useful here: an emphasis on immersion in and interpretation of actual cases and a claim about whether moral judgments or moral theory is a better source of moral knowledge. The three books reviewed are equally casuistic in relation to the first feature. But whereas Zaner and Jonsen and Toulmin seem comfortable with the idea that moral knowledge emerges from well-reasoned judgments about specific cases, Brody appears to hold instead that moral knowledge comes primarily from principles that can be elucidated in advance of cases.

It seems, therefore, that a conversation model may be defended as a reasonable approach to medical ethics and that within that model both formal and narrative reasoning may play a role. I have not been able to illustrate in this book a formal application of the concept of power to cases in medical ethics; the three guidelines for the responsible use of power seem too rough to serve as formal principles without a great deal of interpretation in various case contexts. But so long as narrative reasoning forms a valued component of moral thinking, the concept of power can be a useful guide, helping to isolate pertinent features of cases and to place discrete events and actions in a broader context.

CHAPTER 16

THE

PHYSICIAN'S

CHARACTER

The "new" medical ethics has been dominated by a rights-and-rules approach in which problems are taken one at a time and specific, observable behavior is recommended by way of resolution. What sort of person the physician is, how consistent his views and attitudes are over a lifetime, and the intentions and reflections that accompany his problem-resolving behaviors are all pushed aside as of little ethical interest. As some critics have charged, it is as if we thought we could make medical ethics "doctor-proof" (Smith and Newton 1984).[1]

It has now become more common to include some mention of virtue in medical ethics (Shelp 1985; Brody 1989c).[2] Ethics acquires a dimension of virtue when one is no longer occupied solely with discrete problems and resolutions but also with "practices" as organized, evolving forms of human excellence and with the internal standards that inform such practices (MacIntyre 1981). One can speak of the virtuous person when one views human lives as integrated narratives, from birth to death, and asks what standards of excellence can shape such narratives. One can speak of the

---

1. "Ethics is practiced by medical ethicists as if neither their own characters nor the character of the physician had anything to do with the enterprise" (Drane 1988, p. 139).

2. An interesting effort to derive a comprehensive medical ethics from virtue is Drane 1988. Drane explains the reluctance of the "new" ethics to consider this option: "The very words, virtue and character, have a religious ring to the secular thinker, which is reason enough to consider them out of place. To be seriously considered, these words would have to be 'laundered' and 'operationalized' " (p. 142). Hence the tendency among analytic philosophers of medical ethics to reduce virtue and character to tendencies to behave or decide in certain ways, and to miss the point that these concepts presuppose standards of excellence, rather than rules for minimally acceptable behavior, and the coherence of one's actions over a lifetime, rather than discrete decisions.

virtuous physician when one looks at medicine as a practice and asks what standards of excellence inform and guide that practice, given its particular goals and its history as a human activity carried out by a defined community. It is therefore fitting here to discuss the physician's character—what sort of person the good physician ought to be, not just what rules the good physician ought to follow.

Any listing of virtues is likely to seem an uninspiring and even pointless task both to analytic philosophers and to scientifically minded physicians. To the philosophers, the problem is that there is no *logical* process to be sure that one has supplied an exhaustive list, whereas in the rules-and-rights mode one seems to be able to demonstrate that X or Y are necessary and sufficient conditions for respect for autonomy or for adequately informed consent or whatever. For the physicians, it appears that one can never measure or evaluate virtuous behavior objectively, and so any discussion of the medical virtues is bound to degenerate into a political or "turf" debate over who gets to be the judge. It is therefore of some interest that the American Board of Internal Medicine, not widely regarded as a bastion of subjectivism, has undertaken the ambitious project of identifying a list of virtues ("humanistic qualities"), insisting that residency directors in their specialties can and should evaluate these rigorously and stating that a resident who lacks these virtues should not be granted board certification. Even if the realities within internal-medicine residencies today do not live up to this idealistic statement of goals, the list and definitions of the virtues are still worth exploring for their own sake (Subcommittee 1983).

The subcommittee of the board suggested that the essential humanistic qualities of the internist are integrity, respect, and compassion, which they defined as follows:

> Integrity is the personal commitment to be honest and trustworthy in evaluating and demonstrating one's own skills and abilities.
>
> Respect is the personal commitment to honor others' choices and rights regarding themselves and their medical care.
>
> Compassion is an appreciation that suffering and illness engender special needs for comfort and help without evoking excessive emotional involvement that could undermine professional responsibility for the patient. (Subcommittee 1983, p. 722)

The fear of "excessive emotional involvement" is a key point to which I shall return later. For now, it is important both to note the substance of the list and the degree of commitment to reform suggested by its official adoption. For example, the board subcommittee not only suggests how residents may be systematically observed to see whether they exhibit these virtues but also lists ways in which their faculty and directors may fail to set the proper tone or the proper example to encourage residents in the pursuit of the virtues. Taken seriously, such a list would call for a wholesale housecleaning in many traditional residency programs.

Even though all three virtues are fully consistent with both a power approach to medical ethics and a preference for a conversation model of moral reasoning, there appears little *direct* link between a power approach and the virtues of integrity and respect. The physician motivated by integrity will feel a strong sense of moral accountability and hence an eagerness to engage candidly and nondefensively in productive moral conversation with peers. She will be less interested in justifying her existing behavior than in becoming aware of new perspectives and potential improvements in her behavior. The physician motivated by respect will desire to follow all the relevant rules and respect the rights of patients. Engagement in moral conversation will be more productive because an attitude of respect will cause her to listen attentively to the opinions of even those with whom she disagrees. Ultimately, both virtues will lead to willingness to label and discuss power disparities and to a deeper awareness of how the unthinking use of power can undermine one's integrity as well as violate the rights of patients.

By contrast, the virtue of compassion occupies a key role in any analysis of the physician's character that grows out of the power approach I have advocated. The reasons for this go beyond the crude observation that compassion is an antidote to power abuse: the irresponsible use of power is often preceded by the relegation of the victim to the status of "other" or even "enemy" (see chapter 3). So long as the other party remains someone with whom the physician can identify and sympathize, she is much more likely to use power responsibly. But to see the full range of linkages between compassion and the various issues surrounding power in the medical en-counter will take a deeper and more sophisticated analysis of what com-passion entails.

The Virtue of Compassion

Reich (1989) offers just the sort of sophisticated analysis of compassion that I require here. He begins by suggesting that compassion is intimately bound up with another's suffering and by proposing that the experience of suffering can be seen as occurring in three phases, which in turn generate three reciprocal phases of compassion. The phases of suffering are labeled *mute suffering*, during which the sufferer is overwhelmed by the immensity of the suffering and is unable to find words to express it; *expressive suffering*, during which the sufferer uses language to try to enhance understanding (and hence ultimately control) of his experience; and *new identity in suffering*, during which the sufferer undergoes a profound change by integrating the new understanding of the meaning of his suffering into a new sense of his own identity as a person. In this third stage, the story he has constructed of his suffering is now fully bound up into the story of his life, and he cannot say who he is without including the suffering and the meaning it has come to have for him (Brody 1987d). Reich adds that this third phase generally requires "solidarity with compassionate others" (1989, p. 91).

Reich proceeds to describe three phases of compassion that reflect his account of suffering. In effect, compassion is defined as a virtue in terms of its relationship to the varying needs of the suffering other. The first phase is *silent compassion* or silent empathy; one shows a commitment to be with the sufferer in his anguish without attempting to control, rationalize, or intellectualize the experience by placing a label on it. This silence, as some clinicians have noted, is not a void; it throws the sufferer back upon himself in the search for words and ultimately helps him move to the second phase. It is one thing to try to find words when one is overwhelmed by a sense of social isolation, quite another to find words when a compassionate companion is standing by in an attitude of openness and receptivity.

Expressive compassion involves more active use of clinical skills, but again without taking charge to the extent of putting one's own language and meaning into the mouth of the sufferer. However one does this, Reich notes, "the role is to make some limited attempt to broaden sufferers' perceptions, so that they become conscious of and connected with a wider spectrum of meaning and value" (1989, p. 94). In its simplest form, and when the suffering is tied directly to physical symptoms, the physician may help most by providing an authoritative diagnosis, giving the sufferer both a socially acceptable name for his misery and a corresponding sense of control over it (Cassell 1976; Brody 1980). In more involved cases, the physician and the sufferer may join in a prolonged project amounting to the construction of the new narrative of the patient's life (Brody 1987d; Kleinman 1988).

There are two critical ingredients of a successful story of suffering in this expressive phase. First, the story must appear coherent and relevant to the sufferer himself. It must be comprehensive enough to take into account the suffering experience in its totality, not just particular features of it (hence the inadequacy of medical diagnosis by itself in cases where the suffering is in large part psychological and spiritual). And it must be sufficiently particularized to be recognizable as the sufferer's own story rather than some mass-produced account. But second, the story must help reconnect the sufferer to the broader society and culture (Cassell 1982, Brody 1987d). It must label the experience in ways that indicate how others have shared similar (if not identical) experiences and in ways that help to promote a fellowship among all humans who have suffered. The compassionate presence and participation of the physician symbolizes this two-directional feature of the successful story. On the one hand, the physician attends to the sufferer as a unique person; on the other hand, the physician represents the broader society and culture, the "normal" people, reminding the sufferer that the suffering has not totally cut him off from the "normal" world.

Berger, in his essay on an English country doctor (Berger and Mohr 1967), describes this feature of the compassionate physician more powerfully. He suggests that many people who visit the physician are simply ill, and almost any moderately skilled and decent response will suffice. But a good number are also deeply unhappy, even anguished. The anguished patient is afflicted not only with an illness but also with a crippling and isolating set of beliefs. He sees his experience as unique, unrecognizable to members of the "normal" human community, and hence feels himself to be an outcast among humankind. This conviction of course seems absurd to the rational onlooker; and this attitude indeed further isolates the anguished person from human companionship. Ultimately, he takes his case to the physician. At this point he has no hope whatever that the physician will recognize him, and reach out to him, as a fellow human being. But perhaps the physician will recognize at least his illness and give it a diagnostic label; that would be some small comfort.

The physician then confronts this anguished and well-nigh hopeless person. If the physician is the right sort of individual, something special may happen. The physician may just manage to appear before the patient as a fellow human being enough like him to be able to comprehend, or even to share, the experience of illness, isolation, and hopelessness. As Berger puts it, the physician *recognizes* the patient, in such a way that the patient feels recognized even in the face of his firm conviction that his sickness and isolation have rendered him unrecognizable. Not only does the physician tell the patient that his illness has a name, that his experience has been shared by countless others who have managed to rejoin the human community; the patient *feels* human reconnection in the physician's attentive and compassionate presence.

This task is not easy. The anguished person—who is, after all, totally absorbed in his suffering—all too readily engenders in others impatient irritation instead of compassion. The physician must be a strange amalgam of Everyman and his humble self. He must be enough like the patient so that the patient can truly identify with him, even in the patient's present abnormal state; and yet he must still be himself, not a poseur—a solid human being, not just an image in a mirror held up before the patient's face. The physician will fail if he is tired or preoccupied; if he pays too much attention to the disease and not enough to the patient; if he misinterprets a word, a tone of voice, a glance. So it cannot be, Berger concludes, that his doctor is a good doctor because he invariably succeeds in connecting with the patient emotionally. Instead, Berger observes, he is a good doctor because "there is about him the constant will of a man trying to recognize" (Berger and Mohr 1967, p. 71). Berger's account seems to mesh with Reich's notion of what is required in the expressive phase of compassion.

The third phase, *new identity in compassion*, is the most controversial of Reich's arguments and also the most critical for a power analysis of the medical encounter. Many would argue that compassion must have only two phases: is not the job over when one has helped the sufferer find a new voice, a new story, a new identity in his suffering that has reestablished his link with the rest of humanity? But Reich finds it unthinkable that the compassionate person could experience (empathically) the anguish of the sufferer and go through the difficult process of identification with the sufferer necessary to find the appropriate words for the suffering without being fundamentally changed herself. Reich here takes literally what Richard Selzer, in some of his short stories, expresses symbolically as the idea that the surgeon must heal the patient in order to be healed himself (Selzer 1975; Beppu and Tavormina 1981).

Several considerations support Reich's assertion on this point. For one thing, unless the physician has a genuine openness and vulnerability, it is unlikely that the sufferer will experience the encounter as fully healing. It is hard to identify empathically with the anguish of the sufferer and at the same time maintain a strict guard against any impressions or ideas that might threaten one's current sense of identity. So long as the physician responds to the sufferer as a threat, or as a potential threat, to the physician's own composure and sense of self, she represents those who would cast the sufferer out of the human community rather than those who would bridge the chasm of suffering and reestablish human connections. But the only psychologically realistic alternative to a guarded defensiveness is a genuine vulnerability and openness to change and growth. (This and later points suggest a virtue that accompanies compassion, empathic curiosity, which I discuss in the next section.)

Reich notes further that there are special barriers to compassion among physicians. The traditional reliance on benevolent paternalism urges the physician to respond to the sufferer in a "There, there, it's not so bad" manner that immediately imposes the physician's preferred meaning onto the experience of suffering and cuts off the patient's efforts to find his own voice and his own story. The physician trained to fix things may have a hard time demonstrating empathic silence and engaging in a genuinely mutual search for narrative meaning. And the physician trained to be scientific and objective may find it hard to enter the subjective world of somebody else's anguish.

The obvious implication is that the physician must constantly struggle against such obstacles in order to practice compassion. The whole point of calling compassion a virtue instead of an obligation or duty is to note how it must become internalized as a habit of character before it can truly be called compassion at all. But unless the physician adopts an instinctive attitude of openness and vulnerability, it is difficult to see how these barriers to compassion can successfully be overcome. The physician who is closed and defensive in the face of anguish and suffering will magnify these obstacles rather than overcome them.

We are now in a position to see why the virtue of compassion is integrally linked to the ethical use of power in the physician-patient relationship. Surely, being with the sufferer and helping him find his own story to attach meaning to his experience is a prime example of shared power. Few things that the physician can do have the capacity to empower the patient to a similar degree. Disease may threaten bodily function and bodily integrity; suffering threatens one's connections with humanity and one's ability to make sense of one's own life. If the physician attends only to disease and ignores suffering, he may cure but still fail to heal (Cassell 1982). To be compassionate in response to the suffering of the patient is therefore one of the most powerful things a physician can do; but this is possible only to the extent that the physician is willing to adopt a position of relative powerlessness, to acknowledge that the patient's suffering has incredible power over him and that he cannot remain unchanged in the face of it. This is a major irony of the physician-patient relationship, in which a sense both of one's own healing power and of one's necessary humility forms a synthesis of the apparent contradiction of power and powerlessness.[3]

In chapter 2, I reviewed the story of the healer Snake and discussed the apparent unreality of her lack of charismatic and social power. Her powerlessness seemed an impediment to her carrying out her healing function in the setting in which she found herself. But we can now see a deeper meaning to that aspect of Snake's story. Snake and her teachers seem to have glimpsed the synthesis of power and powerlessness that comes with a proper sense of one's humility as a healer. In a particular social setting, humility and powerlessness may have served Snake poorly. But in the long run, her humility may be her most empowering attribute.

It may be largely out of this dual sense of power and humility that the physician's virtue and character can help insure that power is used responsibly and that its abuses are avoided. Owned, aimed, and shared power each arise naturally from this dual sense of power and humility engendered by the virtue of compassion.

Empathic Curiosity: Not Being Full of Oneself

Are there any additional, specifiable virtues or character traits in the physician that will promote and enhance the exercise of compassion, and thereby the responsible use of power? William Carlos Williams's story "The Use of Force" served earlier as a paradigm case of "the dark side of the force"; so it is fitting that some reflections of Dr. Williams's may help in answering this latest question. Robert Coles has recounted some of Williams's views on medical practice, medical teaching, and medical ethics, taken from tape-recorded interviews of the elder physician when Coles was a medical student:

> Everyone thinks doctors are good people because they help other people who are sick. But if you ask me, the people who are sick are helping us all the time—if we'll let them help us. How many times I've gotten up and felt lousy; [and on starting to hear the patient's story of the illness] the next thing with me is that I've forgotten myself—isn't that an achievement!—because I'm all tied up with

3. McCullough (1989) may be referring to a related irony when he states that so long as medical care involves medical language, the physician's sense of control is threatened, since it is ultimately the patient and not the physician who will attach the final meaning and interpretation to the language in the context of his own life: "The physician, as a consequence of using medical language—which he or she was taught was a means to describe and thus control reality—experiences a threat to his or her control and sense of power and authority" (McCullough 1989, p. 122).

someone else. . . . I can't hear a [patient] talk like that and not be sprung—sprung right out of my own damn self-preoccupations. . . .

You can set rules; you can teach lessons; you can give tests; you can pass them . . . but even so, stubborn human nature is out there, threatening to take charge of the intellect. . . . There's a big difference between our high talk, though, and how we behave ourselves when we're out there on our own. . . . It's too damn easy to teach, to preach, then go off and be your own, full-of-yourself self. . . .

Why should we always be told that the alternative is between a doctor who really knows what he's doing, even if he doesn't have much time to be with patients, to talk with them and be understanding of them, and a doctor who has all the time in the world for his patients, but he's a first-class idiot, and could end up being a threat to your favorite relative's health, even life? I'll answer that. It's not a question; it's a rhetorical statement meant to rationalize callousness and egotism!

For crying out loud: who in hell wants a dope hanging around with a stethoscope? But why is this dope conjured up every time some swaggering tyrant or mean, cold son-of-a-bitch, who happens to have an M.D. after his name, shows up and starts bullying people? I guess it's because the rest of us don't want to see him get what he deserves. And why? Hell, we know our own dark side! We rally around others to protect ourselves! . . .

Who are we, a bunch of moral monsters? Maybe we're tempted to be, sometimes. When people are scared as hell, and death's around the next corner, or maybe facing them, right in front of them, they'll grab at anything there is, and we're what there is, what's available. . . . So, we're gods for others—but we know how tinny we can be, or we damn well should know. I guess the raw truth is that the worst of us don't know: the ones who strut and prance and con themselves and everyone else into thinking they are God's hand-picked emissary, if not chosen successor. (Coles 1989, pp. 104, 108–10)

Williams claims sainthood neither for himself nor for even the best of his fellow physicians. There is always human nature to contend with; there are always those days when one feels lousy, totally caught up with oneself and one's petty or not-so-petty concerns. The virtuous physician, in Williams's account, seems to have two particular qualities: first, a readiness to be drawn out of herself through genuine concern for and involvement with her patients; and second, a self-critical humility that allows her better self to see how silly the "full-of-yourself self" looks. If people seem to worship at the doctor's feet, Williams points out, it is not because of the doctor's divine qualities; it is because the patient is scared and the doctor is "what's available."[4]

Williams warns less of great evils and more of the unavoidable lapses of everyday life. His "dark side," in the above passages, is not the dark side of the force as described in chapters 2 and 3. Using one's power against the patient to enjoy the release that this brings is the cardinal sin. Williams is concerned more with the venial sin of not trying hard enough to shed one's natural self-preoccupations when one is with a patient. In response to venial sin, which is humanly unavoidable, the physician has two characterologic responses. She can chastise herself when she slips, and resolve to try to do better in the future. Or she can adopt the ever-present rationalizations—which would you rather have, me with my flaws, or the idiot with the stethoscope?—and give herself up to self-preoccupation. With that choice invariably comes arrogance. For if she can, day in and day out, be self-preoccupied, and if people nonetheless seek her services and appear grateful, then she must indeed start thinking that she is a superior being, immune to the criticisms that mere mortals earn.

The link between the virtue of compassion, as discussed in the previous section, and Williams's admonition not to be too full of oneself, lies in the way that self-preoccupation distracts the physician from the attitude of humility, of openness and vulnerability, which I have argued is an essential ingredient of compassion. It is worth recalling here Berger's (1967) account of "recognizing," his insistence that the good physician should have "the constant will of a man trying to recognize," even while admitting that he will often fail. He is most likely to fail on those bad days when he is too full of himself and hence unable either to attend carefully to the anguished patient or else too wrapped up in himself to be open to the experience of anguish in the other.

I think that the sort of physician Williams admires is one who would like to have as his epitaph, *There was about him the constant will of a man trying to recognize.* This sentence makes no grandiose claim of success or

---

4. James Drane (1988) seems to allude to this point: "Physicians are vulnerable to self-ignorance and self-deceit because they are persons of power and prestige. People cater to them and infrequently tell them the truth about themselves. . . . As a result, it is easy for doctors to develop a narrow and conceited view of themselves, frankly to become fools when it comes to their own inner truth" (p. 61). Elsewhere (p. 91) Drane urges upon physicians the virtue of friendliness, which encourages one not to take oneself too seriously and constitutes the opposite of pomposity.

superhuman powers. It displays a frank admission of occasional, even frequent failure. The words in their very simplicity bespeak a human task aspired to by those who are humble in the knowledge of their limits. Even when one succeeds in this task, the words will not permit much self-congratulation. The physician who manages to "recognize" is not thereby a great person; both physician and patient are in the presence of a deep human mystery greater than both of them. As Williams would be the first to point out, "recognizing" can occur only when the patient has been open and candid in laying his story before the physician; and it is the physician, not the patient, who should thereby feel privileged.

As *not being full of oneself* is a rather clumsy label, I propose to call this virtue, which contributes to the greater virtue of compassion, *empathic curiosity*. This phrase is suggested in part by Engel's (1988) discussion of the biologically grounded human needs that play themselves out in the clinical encounter. It is a great mystery that a suffering human being will so readily bare her soul to the physician, even as she feels totally cut off from normal human society. It is even more mysterious that this can often occur when the physician is a stranger whom she has known for only five minutes. Engel proposes that this could happen only if the human organism were hard-wired (as it were) with two reciprocal basic needs: the physician's need to know and the patient's need to be understood. The physician is motivated by scientific curiosity in the best and highest sense, because without this type of science, all of the rest of medical science grinds to a halt. As I showed in chapter 4, all scientific reasoning in medicine requires first an accurate data base, and a thorough medical history requires first a patient who feels at ease with the physician and who feels prompted to tell his own story in appropriate detail and with appropriate insight and candor. The physician's attitude of empathic curiosity is what is required to place the patient in this state; being too full of oneself will confuse, inhibit, or antagonize the patient and virtually insure that one collects unsound and unscientific data from the outset. In this way, the virtue of empathic curiosity is as critical for scientific medicine as it is for ethically optimal medicine.

It seems that the physician who can best be trusted to use power re-sponsibly—the physician who has internalized the responsible use of power as a self-imposed standard of scientific as well as behavioral excellence and who need not be exhorted to use power responsibly by a litany of rules and rights—is the one who possesses the virtue of empathic curiosity as an adjunct to compassion. The physician who is painfully aware of how easy it is to be full of oneself is the one who is most likely to be more comfortable when power is shared instead of monopolized. The physician who is inclined to be self-reflective and self-critical about such matters, who knows that the easy rationalizations lead to arrogance, will be more likely to own responsibility for the power that is used and to question carefully the goals toward which that power is applied.[5]

Therapeutic Distance and Fear of Powerlessness

What are we to make of the fact that the subcommittee of the Board of Internal Medicine stated the "humanistic qualities" of integrity and respect straightforwardly and robustly but felt compelled in defining compassion to qualify it, "without invoking excessive emotional involvement that could undermine professional responsibility for the patient" (Subcommittee 1983, p. 722)? Is this a legitimate observation on the nature of effective compassion in medicine? Or is it a reversion to Williams's "idiot with the stethoscope," who in this case is reduced to idiocy because he has identified too closely with the patient and thereby allowed his own emotional turmoil to derail his scientific reasoning skills?

The advice, "Be compassionate and empathic but don't get too involved," seems a stock item in the training of physicians. Even Reich feels constrained to observe, "Because compassion is an altruistic virtue, it easily leads to impossible ideals and over-identification with the suffering person, threatening stress and burn-out" (1989, p. 105). One naturally wonders: where are all the cases of medical disasters that gave rise to this warning, that occurred because the physician became too emotionally involved? The larger portion of Reich's argument certainly suggests that the opposite is true. The cemetery is filled not with the corpses of patients who died because their overinvolved physicians became irrational and ineffective, but rather with those of sufferers whose physicians attended to their diseases but failed to heal because of the multiple characterological barriers that cause physicians *not to get close enough*. If the truly prevalent problem is in not getting close enough to hear empathically and to construct mutually a healing narrative, why the ritual advice against getting too close?[6]

---

5. This further illustrates why virtue cannot be reduced to a mere disposition to behave in a morally correct manner (Childress 1989). We ought to be able, by now, to see clearly the contrast between being disposed to perform healing actions and striving over time to become a healing sort of person.

6. I have seen perhaps two cases in my teaching experience of residents in training who seemed to have such a problem of overinvolvement with patients that it threatened their effectiveness as physicians and caused the patients to develop a dependency that seemed contrary to their own interests. In both cases the overinvolvement seemed to be not an isolated problem but a symptom of a much more global difficulty in carving out an acceptable

My previous analysis offers an answer: the irony of compassion, the synthesis of power and humility, is a subtle point difficult to grasp and internalize. Faced with the apparent contradiction between power and powerlessness, it is tempting to focus on the powerlessness and to recoil from it in fear rather than go on to the more difficult step of acceptance and synthesis. The warning, "Don't get overinvolved," is a form of reassurance (even if ultimately false) that the physician can hang onto the supreme power to heal while at the same time avoiding the felt powerlessness of vulnerability and change. This amounts to denial of the power that the patient and the patient's suffering hold over the physician. Fundamentally, this denial is a rejection of the concept of shared power by reframing the power issue as a zero-sum game. The possibility that the physician's power to heal in some way depends on his vulnerability—that, ironically, powerlessness can empower—is lost sight of.[7]

Can the narrative approach or metaphor help resolve this problem? I believe that one way to make more sense of the advice against overinvolvement is to see it as confusing emotional distance with esthetic distance. There is a type of distance that is desirable (indeed unavoidable) in effective displays of compassion; but it is esthetic distance rather than emotional distance. It is when the concept of distance is extended inappropriately, to try to turn the fear and rejection of powerlessness into a virtue rather than an obstacle to healing, that the damage is done.

Charon (1989) suggests that the proper model for the sensitive clinician is the esthetic distance that ought to mark the reader's approach to fiction. The skill of reading fiction is to be close enough to the subject of the fiction to feel an emotional identification and to experience, not just know about, what is happening, and at the same time to be just far enough away so as to be able to reflect on that experience with some degree of critical detachment. Often this relative distance ebbs and flows. At one point in the narrative

professional self-image. In Williams's terms, these residents were too preoccupied with themselves rather than with their patients; the overinvolvement was generated more by the residents' internal turmoil than by a genuine receptivity to the patients' suffering. Compare the discussion of the "Rabkin explosion" case in chapter 14. More studies of actual cases that fit this description would be very useful for medical education.

7. It is also interesting to review a study of psychological testing in first-year medical students (Gilligan and Pollak 1988). Responding to the thematic apperception test, subjects constructed stories that were analyzed for episodes of danger or violence and for themes of intimacy, isolation, success, and failure. While the males were prone to associate danger with intimacy, women were much more likely to associate danger with isolation. If, as other data show, it is a general masculine trait to fear intimacy more than isolation, it is not hard to see how, in the male-dominated world of medicine, the myth of the need to maintain "therapeutic distance" might have arisen.

one is drawn in so close as almost to fuse with the fiction. At another point one looks down from a higher vantage point and is able to see what is going on with more detachment. (Hence the importance of comic relief within tragedy, such as the graveyard scene in *Hamlet*.) Now, when one reads fiction properly, one maintains the same vulnerability, the same openness to personal change and growth, that marks the proper display of compassion. The reader is able to shed the self-preoccupation that would lead to a fear of loss of power if she opened oneself fully to the text. Yet at the same time she must avoid a fusion of identities with the text; if that occurs, narrative ceases to be narrative: it is no longer a way of attaching meaning to experience if all opportunity to reflect on that experience from an outside vantage point has been lost (Churchill and Churchill 1982).

To suggest, as some literary scholars have, that a suffering patient is a text that the sensitive physician must read is therefore not to advocate emotional distance. On the contrary, it calls for intense emotional engagement. But what is essential to "reading the text" is maintaining in one's imagination that separate vantage point from which the experience of the sufferer can be reinterpreted and reconnected to the broader context of culture and society.

This is what is suggested, in part, by naming the virtue that accompanies and stimulates compassion *empathic curiosity* instead of *empathy*. The good physician should be strongly moved to understand the sufferer's anguish, and that requires the ability to occupy a reflective vantage point. But a full understanding will also require a high degree of emotional identification with the sufferer, as well as the willingness to enter into a mutual relationship for the construction of narrative meaning, or else one's so-called understanding will be a flat representation that does not capture the emotional and human depths of the suffering experience.

The physician can adopt the virtues of compassion and of empathic curiosity only by moving beyond the ritual advice against overinvolvement. On an emotional level, this involves accepting the full irony of power and humility in compassion and overcoming the fear of powerlessness in vulnerability. On an intellectual level, this involves distinguishing between emotional and esthetic distance and cultivating the latter instead of the former.

Finally, there is an important interpersonal and social level to compassion. As Reich notes, "Balance in compassion requires that the subject of compassion become the object of compassion: unless we are compassionate with ourselves and receive compassion from others, we are not able to provide compassion" (1989, p. 105). For physicians to adopt and cultivate compassion as a *professional* virtue requires that they be willing to form themselves into a compassionate community, confident that they will receive empathic compassion and support from each other as they attend to the sufferings of their patients. It is perhaps in this arena that the implicit issues of medical power have most stood in the way of reform. The self-image of the physician as a powerful, scientific, objective individual has worked strongly against the formation of any truly effective peer support system. Given a choice between appearing tough to one's colleagues or entering with them into a network of mutual compassion, toughness usually wins. It is symptomatic that medical educators tell young physicians, "Don't get overinvolved," instead of, "If you find the demands of compassion becoming overwhelming, the rest of us will be here for you, just as you are there for the patient." If medical ethics is to address the physician's character and not only individual actions and rules, then the virtue of compassion will have to become a focus of ethical inquiry. This will in turn require that the professional psychology of power and powerlessness become part of the vocabulary of medical ethics. I believe that substantial progress has been made in recent years; staff support groups in hospice programs and in AIDS clinics are only two examples. Further progress will occur as educators begin to pay more explicit attention to these issues.

CHAPTER 17

CONCLUDING

REMARKS

In this book I have presented an argument for expanding the conversation that makes up the contemporary discipline of medical ethics. The argument may be summarized as follows:

1. The physician's power can be analyzed to show its elements and origins, even though in practice the various elements are intermingled.

2. General guidelines can be provided for the responsible use of power; and those guidelines can be applied to particular cases and topics that commonly arise within medical ethics.

3. The reasons why *power* has generally been excluded from the vocabulary of medical ethics are accidental and historical, not conceptual.

4. The more traditional vocabulary of medical ethics tends to gloss over the power dimensions of ethical issues and interpersonal relationships, therefore painting on occasion an unrealistic picture of the context in which ethical decisions must be made.

5. Power can serve as a bridging metaphor between ethics and the social sciences, allowing insights from the latter to be applied to the former. (The same is true of insights from literature and from feminist philosophy.)

6. There is a variety of reasons why medical ethics ought to develop a greater sensitivity to issues of virtue and character and to contextual approaches to the analysis of cases. These do not entail rejecting the more traditional vocabulary of rights and principles. A power approach fits comfortably within this expanded conception of medical ethics.

This argument has been supported and illustrated by reviewing a number of familiar topics in medical ethics. An effort has been made to include topics that would normally not be mentioned at all within medical ethics (the care-work tension; the physician's income); topics for which a power approach provides fundamentally novel insights (informed consent; the primary-care relationship); and topics for which a power approach coheres rather closely with the guidance gleaned from the more traditional rights-and-principles approach (control of information).

In no sense has this book provided a comprehensive overview of all topics in medical ethics. The ethics of medical research, abortion and reproductive technologies, genetic screening and gene manipulation, brain death and persistent vegetative state, psychiatric ethics, and behavior control are only some of the topics not addressed in any detail. An obvious next step, if the expanded conversation of medical ethics seems worth pursuing, is to try to use the power approach to look at each of those issues in turn.

Another obvious step is to challenge the power approach in a variety of ways, to try further to clarify and strengthen it. Is the centrality of primary care a defensible feature of a power approach, or is it a bit of nostalgia for the old-time family doctor of bygone days? Was the vocabulary of power truly rejected by medical ethics for the reasons cited, or are there better, conceptual reasons to avoid it? (For that matter, are there extended and perceptive discussions of medical power in the existing literature that I missed?) Is it really true that using power responsibly means anything more than, "Don't violate the patient's rights and adhere to sound ethical principles"? Is using power responsibly simply a disingenuous way of re-habilitating the "old" medical paternalism? Does the use of the concept of patient autonomy within the power approach always relegate autonomy to the role of an end constraint and thereby intolerably weaken the importance of the autonomy principle?

A vigorous debate on all of these questions might show that the power conversation is truly a dead end for medical ethics and that we ought to return to other, better-established lines of inquiry. Alternatively, the debate might reveal the strength and depth of the power approach and its connections with other important aspects of ethical theory and practice. The entire point of the conversation metaphor is that it is notoriously hard to predict in advance how a particular conversation will proceed and develop.

Though the questions listed above are all worth debating, an even larger question looms in the background: what is the comprehensive or overarching theory of medical ethics, within which the conversation about power is supposed to find its niche? It might be assumed that to say that we can add power talk to medical ethics without replacing or rejecting other familiar concepts *presupposes* some overarching theory such that talk of power and talk of autonomy, beneficence, and justice are all compatible with the theory and with each other. But if this theory looks like the more standard utilitarian or deontological theories, then it must be the case that power talk is a fifth wheel within it, and whatever can be said about power can easily be rephrased in the vocabulary of rights, duties, maximization of good consequences, or whatever. And if the theory is quite different from all those standard theories, then what must it be like?

It may be, however, that what is presupposed is not some overarching ethical theory but instead an understanding of why no such theory can or need be stated. Following Rorty (1979), one might assert that the felt need for such a comprehensive theory is a symptom of continued attraction to the Cartesian-Kantian mode of conceptualizing philosophy and ethics. That mode, although both interesting and productive, is nevertheless historically limited. It is neither the only way to see the task of ethics nor necessarily the best way in our present age. It may simply be the case that the appreciation of medical-ethics problems, *within the full complexity of the contexts in which they arise*, requires something other than abstraction out of context, which is what is promised by most overarching theories. The proper tools to deal with complex problems in their real-life contexts may come from further developments of casuistic methods, as was discussed in chapter 15.

General ethical theories, on the other hand, have proved excellent at highlighting certain morally relevant features of real-life contexts, but only at the price of obscuring some other features. Up until now, medical ethics has proceeded largely by working on the features that are highlighted by the standard general theories and by taking on faith that the features thereby obscured are of much lesser moral import. This book is an attempt to call that strategy into question and suggest that we must begin systematically to drag some of the obscured features out into the light and examine them afresh.

When medical ethics as we now understand it got off the ground in the late 1960s and early 1970s, it was very much in need of the application of general philosophical-ethical theories. The conversation about ethics in medicine had tended to go on within the medical profession only and had been isolated to a considerable degree from the more general conversation about ethics that had been going on over the centuries in the broader culture. It was therefore an appropriate move to reintroduce into medicine the general ethical theories that serve as distillations of that broad ethical conversation throughout the history of Western culture.

It may be that for the next round within medical ethics, we will need fewer general theories and more reasoning tools to help balance a variety of competing considerations. For example, the "new" medical ethics has been criticized from the standpoint of the "newer" ethics as being too occupied with procedural questions and not occupied sufficiently with substantive questions. Another way of phrasing this same criticism is that medical ethics has focused too much on patient choices and not enough on professional values. Presumably, professional values would lead to the substantive questions about which choices patients ought to make (or ought to be *allowed* to make), whereas the ethical discourse in medicine in the past two decades has tended to focus on the rights of patients to make their own choices or for surrogates to make them on the patient's behalf.

The historical forces discussed in chapter 10, including the Baby Doe debates and the *Cruzan* case, illustrate the turn toward substantive considerations of professional values, as do the many recent books on virtue in medical ethics and on efforts to derive a medical ethics from specifically medical values and presuppositions. What seems evident now is that careful balancing is necessary to do justice to the two competing sets of moral considerations. The delicacy of this balance was probably best reflected in chapter 11. If medical ethics tilts too far in one direction, patients are empowered to demand therapy that medical science holds to be futile on good grounds, and patients are thereby empowered effectively to dismember the practice of medicine. If it tilts too far in the other direction, physicians are empowered to eliminate patients' choices in important ways, on the basis of unexamined professional or even individual biases.

The scholars who developed the field of medical ethics in the 1960s and 1970s worried about unbridled physician paternalism and therefore invented the "new" ethic of patient autonomy. Their successors have found that in throwing out paternalism they may have thrown out some important values that go to shape the very nature of good medical practice, as well as some values that may be essential for our communal existence and well-being more generally. Their predecessors did such a good job of trouncing the "old" paternalism that they need not fear that it will rise up in its original form anytime soon. (At any rate, if they continue to do medical ethics as if they thought that medical paternalism were the major enemy, they run an increasing risk of defending the ramparts at precisely the point that is no longer under attack.) But that still leaves them with the problem of reintroducing some substantive considerations into an ethical framework that has tended to focus solely on procedure. And that means that they will have to confront the sorts of power struggles that are inherent in any such debate.

For the "new" ethic was a struggle to take power away from the physician and profession in order to return some of it to the patient; and the call for new substantive restrictions on patient choice is an effort to take some of that power away from the patient and give it to others in turn—back to the medical profession, or to those who control the purse strings of the health-care budget, or to those who represent various powerful ideological or religious lobbies in society.

My point in this book has been that if one is trying to do ethical analysis responsibly and helpfully, one needs a language that will label these power struggles for what they are and explore all the relevant implications of them.

The quotation from Camus that serves as an epigraph to this book could be taken in several different ways. An obvious meaning is that the "new" ethics is simply wrongheaded, since so long as people can get sick, an ethics based primarily on autonomy is foolish. I hope it has been clear that I reject that particular conclusion. Another meaning is that concepts like *freedom* may be the stuff of elegant philosophical theories, but the real world has a way of being messier than those theories would allow for. A world that contains sicknesses that interfere with peoples' lives in varied and complex ways, and in which medicine has substantial but imperfect power to resolve those sicknesses, is precisely that sort of messy world. We need all the reasoning tools at our disposal to make sense of such a world. We should not lightly cast aside the tools that have served us well in the past, but neither should we be reluctant to test out new tools that may supplement and enhance the old ones.

APPENDIX

VONDA MCINTYRE

OF MIST,

AND GRASS,

AND SAND

The little boy was frightened. Gently, Snake touched his hot forehead. Behind her, three adults stood close together, watching, suspicious, afraid to show their concern with more than narrow lines around their eyes. They feared Snake as much as they feared their only child's death. In the dimness of the tent, the flickering lamplights gave no reassurance.

The child watched with eyes so dark the pupils were not visible, so dull that Snake herself feared for his life. She stroked his hair. It was long and very pale, a striking color against his dark skin, dry and irregular for several inches near the scalp. Had Snake been with these people months ago, she would have known the child was growing ill.

"Bring my case, please," Snake said.

The child's parents started at her soft voice. Perhaps they had expected the screech of a bright jay, or the hissing of a shining serpent. This was the first time Snake had spoken in their presence. She had only watched, when the three of them had come to observe her from a distance and whisper about her occupation and her youth; she had only listened, and then nodded, when finally they came to ask her help. Perhaps they had thought she was mute.

The fair-haired younger man lifted her leather case from the felt floor. He held the satchel away from his body, leaning to hand it to her, breathing shallowly with nostrils flared against the faint smell of musk in the dry desert air. Snake had almost accustomed herself to the kind of uneasiness he showed; she had already seen it often.

From *Analog*, vol. 92, no. 2 (October 1972), pp. 73–91. Copyright © 1973, 1978, by Vonda N. McIntyre. Reprinted by permission of the author.

When Snake reached out, the young man jerked back and dropped the case. Snake lunged and barely caught it, set it gently down, and glanced at him with reproach. His husband and his wife came forward and touched him to ease his fear. "He was bitten once," the dark and handsome woman said. "He almost died." Her tone was not of apology, but of justification.

"I'm sorry," the younger man said. "It's—" He gestured toward her; he was trembling, and trying visibly to control the reactions of his fear. Snake glanced down, to her shoulder, where she had been unconsciously aware of the slight weight and movement. A tiny serpent, thin as the finger of a baby, slid himself around behind her neck to show his narrow head below her short black curls. He probed the air with his trident tongue, in a leisurely manner, out, up and down, in, to savor the taste of the smells.

"It's only Grass," Snake said. "He cannot harm you."

If he were bigger, he might frighten; his color was pale green, but the scales around his mouth were red, as if he had just feasted as a mammal eats, by tearing. He was, in fact, much neater.

The child whimpered. He cut off the sound of pain; perhaps he had been told that Snake, too, would be offended by crying. She only felt sorry that his people refused themselves such a simple way of easing fear. She turned from the adults, regretting their terror of her, but unwilling to spend the time it would take to convince them their reactions were unjustified. "It's all right," she said to the little boy. "Grass is smooth, and dry, and soft, and if I left him to guard you, even death could not reach your bedside." Grass poured himself into her narrow, dirty hand, and she extended him toward the child. "Gently." He reached out and touched the sleek scales with one fingertip. Snake could sense the effort of even such a simple motion, yet the boy almost smiled.

"What are you called?"

He looked quickly toward his parents, and finally they nodded. "Stavin," he whispered. He had no strength or breath for speaking.

"I am Snake, Stavin, and in a little while, in the morning, I must hurt you. You may feel a quick pain, and your body will ache for several days, but you will be better afterwards."

He stared at her solemnly. Snake saw that though he understood and feared what she might do, he was less afraid than if she had lied to him. The pain must have increased greatly as his illness became more apparent, but it seemed that others had only reassured him, and hoped the disease would disappear or kill him quickly.

Snake put Grass on the boy's pillow and pulled her case nearer. The lock opened at her touch. The adults still could only fear her; they had

had neither time nor reason to discover any trust. The wife was old enough that they might never have another child, and Snake could tell by their eyes, their covert touching, their concern, that they loved this one very much. They must, to come to Snake in this country.

It was night, and cooling. Sluggish, Sand slid out of the case, moving his head, moving his tongue, smelling, tasting, detecting the warmth of bodies.

"Is that—?" The older husband's voice was low, and wise, but terrified, and Sand sensed the fear. He drew back into striking position, and sounded his rattle softly. Snake spoke to him and extended her arm. The pit viper relaxed and flowed around and around her slender wrist to form black and tan bracelets. "No," she said. "Your child is too ill for Sand to help. I know it is hard, but please try to be calm. This is a fearful thing for you, but it is all I can do."

She had to annoy Mist to make her come out. Snake rapped on the bag, and finally poked her twice. Snake felt the vibration of sliding scales, and suddenly the albino cobra flung herself into the tent. She moved quickly, yet there seemed to be no end to her. She reared back and up. Her breath rushed out in a hiss. Her head rose well over a meter above the floor. She flared her wide hood. Behind her, the adults gasped, as if physically assaulted by the gaze of the tan spectacle design on the back of Mist's hood. Snake ignored the people and spoke to the great cobra in a singsong voice. "Ah, thou. Furious creature. Lie down; 'tis time for thee to earn thy piglet. Speak to this child, and touch him. He is called Stavin." Slowly, Mist relaxed her hood, and allowed Snake to touch her. Snake grasped her firmly behind the head, and held her so she looked at Stavin. The cobra's silver eyes picked up the yellow of the lamplight. "Stavin," Snake said, "Mist will only meet you now. I promise that this time she will touch you gently."

Still, Stavin shivered when Mist touched his thin chest. Snake did not release the serpent's head, but allowed her body to slide against the boy's. The cobra was four times longer than Stavin was tall. She curved herself in stark white loops across Stavin's swollen abdomen, extending herself, forcing her head toward the boy's face, straining against Snake's hands. Mist met Stavin's frightened stare with the gaze of lidless eyes. Snake allowed her a little closer.

Mist flicked out her tongue to taste the child.

The younger husband made a small, cut-off, frightened sound. Stavin flinched at it, and Mist drew back, opening her mouth, exposing her fangs, audibly thrusting her breath through her throat. Snake sat back on her heels, letting out her own breath. Sometimes, in other places, the kinfolk could stay while she worked. "You must leave," she said gently. "It's dangerous to frighten Mist."

"I won't—"

"I'm sorry. You must wait outside."

Perhaps the younger husband, perhaps even the wife, would have made the indefensible objections and asked the answerable questions, but the older man turned them and took their hands and led them away.

"I need a small animal," Snake said as the man lifted the tent-flap. "It must have fur, and it must be alive."

"One will be found," he said, and the three parents went into the glowing night. Snake could hear their footsteps in the sand outside.

Snake supported Mist in her lap, and soothed her. The cobra wrapped herself around Snake's narrow waist, taking in her warmth. Hunger made her even more nervous than usual, and she was hungry, as was Snake. Coming across the black sand desert, they had found sufficient water, but Snake's traps were unsuccessful. The season was summer, the weather was hot, and many of the furry tidbits Sand and Mist preferred were estivating. When the serpents missed their regular meal, Snake began a fast as well.

She saw with regret that Stavin was more frightened now. "I am sorry to send your parents away," she said. "They can come back soon."

His eyes glistened, but he held back the tears. "They said to do what you told me."

"I would have you cry, if you are able," Snake said. "It isn't such a terrible thing." But Stavin seemed not to understand, and Snake did not press him; she knew that his people taught themselves to resist a difficult land by refusing to cry, refusing to mourn, refusing to laugh. They denied themselves grief, and allowed themselves little joy, but they survived.

Mist had calmed to sullenness. Snake unwrapped her from her waist and placed her on the pallet next to Stavin. As the cobra moved, Snake guided her head, feeling the tension of the striking muscles. "She will touch you with her tongue," she told Stavin. "It might tickle, but it will not hurt. She smells with it, as you do with your nose."

"With her tongue?"

Snake nodded, smiling, and Mist flicked out her tongue to caress Stavin's cheek. Stavin did not flinch; he watched, his child's delight in knowledge briefly overcoming pain. He lay perfectly still as Mist's long tongue brushed his cheeks, his eyes, his mouth. "She tastes the sickness," Snake said. Mist stopped fighting the restraint of her grasp, and drew back her head. Snake sat on her heels and released the cobra, who spiraled up her arm and laid herself across her shoulders.

"Go to sleep, Stavin," Snake said. "Try to trust me, and try not to fear the morning."

Stavin gazed at her for a few seconds, searching for truth in Snake's pale eyes. "Will Grass watch?"

The question startled her, or, rather, the acceptance behind the question. She brushed his hair from his forehead and smiled a smile that was tears just beneath the surface. "Of course." She picked Grass up. "Thou wilt watch this child, and guard him." The snake lay quiet in her hand, and his eyes glittered black. She laid him gently on Stavin's pillow.

"Now sleep."

Stavin closed his eyes, and the life seemed to flow out of him. The alteration was so great that Snake reached out to touch him, then saw that he was breathing, slowly, shallowly. She tucked a blanket around him and stood up. The abrupt change in position dizzied her; she staggered and caught herself. Across her shoulders, Mist tensed.

Snake's eyes stung and her vision was over-sharp, fever-clear. The sound she imagined she heard swooped in closer. She steadied herself against hunger and exhaustion, bent slowly, and picked up the leather case. Mist touched her cheek with the tip of her tongue.

She pushed aside the tent-flap and felt relief that it was still night. She could stand the heat, but the brightness of the sun curled through her, burning. The moon must be full; though the clouds obscured everything, they diffused the light so the sky appeared gray from horizon to horizon. Beyond the tents, groups of formless shadows projected from the ground. Here, near the edge of the desert, enough water existed so clumps and patches of bush grew, providing shelter and sustenance for all manner of creatures. The black sand, which sparkled and blinded in the sunlight, at night was like a layer of soft soot. Snake stepped out of the tent, and the illusion of softness disappeared; her boots slid crunching into the sharp hard grains.

Stavin's family waited, sitting close together between the dark tents that clustered in a patch of sand from which the bushes had been ripped and burned. They looked at her silently, hoping with their eyes, showing no expression in their faces. A woman somewhat younger than Stavin's mother sat with them. She was dressed, as they were, in a long loose robe, but she wore the only adornment Snake had seen among these people: a leader's circle, hanging around her neck on a leather thong. She and the older husband were marked close kin by their similarities: sharp-cut planes of face, high cheekbones, his hair white and hers graying early from deep black, their eyes the dark brown best suited for survival in the sun. On the ground by their feet a small black animal jerked sporadically against a net, and infrequently gave a shrill weak cry.

"Stavin is asleep," Snake said. "Do not disturb him, but go to him if he wakes."

The wife and young husband rose and went inside, but the older man stopped before her. "Can you help him?"

"I hope we may. The tumor is advanced, but it seems solid." Her own voice sounded removed, slightly hollow, as if she were lying. "Mist will be ready in the morning." She still felt the need to give him reassurance, but she could think of none.

"My sister wished to speak with you," he said, and left them alone, without introduction, without elevating himself by saying that the tall woman was the leader of this group. Snake glanced back, but the tent flap fell shut. She was feeling her exhaustion more deeply, and across her shoulders Mist was, for the first time, a weight she thought heavy.

"Are you all right?"

Snake turned. The woman moved toward her with a natural elegance made slightly awkward by advanced pregnancy. Snake had to look up to meet her gaze. She had small fine lines at the corners of her eyes, as if she laughed, sometimes, in secret. She smiled, but with concern. "You seem very tired. Shall I have someone make you a bed?"

"Not now," Snake said, "not yet. I won't sleep until afterwards."

The leader searched her face, and Snake felt a kinship with her, in their shared responsibility.

"I understand, I think. Is there anything we can give you? Do you need aid with your preparations?"

Snake found herself having to deal with the questions as if they were complex problems. She turned them in her tired mind, examined them, dissected them, and finally grasped their meanings. "My pony needs food and water—"

"It is taken care of."

"And I need someone to help me with Mist. Someone strong. But it's more important that he is not afraid."

The leader nodded. "I would help you," she said, and smiled again, a little. "But I am a bit clumsy of late. I will find someone."

"Thank you."

Somber again, the older woman inclined her head and moved slowly toward a small group of tents. Snake watched her go, admiring her grace. She felt small and young and grubby in comparison.

Sand began to unwrap himself from her wrist. Feeling the anticipatory slide of scales on her skin, she caught him before he could drop to the ground. Sand lifted the upper half of his body from her hands. He flicked out his tongue, peering toward the little animal, feeling its body heat, smelling its fear. "I know thou art hungry," Snake said, "but that creature is not for thee." She put Sand in the case, lifted Mist from her shoulder, and let her coil herself in her dark compartment.

The small animal shrieked and struggled again when Snake's diffuse shadow passed over it. She bent and picked it up. The rapid series of terrified cries slowed and diminished and finally stopped as she stroked it. Finally it lay still, breathing hard, exhausted, staring up at her with yellow eyes. It had long hind legs and wide pointed ears, and its nose twitched at the serpent smell. Its soft black fur was marked off in skewed squares by the cords of the net.

"I am sorry to take your life," Snake told it. "But there will be no more fear, and I will not hurt you." She closed her hand gently around it, and, stroking it, grasped its spine at the base of its skull. She pulled, once, quickly. It seemed to struggle, briefly, but it was already dead. It convulsed; its legs drew up against its body, and its toes curled and quivered. It seemed to stare up at her, even now. She freed its body from the net.

Snake chose a small vial from her belt pouch, pried open the animal's clenched jaws, and let a single drop of the vial's cloudy preparation fall into its mouth. Quickly she opened the satchel again, and called Mist out. She came slowly, slipping over the edge, hood closed, sliding in the sharp-grained sand. Her milky scales caught the thin light. She smelled the animal, flowed to it, touched it with her tongue. For a moment Snake was afraid she would refuse dead meat, but the body was still warm, still twitching reflexively, and she was very hungry. "A tidbit for thee," Snake said. "To whet thy appetite." Mist nosed it, reared back, and struck, sinking her short fixed fangs into the tiny body, biting again, pumping out her store of poison. She released it, took a better grip, and began to work her jaws around it; it would hardly distend her throat. When Mist lay quiet, digesting the small meal, Snake sat beside her and held her, waiting.

She heard footsteps in the coarse sand.

"I'm sent to help you."

He was a young man, despite a scatter of white in his dark hair. He was taller than Snake, and not unattractive. His eyes were dark, and the sharp planes of his face were further hardened because his hair was pulled straight back and tied. His expression was neutral.

"Are you afraid?"

"I will do as you tell me."

Though his body was obscured by his robe, his long fine hands showed strength.

"Then hold her body, and don't let her surprise you." Mist was beginning to twitch from the effects of the drugs Snake had put in the small animal's body. The cobra's eyes stared, unseeing.

"If it bites—"

"Hold, quickly!"

The young man reached, but he had hesitated too long. Mist writhed, lashing out, striking him in the face with her tail. He staggered back, at least as surprised as hurt. Snake kept a close grip behind Mist's jaws, and struggled to catch the rest of her as well. Mist was no constrictor, but she was smooth and strong and fast. Thrashing, she forced out her breath in a long hiss. She would have bitten anything she could reach. As Snake fought with her, she managed to squeeze the poison glands and force out the last drops of venom. They hung from Mist's fangs for a moment, catching light as jewels would; the force of the serpent's convulsions flung them away into the darkness. Snake struggled with the cobra, speaking softly, aided for once by the sand, on which Mist could get no purchase. Snake felt the young man behind her, grabbing for Mist's body and tail. The seizure stopped abruptly, and Mist lay limp in their hands.

"I am sorry—"

"Hold her," Snake said. "We have the night to go."

During Mist's second convulsion, the young man held her firmly and was of some real help. Afterward, Snake answered his interrupted question. "If she were making poison and she bit you, you would probably die. Even now her bite would make you ill. But unless you do something foolish, if she manages to bite, she will bite me."

"You would benefit my cousin little, if you were dead or dying."

"You misunderstand. Mist cannot kill me." She held out her hand, so he could see the white scars of slashes and punctures. He stared at them, and looked into her eyes for a long moment, then looked away.

The bright spot in the clouds from which the light radiated moved westward in the sky; they held the cobra like a child. Snake found herself half-dozing, but Mist moved her head, dully attempting to evade restraint, and Snake woke herself abruptly. "I must not sleep," she said to the young man. "Talk to me. What are you called?"

As Stavin had, the young man hesitated. He seemed afraid of her, or of something. "My people," he said, "think it unwise to speak our names to strangers."

"If you consider me a witch you should not have asked my aid. I know no magic, and I claim none. I can't learn all the customs of all the people on this earth, so I keep my own. My custom is to address those I work with by name."

"It's not a superstition," he said. "Not as you might think. We're not afraid of being bewitched."

Snake waited, watching him, trying to decipher his expression in the dim light.

"Our families know our names, and we exchange names with those we would marry."

Snake considered that custom, and thought it would fit badly on her. "No one else? Ever?"

"Well . . . a friend might know one's name."

"Ah," Snake said. "I see. I am still a stranger, and perhaps an enemy."

"A *friend* would know my name," the young man said again. "I would not offend you, but now you misunderstand. An acquaintance is not a friend. We value friendship highly."

"In this land one should be able to tell quickly if a person is worth calling 'friend'."

"We make friends seldom. Friendship is a commitment."

"It sounds like something to be feared."

He considered that possibility. "Perhaps it's the betrayal of friendship we fear. That is a very painful thing."

"Has anyone ever betrayed you?"

He glanced at her sharply, as if she had exceeded the limits of propriety. "No," he said, and his voice was as hard as his face. "No friend. I have no one I call friend."

His reaction startled Snake. "That's very sad," she said, and grew silent, trying to comprehend the deep stresses that could close people off so far, comparing her loneliness of necessity and theirs of choice. "Call me Snake," she said finally, "if you can bring yourself to pronounce it. Speaking my name binds you to nothing."

The young man seemed about to speak; perhaps he thought again that he had offended her, perhaps he felt he should further defend his customs. But Mist began to twist in their hands, and they had to hold her to keep her from injuring herself. The cobra was slender for her length, but powerful, and the convulsions she went through were more severe than any she had ever had before. She thrashed in Snake's grasp, and almost pulled away. She tried to spread her hood, but Snake held her too tightly. She opened her mouth and hissed, but no poison dripped from her fangs.

She wrapped her tail around the young man's waist. He began to pull her and turn, to extricate himself from her coils.

"She's not a constrictor," Snake said. "She won't hurt you. Leave her—"

But it was too late; Mist relaxed suddenly and the young man lost his balance. Mist whipped herself away and lashed figures in the sand. Snake wrestled with her alone while the young man tried to hold her, but she curled herself around Snake and used the grip for leverage. She started to pull herself from Snake's hands. Snake threw them both backward into the sand; Mist rose above her, openmouthed, furious, hissing. The young man lunged and grabbed her just beneath her hood. Mist struck at him, but Snake, somehow, held her back. Together they deprived Mist of her hold, and regained control of her. Snake struggled up, but Mist suddenly went quite still and lay almost rigid between them. They were both sweating; the young man was pale under his tan, and even Snake was trembling.

"We have a little while to rest," Snake said. She glanced at him and noticed the dark line on his cheek where, earlier, Mist's tail had slashed him. She reached up and touched it. "You'll have a bruise, no more," she said. "It will not scar."

"If it were true that serpents sting with their tails, you would be restraining both the fangs and the stinger, and I'd be of little use."

"Tonight I'd need someone to keep me awake, whether or not he helped me with Mist." Fighting the cobra had produced adrenaline, but now it ebbed, and her exhaustion and hunger were returning, stronger.

"Snake . . ."

"Yes?"

He smiled, quickly, half-embarrassed. "I was trying the pronunciation."

"Good enough."

"How long did it take you to cross the desert?"

"Not very long. Too long. Six days."

"How did you live?"

"There is water. We traveled at night, except yesterday, when I could find no shade."

"You carried all your food?"

She shrugged. "A little." And wished he would not speak of food.

"What's on the other side?"

"More sand, more bush, a little more water. A few groups of people, traders, the station I grew up and took my training in. And farther on, a mountain with a city inside."

"I would like to see a city. Someday."

"The desert can be crossed."

He said nothing, but Snake's memories of leaving home were recent enough that she could imagine his thoughts.

The next set of convulsions came, much sooner than Snake had expected. By their severity, she gauged something of the stage of Stavin's illness, and wished it were morning. If she were to lose him, she would have it done, and grieve, and try to forget. The cobra would have battered herself to death against the sand if Snake and the young man had not been holding her. She suddenly went completely rigid, with her mouth clamped shut and her forked tongue dangling.

She stopped breathing.

"Hold her," Snake said. "Hold her head. Quickly, take her, and if she gets away, run. Take her! She won't strike at you now, she could only slash you by accident."

He hesitated only a moment, then grasped Mist behind the head. Snake ran, slipping in the deep sand, from the edge of the circle of tents to a place where bushes still grew. She broke off dry thorny branches that tore her scarred hands. Peripherally she noticed a mass of horned vipers, so ugly they seemed deformed, nesting beneath the clump of dessicated veg- etation; they hissed at her: she ignored them. She found a narrow hollow stem and carried it back. Her hands bled from deep scratches.

Kneeling by Mist's head, she forced open the cobra's mouth and pushed the tube deep into her throat, through the air passage at the base of Mist's tongue. She bent close, took the tube in her mouth, and breathed gently into Mist's lungs.

She noticed: the young man's hands, holding the cobra as she had asked; his breathing, first a sharp gasp of surprise, then ragged; the sand scraping her elbows where she leaned; the cloying smell of the fluid seeping from Mist's fangs; her own dizziness, she thought from exhaustion, which she forced away by necessity and will.

Snake breathed, and breathed again, paused, and repeated, until Mist caught the rhythm and continued it unaided.

Snake sat back on her heels. "I think she'll be all right," she said. "I hope she will." She brushed the back of her hand across her forehead. The touch sparked pain: she jerked her hand down and agony slid along her bones, up her arm, across her shoulder, through her chest, enveloping her heart. Her balance turned on its edge. She fell, tried to catch herself but moved too slowly, fought nausea and vertigo and almost succeeded, until the pull of the earth seemed to slip away in pain and she was lost in darkness with nothing to take a bearing by.

She felt sand where it had scraped her cheek and her palms, but it was soft. "Snake, can I let go?" She thought the question must be for someone else, while at the same time she knew there was no one else to answer it, no one else to reply to her name. She felt hands on her, and they were gentle; she wanted to respond to them, but she was too tired. She needed sleep more, so she pushed them away. But they held her head and put dry leather to her lips and poured water into her throat. She coughed and choked and spat it out.

She pushed herself up on one elbow. As her sight cleared, she realized she was shaking. She felt as she had the first time she was snake-bit, before her immunities had completely developed. The young man knelt over her, his water flask in his hand. Mist, beyond him, crawled toward the darkness. Snake forgot the throbbing pain. "Mist!"

The young man flinched and turned, frightened; the serpent reared up, her head nearly at Snake's standing eye level, her hood spread, swaying, watching, angry, ready to strike. She formed a wavering white line against black. Snake forced herself to rise, feeling as though she were fumbling with the control of some unfamiliar body. She almost fell again, but held herself steady. "Thou must not go to hunt now," she said. "There is work for thee to do." She held out her right hand, to the side, a decoy, to draw Mist if she struck. Her hand was heavy with pain. Snake feared, not being bitten, but the loss of the contents of Mist's poison sacs. "Come here," she said. "Come here, and stay thy anger." She noticed blood flowing down between her fingers, and the fear she felt for Stavin was intensified. "Didst thou bite me, creature?" But the pain was wrong: poison would numb her, and the new serum only sting . . .

"No," the young man whispered, from behind her.

Mist struck. The reflexes of long training took over. Snake's right hand jerked away, her left grabbed Mist as she brought her head back. The cobra writhed a moment, and relaxed. "Devious beast," Snake said. "For shame." She turned, and let Mist crawl up her arm and over her shoulder, where she lay like the outline of an invisible cape and dragged her tail like the edge of a train.

"She did not bite me?"

"No," the young man said. His contained voice was touched with awe. "You should be dying. You should be curled around the agony, and your arm swollen purple. When you came back—" He gestured toward her hand. "It must have been a bush viper."

Snake remembered the coil of reptiles beneath the branches, and touched the blood on her hand. She wiped it away, revealing the double puncture of a snakebite among the scratches of the thorns. The wound was slightly swollen. "It needs cleaning," she said. "I shame myself by falling to it." The pain of it washed in gentle waves up her arm, burning no longer. She stood looking at the young man, looking around her, watching the landscape shift and change as her tired eyes tried to cope with the low light of setting moon and false dawn. "You held Mist well, and bravely," she said to the young man. "Thank you."

He lowered his gaze, almost bowing to her. He rose, and approached her. Snake put her hand gently on Mist's neck so she would not be alarmed.

"I would be honored," the young man said, "if you would call me Arevin."

"I would be pleased to."

Snake knelt down and held the winding white loops as Mist crawled slowly into her compartment. In a little while, when Mist had stabilized, by dawn, they could go to Stavin.

The tip of Mist's white tail slid out of sight. Snake closed the case and would have risen, but she could not stand. She had not yet quite shaken off the effects of the new venom. The flesh around the wound was red and tender, but the hemorrhaging would not spread. She stayed where she was, slumped, staring at her hand, creeping slowly in her mind toward what she needed to do, this time for herself.

"Let me help you. Please."

He touched her shoulder and helped her stand. "I'm sorry," she said. "I'm so in need of rest . . ."

"Let me wash your hand," Arevin said. "And then you can sleep. Tell me when to waken you—"

"No. I can't sleep yet." She pulled together the skeins of her nerves, collected herself, straightened, tossed the damp curls of her short hair off her forehead. "I'm all right now. Have you any water?"

Arevin loosened his outer robe. Beneath it he wore a loincloth and a leather belt that carried several leather flasks and pouches. The color of his skin was slightly lighter than the sun-darkened brown of his face. He brought out his water flask, closed his robe around his lean body, and reached for Snake's hand.

"No, Arevin. If the poison gets in any small scratch you might have, it could infect."

She sat down and sluiced lukewarm water over her hand. The water dripped pink to the ground and disappeared, leaving not even a damp spot visible. The wound bled a little more, but now it only ached. The poison was almost inactivated.

"I don't understand," Arevin said, "how it is that you're unhurt. My younger sister was bitten by a bush viper." He could not speak as uncaringly as he might have wished. "We could do nothing to save her—nothing we had would even lessen her pain."

Snake gave him his flask and rubbed salve from a vial in her belt pouch across the closing punctures. "It's a part of our preparation," she said. "We work with many kinds of serpents, so we must be immune to as many as possible." She shrugged. "The process is tedious and somewhat painful." She clenched her fist; the film held, and she was steady. She leaned toward Arevin and touched his abraded cheek again. "Yes . . ." She spread a thin layer of the salve across it. "That will help it heal."

"If you cannot sleep," Arevin said, "can you at least rest?"

"Yes," she said. "For a little while."

Snake sat next to Arevin, leaning against him, and they watched the sun turn the clouds to gold and flame and amber. The simple physical contact with another human being gave Snake pleasure, though she found it unsatisfying. Another time, another place, she might do something more, but not here, not now.

When the lower edge of the sun's bright smear rose above the horizon, Snake rose and teased Mist out of the case. She came slowly, weakly, and crawled across Snake's shoulders. Snake picked up the satchel, and she and Arevin walked together back to the small group of tents.

Stavin's parents waited, watching for her, just outside the entrance of their tent. They stood in a tight, defensive, silent group. For a moment Snake thought they had decided to send her away. Then, with regret and fear like hot iron in her mouth, she asked if Stavin had died. They shook their heads, and allowed her to enter.

Stavin lay as she had left him, still asleep. The adults followed her with their stares, and she could smell fear. Mist flicked out her tongue, growing nervous from the implied danger.

"I know you would stay," Snake said. "I know you would help, if you could, but there is nothing to be done by any person but me. Please go back outside."

They glanced at each other, and at Arevin, and she thought for a moment that they would refuse. Snake wanted to fall into the silence and sleep. "Come, cousins," Arevin said. "We are in her hands." He opened the tent flap and motioned them out. Snake thanked him with nothing more than a glance, and he might almost have smiled. She turned toward Stavin, and knelt beside him. "Stavin—" She touched his forehead; it was very hot. She noticed that her hand was less steady than before. The slight touch awakened the child. "It's time," Snake said.

He blinked, coming out of some child's dream, seeing her, slowly re-cognizing her. He did not look frightened. For that Snake was glad; for some other reason she could not identify she was uneasy.

"Will it hurt?"

"Does it hurt now?"

He hesitated, looked away, looked back. "Yes."

"It might hurt a little more. I hope not. Are you ready?"

"Can Grass stay?"

"Of course," she said.

And realized what was wrong.

"I'll come back in a moment." Her voice changed so much, she had pulled it so tight, that she could not help but frighten him. She left the tent, walking slowly, calmly, restraining herself. Outside, the parents told her by their faces what they feared.

"Where is Grass?" Arevin, his back to her, started at her tone. The younger husband made a small grieving sound, and could look at her no longer.

"We were afraid," the older husband said. "We thought it would bite the child."

"I thought it would. It was I. It crawled over his face, I could see its fangs—" The wife put her hands on the younger husband's shoulders, and he said no more.

"Where is he?" She wanted to scream; she did not.

They brought her a small open box. Snake took it, and looked inside.

Grass lay cut almost in two, his entrails oozing from his body, half turned over, and as she watched, shaking, he writhed once, and flicked his tongue out once, and in. Snake made some sound, too low in her throat to be a cry. She hoped his motions were only reflex, but she picked him up as gently as she could. She leaned down and touched her lips to the smooth green scales behind his head. She bit him quickly, sharply, at the base of the skull. His blood flowed cool and salty in her mouth. If he were not dead, she had killed him instantly.

She looked at the parents, and at Arevin; they were all pale, but she had no sympathy for their fear, and cared nothing for shared grief. "Such a small creature," she said. "Such a small creature, who could only give pleasure and dreams." She watched them for a moment more, then turned toward the tent again.

"Wait—" She heard the older husband move up close behind her. He touched her shoulder; she shrugged away his hand. "We will give you anything you want," he said, "but leave the child alone."

She spun on him in a fury. "Should I kill Stavin for your stupidity?" He seemed about to try to hold her back. She jammed her shoulder hard into his stomach, and flung herself past the tent flap. Inside, she kicked over the satchel. Abruptly awakened, and angry, Sand crawled out and coiled himself. When the younger husband and the wife tried to enter, Sand hissed and rattled with a violence Snake had never heard him use before. She did not even bother to look behind her. She ducked her head and wiped her tears on her sleeve before Stavin could see them. She knelt beside him.

"What's the matter?" He could not help but hear the voices outside the tent, and the running.

"Nothing, Stavin," Snake said. "Did you know we came across the desert?"

"No," he said, with wonder.

"It was very hot, and none of us had anything to eat. Grass is hunting now. He was very hungry. Will you forgive him and let me begin? I will be here all the time."

He seemed so tired; he was disappointed, but he had no strength for arguing. "All right." His voice rustled like sand slipping through the fingers.

Snake lifted Mist from her shoulders, and pulled the blanket from Stavin's small body. The tumor pressed up beneath his rib cage, distorting his form, squeezing his vital organs, sucking nourishment from him for its own growth. Holding Mist's head, Snake let her flow across him, touching and tasting him. She had to restrain the cobra to keep her from striking; the excitement had agitated her. When Sand used his rattle, she flinched. Snake spoke to her softly, soothing her; trained and bred-in responses began to return, overcoming the natural instincts. Mist paused when her tongue flicked the skin above the tumor, and Snake released her.

The cobra reared, and struck, and bit as cobras bite, sinking her fangs their short length once, releasing, instantly biting again for a better purchase, holding on, chewing at her prey. Stavin cried out, but he did not move against Snake's restraining hands.

Mist expended the contents of her venom sacs into the child, and released him. She reared up, peered around, folded her hood, and slid across the mats in a perfectly straight line toward her dark, close compartment.

"It is all finished, Stavin."

"Will I die now?"

"No," Snake said. "Not now. Not for many years, I hope." She took a vial of powder from her belt pouch. "Open your mouth." He complied, and she sprinkled the powder across his tongue. "That will help the ache."

She spread a pad of cloth across the series of shallow puncture wounds, without wiping off the blood.

She turned from him.

"Snake? Are you going away?"

"I will not leave without saying good-bye. I promise."

The child lay back, closed his eyes, and let the drug take him.

Sand coiled quiescently on the dark matting. Snake called him. He moved toward her, and suffered himself to be replaced in the satchel. Snake closed it, and lifted it, and it still felt empty. She heard noises outside the tent. Stavin's parents and the people who had come to help them pulled open the tent flap and peered inside, thrusting sticks in even before they looked.

Snake set down her leather case. "It's done."

They entered. Arevin was with them too; only he was emptyhanded. "Snake—" He spoke through grief, pity, confusion, and Snake could not tell what he believed. He looked back. Stavin's mother was just behind him. He took her by the shoulder. "He would have died without her. Whatever has happened now, he would have died."

The woman shook his hand away. "He might have lived. It might have gone away. We—" She could not speak for hiding tears.

Snake felt the people moving, surrounding her. Arevin took one step toward her and stopped, and she could see he wanted her to defend herself. "Can any of you cry?" she said. "Can any of you cry for me and my despair, or for them and their guilt, or for small things and their pain?" She felt tears slip down her cheeks.

They did not understand her; they were offended by her crying. They stood back, still afraid of her, but gathering themselves. She no longer needed the pose of calmness she had used to deceive the child. "Ah, you fools." Her voice sounded brittle. "Stavin—"

Light from the entrance struck them. "Let me pass." The people in front of Snake moved aside for their leader. She stopped in front of Snake, ignoring the satchel her foot almost touched. "Will Stavin live?" Her voice was quiet, calm, gentle.

"I cannot be certain," Snake said, "but I feel that he will."

"Leave us." The people understood Snake's words before they did their leader's; they looked around and lowered their weapons, and finally, one by one, they moved out of the tent. Arevin remained. Snake felt the strength that came from danger seeping from her. Her knees collapsed. She bent over the satchel with her face in her hands. The older woman knelt in front of her, before Snake could notice or prevent her. "Thank you," she said. "Thank you. I am so sorry . . ." She put her arms around Snake, and drew her toward her, and Arevin knelt beside them, and he embraced Snake too. Snake began to tremble again, and they held her while she cried.

Later she slept, exhausted, alone in the tent with Stavin, holding his hand. They had given her food, and small animals for Sand and Mist, and supplies for her journey, and sufficient water for her to bathe, though that must have strained their resources. About that, Snake no longer cared.

When she awakened, she felt the tumor, and found that it had begun to dissolve and shrivel, dying, as Mist's changed poison affected it. Snake felt little joy. She smoothed Stavin's pale hair back from his face. "I would not lie to you again, little one," she said, "but I must leave soon. I cannot stay here." She wanted another three days' sleep, to finish fighting off the effects of the bush viper's poison, but she would sleep somewhere else. "Stavin?"

He half woke, slowly. "It doesn't hurt any more," he said.

"I am glad."

"Thank you . . ."

"Good-bye, Stavin. Will you remember later on that you woke up, and that I did stay to say goodbye?"

"Good-bye," he said, drifting off again. "Good-bye, Snake. Good-bye, Grass." He closed his eyes, and Snake picked up the satchel and left the tent. Dusk cast long indistinct shadows; the camp was quiet. She found her tiger-striped pony, tethered with food and water. New, full water-skins lay on the ground next to the saddle. The tiger pony whickered at her when she approached. She scratched his striped ears, saddled him, and strapped the case on his back. Leading him, she started west, the way she had come.

"Snake—"

She took a breath, and turned back to Arevin. He faced the sun, and it turned his skin ruddy and his robe scarlet. His streaked hair flowed loose to his shoulders, gentling his face. "You will not stay?"

"I cannot."

"I had hoped . . ."

"If things were different, I might have stayed."

"They were frightened. Can't you forgive them?"

"I can't face their guilt. What they did was my fault. I said he could not hurt them, but they saw his fangs and they didn't know his bite only gave dreams and eased dying. They couldn't know; I didn't understand them until too late."

"You said it yourself, you can't know all the customs and all the fears."

"I'm crippled," she said. "Without Grass, if I cannot heal a person, I cannot help at all. I must go home. Perhaps my teachers will forgive me my stupidity, but I am afraid to face them. They seldom give the name I bear, but they gave it to me, and they'll be disappointed."

"Let me come with you."

She wanted to; she hesitated, and cursed herself for that weakness. "They may cast me out, and you would be cast out too. Stay here, Arevin."

"It wouldn't matter."

"It would. After a while, we would hate each other. I don't know you, and you don't know me. We need calmness, and quiet, and time to understand each other."

He came toward her, and put his arms around her, and they stood together for a moment. When he raised his head, he was crying. "Please come back," he said. "Whatever happens, please come back."

"I will try," Snake said. "Next spring, when the winds stop, look for me. And the spring after that, if I do not come, forget me. Wherever I am, if I live, I will forget you."

"I will look for you," Arevin said, and he would promise no more.

Snake picked up the pony's lead, and started across the desert.

REFERENCES

Ackerman, T. F. 1982. Why doctors should intervene. *Hastings Center Report* 12 (4): 14–17.

Allen, R. W. 1976. Informed consent: a medical decision. *Radiology* 119:233–34.

American Medical Association. 1848. *Code of ethics of the American Medical Association*. Philadelphia: T. K. and P. G. Collins.

Angell, M. 1982. The quality of mercy. *The New England Journal of Medicine* 306: 98–99.

———. 1985. Cost containment and the physician. *Journal of the American Medical Association* 254:1203–07.

Annas, G. J. 1988a. Precatory prediction and mindless mimicry: the case of Mary O' Connor. *Hastings Center Report* 18 (6): 31–33.

———. 1988b. She's going to die: the case of Angela C. *Hastings Center Report* 18 (1): 23–25.

———. 1989. The insane root takes reason prisoner. *Hastings Center Report* 19 (1): 29–31.

Appelbaum, P. S., and Roth, L. H. 1983. Patients who refuse treatment in medical hospitals. *Journal of the American Medical Association* 250:1296–1301.

Arras, J. D. 1984. Toward an ethic of ambiguity. *Hastings Center Report* 14 (2): 25–33.

Barnard, D. 1986. A case of amyotrophic lateral sclerosis. *Literature and Medicine* 5:27–42.

Barsky, A. J. 1988. The paradox of health. *New England Journal of Medicine* 318: 414–18.

Bass, M. J., Buck, C., Turner, L., et al. 1986. The physician's actions and the outcome of illness in family practice. *Journal of Family Practice* 23:43–47.

Bass, M. J., McWhinney, I. R., Dempsey, J. B., et al. 1986. Predictors of outcome in headache patients presenting to family physicians—a one year prospective study. *Headache Journal* 26:285–94.

Beauchamp, T. L., and Childress, J. F. 1983. *Principles of biomedical ethics.* 2d ed. New York: Oxford University Press.

———. 1989. *Principles of biomedical ethics.* 3d ed. New York: Oxford University Press.

Beauchamp, T. L., and McCullough, L. B. 1984. *Medical ethics: The moral responsibilities of physicians.* Englewood Cliffs, N.J.: Prentice-Hall.

Bedell, S. E., and Delbanco, T. L. 1984. Choices about cardiopulmonary resuscitation in the hospital: When do physicians talk with patients? *New England Journal of Medicine* 310:1089–93.

Bedell, S. E., Delbanco, T. L., Cook, E. F., and Epstein, F. H. 1983. Survival after cardiopulmonary resuscitation in the hospital. *New England Journal of Medicine* 309:569–76.

Bell, B. C. 1984. Williams' "The Use of Force" and first principles in medical ethics. *Literature and Medicine* 3:143–51.

Benjamin, M. 1985. Lay obligations in professional relations. *Journal of Medicine and Philosophy* 10:85–103.

Benjamin, M., and Curtis, J. 1986. *Ethics in Nursing.* 2d ed. New York: Oxford University Press.

Benjamin, W. W. 1989. Will centrifugal forces destroy the medical profession? *New England Journal of Medicine* 321:1191–92.

Beppu, K., and Tavormina, M. T. 1981. The healer's art: An interview with Richard Selzer. *Centennial Review* 25:20–40.

Berger, J., and Mohr, J. 1967. *A fortunate man.* New York: Holt, Rinehart and Winston.

Bertakis, K. D., and Robbins, J. A. 1989. Utilization of hospital services: a comparison of internal medicine and family practice. *Journal of Family Practice* 28:91–96.

Blackhall, L. J. 1987. Must we always use CPR? *New England Journal of Medicine* 317:1281–85.

Blanton, W. B. 1931. *Medicine in Virginia in the eighteenth century.* Richmond: Garrett and Massie.

Boyle, J. F., et al. 1987. Health policy agenda for the American people. *Journal of the American Medical Association* 257:1199–1210.

Brett, A. S., and McCullough, L. B. 1986. When patients request specific interventions: defining the limits of the physician's obligation. *New England Journal of Medicine* 315:1347–51.

Brock, D. H., and Ratzan, R. M., eds. 1988. Literature and bioethics. *Literature and Medicine* 7:1–194.

Brody, B. A. 1988a. Ethical questions raised by the persistent vegetative state. *Hastings Center Report* 18 (1): 33–37.

———. 1988b. *Life and death decision making.* New York: Oxford University Press.

Brody, H. 1980. *Placebos and the philosophy of medicine: Clinical, conceptual and ethical issues.* Chicago: University of Chicago Press.

———. 1985. Autonomy revisited: progress in medical ethics. *Journal of the Royal Society of Medicine* 78:380–86.

———. 1986. The placebo response. Part 1. Exploring the myths. Part 2. Use in clinical practice. *Drug Therapy* 16 (7): 106–31.

———. 1987a. Cost containment as professional challenge. *Theoretical Medicine* 8:5–17.

———. 1987b. The physician-patient relationship: Models and criticisms. *Theoretical Medicine* 8:205–20.

———. 1987c. The role of the family in medical decisions: Introductory guest editorial. *Theoretical Medicine* 8:253–57.

———. 1987d. *Stories of sickness*. New Haven: Yale University Press.

———. 1988a. Contested terrain: In the best interests of. *Hastings Center Report* 18 (6): 37–39.

———. 1988b. The symbolic power of the modern personal physician: The placebo effect under challenge. *Journal of Drug Issues* 18:149–61.

———. 1989a. Applied ethics: Don't change the subject. In *Clinical ethics: The nature of applied ethics in medicine*, edited by B. Hoffmaster, B. Freedman, and G. Fraser. Clifton, N.J.: Humana.

———. 1989b. Ethics of gatekeeper role (letter). *Journal of Family Practice* 29:443.

———. 1989c. The physician-patient relationship. In *Medical ethics*, edited by R. M. Veatch. Boston: Jones and Bartlett.

———. 1989d. Transparency: Informed consent in primary care. *Hastings Center Report* 19 (5): 5–9.

———. 1990a. The better half of the resource-based relative value scale. *Journal of Family Practice* 30:190–92.

———. 1990b. A policy imperative for primary care: Reflections on Keystone II. *Family Medicine* 22:42–45.

Cabot, R. C. 1903. The use of truth and falsehood in medicine: an experimental study. *American Medicine* 5:344–49. Reprinted in Reiser, Dyck, and Curran 1977, pp. 213–20.

Callahan, D. 1984. Autonomy: A moral good, not a moral obsession. *Hastings Center Report* 14 (5): 40–42.

———. 1989. Can we return death to disease? *Hastings Center Report* 19 (3 suppl.): 4–6.

Campbell, A. V., and Higgs, R. 1982. *In that case: Medical ethics in everyday practice*. London: Darton, Longman and Todd.

Caplan, A. L. 1983. Can applied ethics be effective in health care and should it strive to be? *Ethics* 93:311–19.

Caplan, A. L., Engelhardt, H. T., and McCartney, J. J., eds. 1981. *Concepts of health and disease: Interdisciplinary perspectives*. Reading, Mass.: Addison-Wesley.

Cassel, C. K. 1985. Doctors and allocation decisions: A new role in the new Medicare. *Journal of Health Politics, Policy and Law* 10:549–64.

Cassell, E. J. 1976. *The healer's art*. Philadelphia: Lippincott.

———. 1982. The nature of suffering and the goals of medicine. *New England Journal of Medicine* 306:639–45.

Charon, R. 1989. Doctor-patient / reader-writer: Learning to find the text. *Soundings* 72:137–52.

Childress, J. F. 1982. *Who shall decide? Paternalism in health care*. New York: Oxford University Press.

———. 1989. The normative principles of medical ethics. In *Medical Ethics*, edited by R. M. Veatch. Boston: Jones and Bartlett.

Chiswick, D. 1985. Use and abuse of psychiatric testimony. *British Medical Journal* 290:975–77.

Christie, R. J., and Hoffmaster, C. B. 1986. *Ethical issues in family medicine*. New York: Oxford University Press.

Churchill, L. R. 1978. The ethicist in professional education. *Hastings Center Report* 8 (6): 13–15.

Churchill, L. R., and Churchill, S. W. 1982. Storytelling in medical arenas: The art of self-determination. *Literature and Medicine* 1:73–79.

Clouser, K. D. 1973. Some things medical ethics is not. *Journal of the American Medical Association* 223:787–89.

———. 1975. Medical ethics: Some uses, abuses, and limitations. *New England Journal of Medicine* 293:384–87.

Clouser, K. D., Culver, C. M., and Gert, B. 1981. Malady: A new treatment of disease. *Hastings Center Report* 11 (3): 29–37.

Coles, R. 1989. *The call of stories: Teaching and the moral imagination*. Boston: Houghton Mifflin.

Coles, W. H., Bono, J. J., Lenkei, E. J., et al. 1987. Teaching informed consent. In *Further developments in assessing clinical competence*, edited by I. R. Hart and R. M. Harden. Montreal: Can-Heal Publications.

Cousins, N. 1980. A layman looks at truth-telling in medicine. *Journal of the American Medical Association* 244:1929–30.

Cranford, R. E., and Doudera, A. E., eds. 1984. *Institutional Ethics Committees and Health Care Decision Making*. Ann Arbor, Mich.: AUPHA Press.

Culver, C. M., Clouser, K. D., Gert, B., et al. 1985. Basic curricular goals in medical ethics. *New England Journal of Medicine* 312:253–56.

Curran, W. J. 1986. Informed consent in malpractice cases: A turn toward reality. *New England Journal of Medicine* 314:429–31.

Daniels, N. 1979. Wide reflective equilibrium and theory acceptance in ethics. *Journal of Philosophy* 76:256–82.

———. 1980. Reflective equilibrium and Archimedean points. *Canadian Journal of Philosophy* 10:83–103.

———. 1984. Understanding physician power: A review of *The social transformation of American medicine*. *Philosophy and Public Affairs* 13:353–58.

———. 1986. Why saying no to patients in the United States is so hard. *New England Journal of Medicine* 314:1380–83.

Dessaur, C. I., and Rutenfrans, C. J. C. 1988. The present day practice of euthanasia. *Issues in Law and Medicine* 3:399–405.

Dickens, B. M. 1988. Legal limits of AIDS confidentiality. *Journal of the American Medical Association* 259:3449–51.

Dickman, R. L., Ford, A. B., Liebman, J., et al. 1987. An end to patchwork reform of health care. *New England Journal of Medicine* 317:1086–89.

Dillon, W. P., Lee, R. V., Buckwald, S., et al. 1982. Life support and maternal brain death during pregnancy. *Journal of the American Medical Association* 248:1089–91.

Doerflinger, R. 1989. Assisted suicide: pro-choice or anti-life? *Hastings Center Report* 19 (3 suppl.): 16–19.

Dostoyevsky, F. (1880) 1950. *The Brothers Karamazov*. Translated by C. Garnett, New York: Modern Library.

Doukas, D. J., and McCullough, L. B. 1988. Assessing the values history of the elderly patient regarding critical and chronic care. In *Handbook of geriatric assessment*, edited by J. Gallo, W. Reichel, and L. Andersen. Rockville, Md.: Aspen Press.

Drane, J. F. 1988. *Becoming a good doctor: The place of virtue and character in medical ethics*. Kansas City, Mo.: Sheed and Ward / The Catholic Health Association.

Duff, R. S., and Campbell, A. G. M. 1976. On deciding the care of severely handicapped or dying persons: With particular reference to infants. *Pediatrics* 57:487–93.

Eaddy, J. A., and Graber, G. C. 1982. Confidentiality and the family physician. *American Family Physician* 25 (1): 141–45.

Elias, P. H. 1986. Physicians who limit their office practice to insured and paying patients (letter). *New England Journal of Medicine* 314:391.

Ellsbury, K. E. 1989. Can the family physician avoid conflict of interest in the gatekeeper role? An affirmative view. *Journal of Family Practice* 28:698–701.

Engel, G. L. 1977. The need for a new medical model: A challenge for biomedicine. *Science* 196:129–36.

———. 1988. How long must medicine's science be bound by a seventeenth century world view? In *The task of medicine: Dialogue at Wickenburg*, edited by K. L. White. Menlo Park, Calif.: Henry J. Kaiser Family Foundation.

Enthoven, A., and Kronick, R. 1989. A consumer-choice health plan for the 1990s: Universal health insurance in a system designed to promote quality and economy. *New England Journal of Medicine* 320:29–37, 94–101.

Erde, E. L. 1980. Involuntary civil commitment: Concerning the grounds of ethics. In *Mental illness: Law and public policy*, edited by B. A. Brody and H. T. Engelhardt. Boston: Reidel.

———. 1989. Studies in the explanation of issues in biomedical ethics: (11) On "on play[ing] God," etc. *Journal of Medicine and Philosophy* 6: 593–615.

Evans, R. G., Lomas, J., Barer, M. L., et al. 1989. Controlling health expenditures—the Canadian reality. *New England Journal of Medicine* 320:571–77.

Ewing, C. P. 1983. "Dr. Death" and the case for an ethical ban on psychiatric and psychological predictions of dangerousness in capital sentencing proceedings. *American Journal of Law and Medicine* 8:407–28.

Faden, R. R., and Beauchamp, T. L. 1986. *A history and theory of informed consent*. New York: Oxford University Press.

Farber, S. J. 1988. Ethics of life support and resuscitation (letter). *New England Journal of Medicine* 318:1757.

Fenigsen, R. 1989. A case against Dutch euthanasia. *Hastings Center Report* 19 (3 suppl.): 22–30.

Field, D. R., Gates, E. A., Creasy, R. K., et al. 1988. Maternal brain death during pregnancy: Medical and ethical issues. *Journal of the American Medical Association* 260:816–22.

Freidson, E. 1970. *Profession of medicine: A study of the sociology of applied knowledge.* New York: Harper and Row.

Fried, C. 1974. *Medical experimentation: Personal integrity and social policy.* New York: American Elsevier.

Fuchs, V. R. 1974. *Who shall live? Health, economics and social choice.* New York: Basic Books.

———. 1984. The rationing of medical care. *New England Journal of Medicine* 311:1572–73.

Gadow, S. 1981. Truth: Treatment of choice, scarce resource, or patient's right? *Journal of Family Practice* 13:857–60.

Gartrell, N., Herman, J., Olarte, S., et al. 1986. Psychiatrist-patient sexual contact: Results of a national survey. Part 1. Prevalence. *American Journal of Psychiatry* 143:1126–31.

Gaylin, W., et al. 1988. Doctors must not kill. *Journal of the American Medical Association* 259:2139–40.

Gilligan, C. 1982. *In a different voice: Psychological theory and women's development.* Cambridge, Mass.: Harvard University Press.

Gilligan, C., and Pollak, S. 1988. The vulnerable and invulnerable physician. Chapter 12 of *Mapping the moral domain: A contribution of women's thinking to psychological theory and education,* edited by C. Gilligan. Cambridge, Mass.: Harvard University Press.

Gillon, R. 1988. Ethics, economics, and general practice. In *Medical ethics and economics in health care,* edited by G. Mooney and A. McGuire. Oxford: Oxford University Press.

Ginzberg, E. 1986. The destabilization of health care. *New England Journal of Medicine* 315:757–61.

———. 1988. For-profit medicine: A reassessment. *New England Journal of Medicine* 319:757–61.

Gonzalez, M. L., and Emmons, D. W., eds. 1988. *Socioeconomic Characteristics of Medical Practice 1988.* Chicago: AMA Center for Health Policy Research.

Graber, G. C., Beasley, A. D., and Eaddy, J. A. 1985. *Ethical analysis of clinical medicine: A guide to self-evaluation.* Baltimore: Urban and Schwarzenberg.

Graham, R. C. 1988. Decisions about CPR. *New England Journal of Medicine* 318:1273.

Green, J. A. 1988. Minimizing malpractice risks by role clarification: The confusing transition from tort to contract. *Annals of Internal Medicine* 109:234–41.

Greenfield, S., Kaplan, S., and Ware, J. E. 1985. Expanding patient involvement in care: Effects on patient outcomes. *Annals of Internal Medicine* 102:520–28.

Guidelines Committee. 1987. *Guidelines on the termination of life-sustaining treatment and the care of the dying. A report of the Hastings Center.* Briarcliff Manor, N.Y.: Hastings Center.

Gustafson, J. M. 1973. Mongolism, parental desires, and the right to life. *Perspectives in Biology and Medicine* 16:529–57.

Gutheil, T. G., and Appelbaum, P. S. 1983. Substituted judgment: Best interests in disguise. *Hastings Center Report* 13 (3): 8–11.

Halper, T. 1985. Life and death in a welfare state: End-stage renal disease in the United Kingdom. *Milbank Memorial Fund Quarterly* 63:52–93.

Hampshire, S. 1983. *Morality and conflict*. Cambridge, Mass.: Harvard University Press.

High, D. M., and Turner, H. B. 1987. Surrogate decision-making: The elderly's familial expectations. *Theoretical Medicine* 8:303–20.

Hilfiker, D. 1985. *Healing the wounds: A physician looks at his work*. New York: Pantheon Books.

Himmelstein, D. U., and Woolhandler, S. 1986. Cost without benefit: Administrative waste in U.S. health care. *New England Journal of Medicine* 314:441–45.

Himmelstein, D. U., Woolhandler, S., et al. 1989. A national health program for the United States: A physicians' proposal. *New England Journal of Medicine* 320:102–08.

Hobbes, T. (1651) 1962. *Leviathan*. Oxford: Clarendon Press.

Holmes, O. W. 1883. The young practitioner. In *Medical essays*. Boston: Houghton Mifflin.

Hooker, W. 1849. Truth in our intercourse with the sick. In *Physician and patient*. New York: Baker and Scribner. Reprinted in Reiser, Dyck, and Curran 1977, pp. 206–12.

Hsiao, W. C., Braun, P., Dunn, D., et al. 1988. Results and policy implications of the resource-based relative-value study. *New England Journal of Medicine* 319:881–88.

Hudson, J. W., and Brody, H. 1989. Hired help: A physician's experiences in a for-profit staff-model HMO (letter). *New England Journal of Medicine* 320:185.

Illich, I. 1976. *Medical nemesis: The expropriation of health*. New York: Pantheon.

International Working Conference. 1989. The Appleton consensus: Suggested international guidelines for decisions to forgo medical treatment. *Journal of the Danish Medical Association* 151:700–706.

It's over, Debbie. 1988. *Journal of the American Medical Association* 259:272.

Jones, A. 1981. *Women who kill*. New York: Fawcett Columbine.

Jones, A. H. 1983. The healer-patient/family relationship in Vonda N. McIntyre's "Of Mist, and Grass, and Sand." *Perspectives in Biology and Medicine* 26:274–80.

Jonsen, A. R. 1982. Ethics, the law, and the treatment of seriously ill newborns. In *Legal and Ethical Aspects of Treating Critically and Terminally ill Patients*, edited by A. E. Doudera and J. D. Peters. Ann Arbor, Mich.: AUPHA Press.

———. 1986a. Bentham in a box: Technology assessment and health care allocation. *Law, Medicine and Health Care* 14 (November): 172–74.

———. 1986b. Casuistry and clinical ethics. *Theoretical Medicine* 7:65–74.

Jonsen, A. R., Jameton, A. L., and Lynch, A. 1978. Medical ethics, history of: North America in the twentieth century. In *Encyclopedia of bioethics*, edited by W. T. Reich. New York: Free Press.

Jonsen, A. R., Siegler, M., and Winslade, W. J. 1986. *Clinical ethics*. 2d ed. New York: Macmillan.

Jonsen, A. R., and Toulmin, S. 1988. *The abuse of casuistry: A history of moral reasoning*. Berkeley and Los Angeles: University of California Press.

Kanoti, G. A., and Vinicky, J. K. 1987. The role and structure of hospital ethics committees. In *Health care ethics: A guide for decision makers*, edited by G. Anderson and V. Glesnes-Anderson. Rockville, Md.: Aspen Press.

Karasu, T. B. 1980. The ethics of psychotherapy. *American Journal of Psychiatry* 137:1502–12.

Kass, L. R. 1989. Neither for love nor money: Why doctors must not kill. *The Public Interest* 94:25–46.

Katz, J. 1984. *The silent world of doctor and patient.* New York: Free Press.

Ketchum, S. A., and Pierce, C. 1981. Rights and responsibilities. *Journal of Medicine and Philosophy* 6:271–79.

Klein, D., Najman, J., Kohrman, A. F., and Munro, C. 1982. Patient characteristics that elicit negative responses from family physicians. *Journal of Family Practice* 14:881–88.

Kleinman, A. 1988. *The illness narratives: Suffering, healing and the human condition.* New York: Basic Books.

Kliever, L. D., ed. 1989. *Dax's case: Essays in medical ethics and human meaning.* Dallas: Southern Methodist University Press.

Komrad, M. S. 1983. A defense of medical paternalism: Maximizing patients' autonomy. *Journal of Medical Ethics* 9:38–44.

Kopelman, L. M., Irons, T. G., and Kopelman, A. E. 1988. Neonatologists judge the "Baby Doe" regulations. *New England Journal of Medicine* 318:667–83.

Kruse, J. A., Thill-Baharozian, M. C., and Carlson, R. W. 1988. Comparison of clinical assessment with APACHE II for predicting mortality risk in patients admitted to a medical intensive care unit. *Journal of the American Medical Association* 260:1739–42.

Ladd, J. 1979. Legalism and medical ethics. *Journal of Medicine and Philosophy* 4: 70–80.

———. 1980. Medical ethics: Who knows best? *Lancet,* no. 2:1127–29.

———. 1981. Physicians and society: Tribulations of power and responsibility. In *The law-medicine relation: A philosophical exploration,* edited by S. F. Spicker, J. M. Healey, and H. T. Engelhardt. Boston: Reidel.

———. 1982. Concepts of health and disease and their ethical implications. In *Value conflicts in health care delivery,* edited by K. Nelson and B. Gruzalski. Boston: Ballinger Press.

Lasch, C. 1979. *The culture of narcissism.* New York: Norton.

Levenstein, J. H., McCracken, E. C., McWhinney, I. R., et al. 1986. The patient-centred clinical method. Part 1. A model for the doctor-patient interaction in family medicine. *Family Practice* 3:24–30.

Levinsky, N. G. 1984. The doctor's master. *New England Journal of Medicine* 311:1573–75.

Levinson, D. F. 1987. Toward full disclosure of referral restrictions and financial incentives by prepaid health plans. *New England Journal of Medicine* 317:1729–31.

Lidz, C. W., Meisel, A., Osterweis, M., et al. 1983. Barriers to informed consent. *Annals of Internal Medicine* 99:539–43.

Like, R. C. 1988. Commentary: Primary care case management: A family physician's perspective. *Quality Review Bulletin* 14:174–78.

Lincourt, J. M., and Sanchez, A. F. 1984. Benevolent deception in family medicine. *Family Medicine* 16:47–49.

Lo, B. 1987. Behind closed doors: promises and pitfalls of ethics committees. *New England Journal of Medicine* 317:46–50.

Lomas, J., Fooks, C., Rice, T., and Labelle, R. J. 1989. Paying physicians in Canada: Minding our P's and Q's. *Health Affairs* 8 (1): 80–102.

Lundberg, G. D. 1988. The debate over the ethics of euthanasia. *Journal of the American Medical Association* 259:2143.

McCullough, L. B. 1978. Historical perspectives on the ethical dimensions of the patient-physician relationship: The medical ethics of Dr. John Gregory. *Ethics in Science and Medicine* 5:47–53.

———. 1988. An ethical model for improving the physician-patient relationship. *Inquiry* 25:454–68.

———. 1989. The abstract character and transforming power of medical language. *Soundings* 72:111–25.

MacIntyre, A. 1981. *After virtue.* South Bend, Ind.: Notre Dame University Press.

Marsh, F. H. 1985. Health care cost containment and the duty to treat. *Journal of Legal Medicine* 6:157–90.

May, R. 1972. *Power and innocence: A search for the sources of violence.* New York: Norton.

May, W. E., Barry, R., Griese, O., et al. 1987. Feeding and hydrating the permanently unconscious and other vulnerable persons. *Issues in Law and Medicine* 3:203–20.

Mechanic, D. 1978. *Medical sociology.* New York: Free Press.

Mehlman, M. J. 1985. Rationing expensive lifesaving medical treatments. *Wisconsin Law Review* 1985:239–303.

Mellinkoff, S. 1987. The medical clerkship. *New England Journal of Medicine* 317:1089–91.

Menzel, P. T. 1979. Are killing and letting die morally different in medical contexts? *Journal of Medicine and Philosophy* 4:269–93.

———. 1983. *Medical costs, moral choices.* New Haven: Yale University Press.

Merenstein, J. H. 1984. A comparison of residency trained family physicians and internists. *Family Medicine* 16:165–69.

Miller, A. 1985. *The price.* New York: Penguin.

Mills, C. W. 1959. *The causes of World War Three.* New York: Simon and Schuster.

Monahan, J. 1984. The prediction of violent behavior: Toward a second generation of theory and policy. *American Journal of Psychiatry* 141:10–15.

Moskop, J. C. 1981. The nature and limits of the physician's authority. In *Doctors, patients, and society: Power and authority in medical care,* edited by M. S. Staum and D. E. Larsen. Waterloo, Ont.: Wilfrid Laurier University Press.

Moss, A. H. 1989. Informing the patient about cardiopulmonary resuscitation: When the risks outweigh the benefits. *Journal of General Internal Medicine* 4:349–55.

Mulhausen, R., and McGee, J. 1989. Physician need: An alternative projection from a study of large, prepaid group practices. *Journal of the American Medical Association* 261:1930–34.

Murphy, D. J. 1988. Do-not-resuscitate orders: Time for reappraisal in long-term-care institutions. *Journal of the American Medical Association* 260:2098–2101.

Murphy, J. S. 1989. Should pregnancies be sustained in brain-dead women? A philosophical discussion of postmortem pregnancy. In *Healing technology: Feminist perspectives*, edited by K. S. Ratcliff, M. M. Ferree, G. O. Mellow, et al. Ann Arbor: University of Michigan Press.

Murray, T. H. 1987. Medical ethics, moral philosophy and moral tradition. *Social Science in Medicine* 25:637–44.

Nelson, L. J. 1988. Neonatology and the law: Looking beyond Baby Doe. In *Year Book of Perinatal/Neonatal Medicine*, edited by M. Klaus and A. Faranoff. Chicago: Year Book Medical Publishers.

Novack, D. H. 1987. Therapeutic aspects of the clinical encounter. *Journal of General Internal Medicine* 2:346–55.

Novack, D. H., Detering, B. J., Arnold, R., et al. 1989. Physicians' attitudes toward using deception to resolve difficult ethical problems. *Journal of the American Medical Association* 261:2980–85.

Novack, D. H., Plumer, R., Smith, R. L., et al. 1979. Changes in physicians' attitudes toward telling the cancer patient. *Journal of the American Medical Association* 241:897–900.

Nozick, R. 1974. *Anarchy, state and utopia*. New York: Basic Books.

Oken, D. 1961. What to tell cancer patients. *Journal of the American Medical Association* 175:1120–28.

Parsons, T. 1978. Health and disease: A sociological and action perspective. In *Encyclopedia of Bioethics*, edited by W. T. Reich. New York: Free Press.

Paterson, T. T. 1966. *Management Theory*. London: Business Publications.

Pellegrino, E. D. 1979. Toward a reconstruction of medical morality: The primacy of the act of profession and the fact of illness. *Journal of Medicine and Philosophy* 4: 32–56.

———. 1986. Rationing health care: The ethics of medical gatekeeping. *Journal of Contemporary Health Law and Policy* 2:23–45.

Pellegrino, E. D., and Thomasma, D. C. 1981. *A Philosophical Basis of Medical Practice*. New York: Oxford University Press.

———. 1988. *For the patient's good: The restoration of beneficence in health care*. New York: Oxford University Press.

Pence, G. E. 1988. Do not go slowly into that dark night: Mercy killing in Holland. *American Journal of Medicine* 84:139–41.

Peszke, M. A. 1975. Is dangerousness an issue for physicians in emergency commitment? *American Journal of Psychiatry* 132:825–28.

Plato. 1945. *The Republic*. Translated by F. M. Cornford. New York: Oxford University Press.

Platt, M. 1975. Commentary: On asking to die. *Hastings Center Report* 5 (6): 9–12.

Pless, J. E. 1983. The story of Baby Doe. *New England Journal of Medicine* 309:664.

Poole, S. R., and Anstett, R. E. 1983. Patients who request alternative (non-medical) health care. *Journal of Family Practice* 16:767–72.

President's Commission for the Study of Ethical Problems in Medicine and Biomedical and Behavioral Research. 1982. *Making health care decisions*. Volume 1. *Report*. Washington, D.C.: U.S. Government Printing Office.

———. 1983. *Deciding to forego life-sustaining treatment*. Washington, D.C.: U.S. Government Printing Office.

Rabkin, E. 1986. A case of self defense. *Literature and Medicine* 5:43–53.

Rachels, J. 1986. *The end of life: Euthanasia and morality*. New York: Oxford University Press.

Ramsey, P. 1978. The Saikewicz precedent: The courts and incompetent patients. *Hastings Center Report* 8 (6): 36–42.

Ratcliff, K. S., et al., eds. 1989. *Healing technology: Feminist perspectives*. Ann Arbor: University of Michigan Press.

Rawls, J. 1971. *A theory of justice*. Cambridge, Mass.: Harvard University Press.

Reich, W. T. 1989. Speaking of suffering: A moral account of compassion. *Soundings* 72:83–108.

Reiser, S. J. 1980. Words as scalpels: Transmitting evidence in the clinical dialogue. *Annals of Internal Medicine* 92:837–42.

Reiser, S. J., Dyck, A. J., and Curran, W. J., eds. 1977. *Ethics in medicine: Historical perspectives and contemporary concerns*. Cambridge, Mass.: MIT Press.

Reitemeier, R. J. 1985. 1985–2000: For medicine, challenges and opportunities. *ACP Newsletter* 5 (10, November): 1.

Relman, A. S. 1989. Universal health insurance: Its time has come. *New England Journal of Medicine* 320:117–18.

Rhoden, N. K. 1988. Litigating life and death. *Harvard Law Review* 102:375–446.

Rhoden, N. K., and Arras, J. D. 1985. Withholding treatment from Baby Doe: From discrimination to child abuse. *Milbank Memorial Fund Quarterly* 63:18–51.

Rigter, H. 1989. Euthanasia in the Netherlands: distinguishing fact from fiction. *Hastings Center Report* 19 (3 suppl.): 31–32.

Rorty, R. 1979. *Philosophy and the mirror of nature*. Princeton, N.J.: Princeton University Press.

———. 1982. *Consequences of pragmatism*. Minneapolis: University of Minnesota Press.

Ross, J. W. 1989. The militarization of disease: Do we really want a war on AIDS? *Soundings* 72:39–58.

Schieber, G. J., and Poullier, J. P. 1988. International health spending and utilization trends. *Health Affairs* 7 (3): 105–12.

Schiedermayer, D. L. 1988. The decision to forgo CPR in the elderly patient. *Journal of the American Medical Association* 260:2096–97.

Schwartz, W. B. 1987. The inevitable failure of current cost-containment strategies: Why they can provide only temporary relief. *Journal of the American Medical Association* 257:220–24.

Schwartz, W. B., and Aaron, H. J. 1984. Rationing hospital care: Lessons from Britain. *New England Journal of Medicine* 310:52–56.

Scovern, H. 1988. Hired help: A physician's experiences in a for-profit staff-model HMO. *New England Journal of Medicine* 319:787–90.

———. 1989. Hired help: A physician's experiences in a for-profit, staff-model HMO (reply). *New England Journal of Medicine* 320:187.

Selker, H. P., Griffith, J. L., Dorey, F. J., and D'Agostino, R. B. 1987. How do physicians adapt when the coronary care unit is full? A prospective multicenter study. *Journal of the American Medical Association* 257:1181–85.

Selzer, R. 1975. *Mortal lessons: Notes on the art of surgery*. New York: Simon and Schuster.

————. 1982. Brute. In *Letters to a young doctor*. New York: Simon and Schuster.

Shelp, E. E., ed. 1985. *Virtue and medicine*. Boston: Reidel.

Shem, S. 1978. *The house of God*. New York: Dell.

Siegel, B. S. 1986. *Love, medicine and miracles*. New York: Harper and Row.

————. 1989. *Peace, love and healing*. New York: Harper and Row.

Siegler, Mark. 1982a. Confidentiality in medicine: A decrepit concept. *New England Journal of Medicine* 307:1518–21.

————. 1982b. The physician-patient accomodation: A central event in clinical medicine. *Archives of Internal Medicine* 142:1899–1902.

Siegler, Mark, and Weisbard, A. J. 1985. Against the emerging stream: Should fluids and nutritional support be discontinued? *Archives of Internal Medicine* 145:129–31.

Siegler, Miriam, and Osmond, H. 1973. Aesculapian authority. *Hastings Center Studies* 1 (2): 41–52.

Singer, D. E., Carr, P. L., Mulley, A. G., and Thibault, G. E. 1983. Rationing intensive care—physician responses to a resource shortage. *New England Journal of Medicine* 309:1155–60.

Smith, D. G., and Newton, L. 1984. Physician and patient: Respect for mutuality. *Theoretical Medicine* 5:43–60.

Smith, D. H. 1986. The limits of narrative. *Literature and Medicine* 5:54–57.

Smith, H. L., and Churchill, L. R. 1986. *Professional ethics and primary health care*. Durham, N.C.: Duke University Press.

Smith, R. C., and Zimny, G. H. 1988. Physicians' emotional reaction to patients. *Psychosomatics* 29:392–97.

Solzhenitsyn, A. I. 1968. *The cancer ward*. Translated by R. Frank. New York: Dell.

Springarn, N. D. 1978. Doctors who tell all. *Washington Post*, 30 July: B8.

Starr, P. 1982. *The social transformation of American medicine*. New York: Basic Books.

Staum, M. S., and Larsen, D. E., eds. 1981. *Doctors, patients, and society: Power and authority in medical care*. Waterloo, Ont.: Wilfrid Laurier University Press.

Stephens, G. G. 1989a. Any more cordials to the drooping spirit? Professional ethics, 1847–1989. *Journal of the American Board of Family Practice* 2:212–15.

————. 1989b. Can the family physician avoid conflict of interest in the gatekeeper role? An opposing view. *Journal of Family Practice* 28:701–04.

Stewart, W. L. 1985. The public perception of physicians. *Journal of Family Practice* 21:335–36.

Strong, C. 1983a. Defective newborns and their impact on families: Ethical and legal considerations. *Law, Medicine and Health Care* 11:168–81.

————. 1983b. The tiniest newborns. *Hastings Center Report* 13 (1): 14–19.

Strull, W. M., Lo, B., and Charles, G. 1984. Do patients want to participate in medical decision making? *Journal of the American Medical Association* 252:2990–94.

Subcommittee on Evaluation of Humanistic Qualities in the Internist, American Board of Internal Medicine. 1983. Evaluation of humanistic qualities in the internist. *Annals of Internal Medicine* 99:720–24.

Szasz, T. S. 1974. *The myth of mental illness*. New York: Harper and Row.

Taffet, G. E., Teasdale, T. A., and Luchi, R. J. 1988. In-hospital cardiopulmonary resuscitation. *Journal of the American Medical Association* 260:2069–72.

Terry, J. S., and Williams, P. C. 1988. Literature and bioethics: The tension in goals and styles. *Literature and Medicine* 7:1–21.

Thomas, K. B. 1987. General practice consultations: Is there any point in being positive? *British Medical Journal* 294:1200–1202.

Thurow, L. C. 1984. Learning to say no. *New England Journal of Medicine* 311: 1569–72.

Todres, I. D., Guillemin, J., Grodin, M. A., and Batten, D. 1988. Life-saving therapy for newborns: A questionnaire survey in the state of Massachusetts. *Pediatrics* 81:643–49.

Tomlinson, T. 1986. The physician's influence on patients' choices. *Theoretical Medicine* 7:105–21.

Tomlinson, T., and Brody, H. 1988. Ethics and communication in do-not-resuscitate orders. *New England Journal of Medicine* 318:43–46.

Tomlinson, T., Howe, K., Notman, M., and Rossmiller, D. 1990. An empirical study of proxy consent for the elderly. *The Gerontologist* 30:54–64.

Tronto, J. C. 1987. Beyond gender difference to a theory of care. *Signs: Journal of Women in Culture and Society* 12:644–63.

U.S. Commission on Civil Rights. 1989. *Medical discrimination against children with disabilities*. Washington, D.C.: U.S. Government Printing Office.

Vaux, K. L. 1988. Debbie's dying: Mercy killing and the good death. *Journal of the American Medical Association* 259:2140–41.

Veatch, R. M. 1977. *Case studies in medical ethics*. Cambridge, Mass.: Harvard University Press.

———. 1981. *A theory of medical ethics*. New York: Basic Books.

———. 1984. Autonomy's temporary triumph. *Hastings Center Report* 14 (5): 38–40.

———. 1986. DRGs and the ethical allocation of resources. *Hastings Center Report* 16 (3): 32–40.

Waitzkin, H., and Stoeckle, J. D. 1972. The communication of information about illness. *Advances in Psychosomatic Medicine* 8:185–89.

Wanzer, S. H., Federman, D. D., Adelstein, S. J., et al. 1989. The physician's responsibility toward hopelessly ill patients: A second look. *New England Journal of Medicine* 320:844–49.

Webb, W. L. 1986. The doctor-patient covenant and the threat of exploitation. *American Journal of Psychiatry* 143:1149–50.

Weir, R. F., and Gostin, L. 1990. Decisions to abate life-sustaining treatment for nonautonomous patients. *Journal of the American Medical Association* 264:1846–53.

Weiss, B. D. 1982. Confidentiality expectations of patients, physicians, and medical students. *Journal of the American Medical Association* 247:2695–97.

Welch, D. D. 1989. Walking in their shoes: Paying respect to incompetent patients. *Vanderbilt Law Review* 42:1617–40.

Welch, H. G., and Larson, E. B. 1988. Dealing with limited resources: The Oregon decision to curtail funding for organ transplantation. *New England Journal of Medicine* 319:171–73.

White, K. L., ed. 1988. *The task of medicine: Dialogue at Wickenburg*. Menlo Park, Calif.: Henry J. Kaiser Family Foundation.

White, R. B., and Engelhardt, H. T. 1975. A demand to die. *Hastings Center Report* 5 (3): 9–10.

Wikler, D. 1988. Not dead, not dying? Ethical categories and the persistent vegetative state. *Hastings Center Report* 18 (1): 41–47.

Williams, M. E., and Hadler, N. M. 1983. The illness as the focus of geriatric medicine. *New England Journal of Medicine* 308:1357–60.

Williams, W. C. [1933] 1984. The use of force. In *William Carlos Williams: The doctor stories*, edited by R. Coles. New York: New Directions.

Youngner, S. J. 1988. Who defines futility? *Journal of the American Medical Association* 260:2094–95.

Zaner, R. M. 1988. *Ethics and the clinical encounter*. Englewood Cliffs, N.J.: Prentice-Hall.